THE PATIENTS' DESK REFERENCE

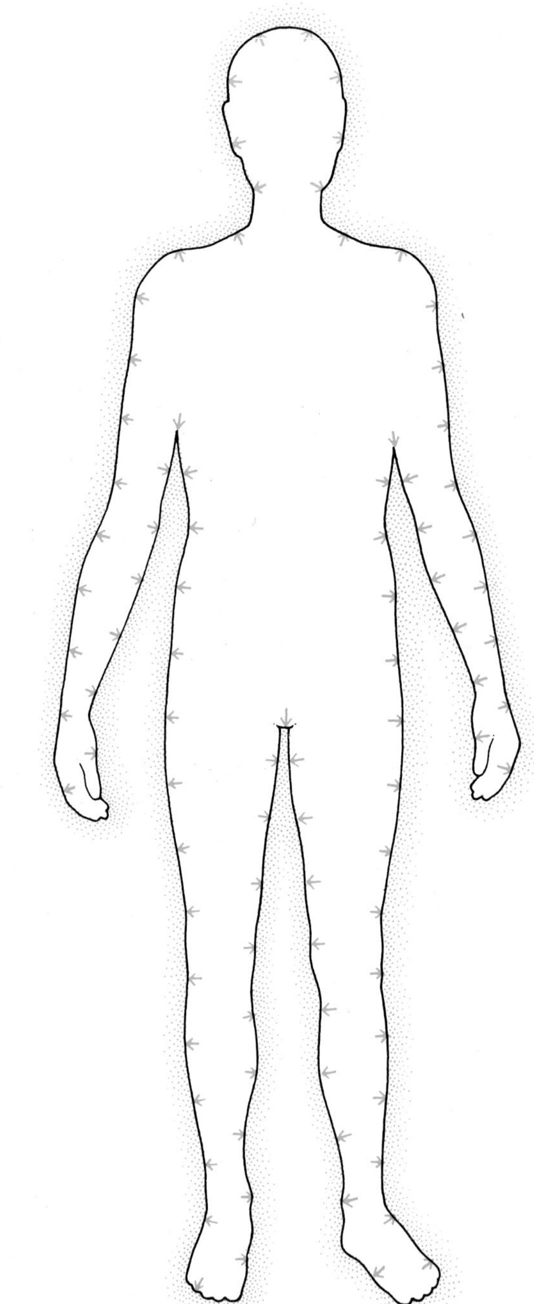

THE PATIENTS' DESK REFERENCE

Thousands of Medications Indexed By Illness

Matthew Conolly, M.D. and Michael Orme, M.D.

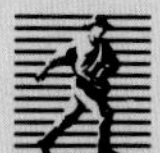

Prentice Hall Press

New York London Toronto Sydney Tokyo

Published in 1988 by Prentice Hall Press
A Division of Simon & Schuster, Inc.
Gulf + Western Building
One Gulf + Western Plaza
New York, NY 10023

Conceived, edited and designed by
Duncan Petersen Publishing Ltd,
5, Botts Mews,
London, W2 5AG

PRENTICE HALL PRESS is a trademark of Simon & Schuster, Inc.
Library of Congress Cataloging-in-Publication Data
#87-043146

ISBN 0-13-573551-3
Manufactured in Hong Kong
10 9 8 7 6 5 4 3 2 1
First Prentice Hall Press Edition

The ideas, procedures, and suggestions contained in this book are not intended to replace the services of a trained health professional. All matters regarding your health require medical supervision. You should consult your physician before adopting the procedures in this book. Any applications of the treatments set forth in this book are at the reader's discretion.

The drug lists in this book are designed for use all over the English-speaking world. Drug names specific to the United States are mentioned first, but the lists also give, where necessary, additional trade names encountered in Britain, Australia, Canada and South Africa. Some of these include medications not available in the United States.

THE CONTRIBUTORS

The consultant editors and publishers are grateful to the many doctors who have contributed to *The Patients' Desk Reference* – all are listed on page 303.

Many are colleagues of Professor Orme and Dr. Graham-Jones at Liverpool University, and at the Royal Liverpool and other local hospitals. Just as many are in hospital posts and general practice all round Britain.

Besides Michael Orme and Susanna Graham-Jones, Dr. Mary Belshaw, Dr. Peter Campion, Dr. P. Carey, Dr. J.M. Carey, Dr. Peter Elliot, Dr. R.M. Graham and Dr. Denise Kitchener made particularly extensive contributions.

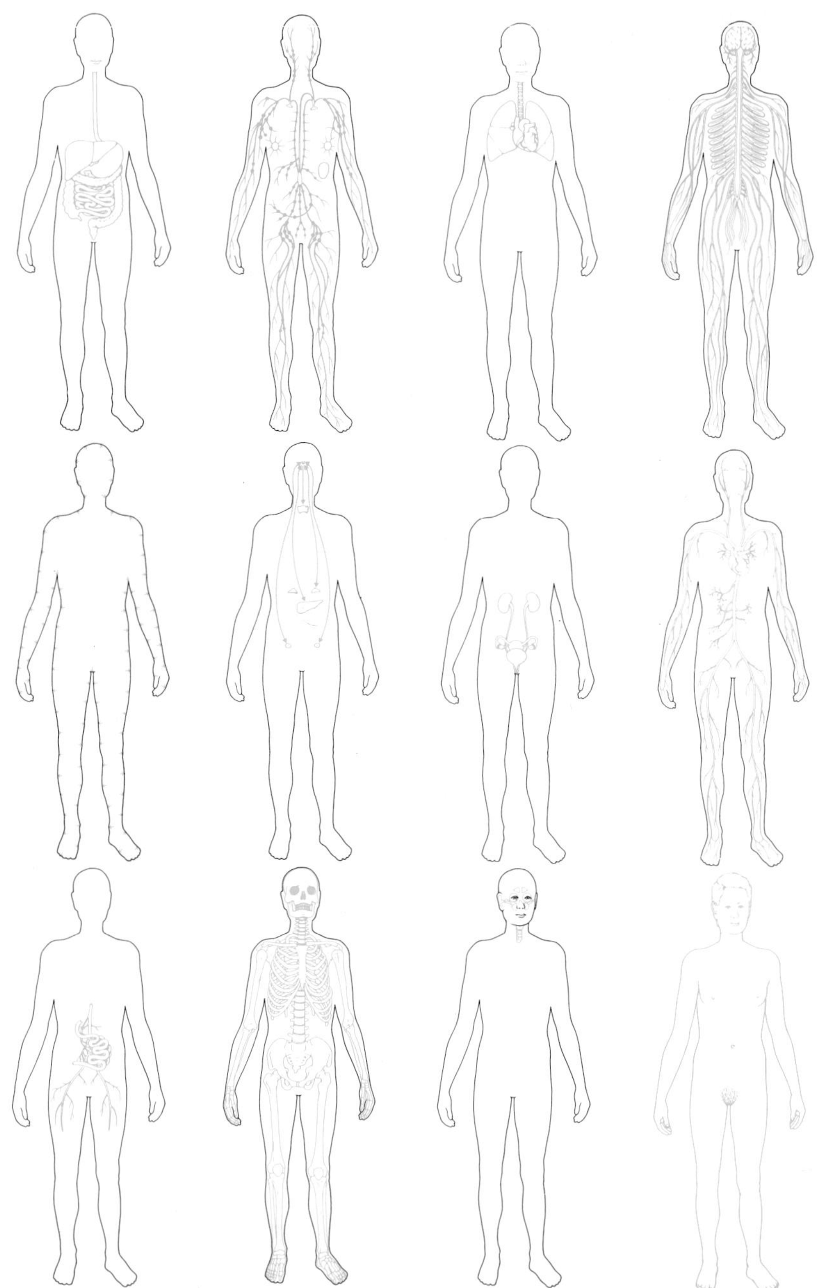

CONTENTS

The Patients' Desk Reference has 12 sections, corresponding to the main branches of medicine. For a detailed breakdown of illnesses covered, plus their page numbers, see the section opener pages listed below.

INTRODUCTION Michael Orme

The ultimate purpose of this book is to increase the understanding of medicine. All the doctors who have contributed believe that a suitably informed patient is generally happier with the treatment and perhaps more able to cope with illness. Certainly the medications in question are more likely to give a beneficial result. But medicine is, of course, a complex subject; it is difficult, if not impossible, to understand about the treatment for an illness unless one first understands the illness itself. For this reason, *The Patients' Desk Reference* is organized by illnesses, rather than the daunting chemical classifications of modern medicine.

Each of the 90-odd sections is devoted to an illness, or group of similar illnesses or diseases. Each begins with a clear definition of what the illness or disease actually is; then moves on to describe the drugs used and how they work. This approach involves some repetition, but this is worth it for the sake of clarity and easy reference.

Of course, treatment of illness or disease does not always involve drugs. In many cases non-drug treatment is highly effective. Dietary treatment of, for example, diabetes or disorders of fat metabolism is often at least as important as the use of drugs. In some cases treatment requires the removal of some insult to your system. So, working alongside the mainstream drug information are sections on how to stop smoking; how to lose weight; how to relax more effectively and thus give up tranquillizers; how to cope with fatigue and stress in general.

Not all drug treatment involves the use of prescribed medicines. For many conditions there are treatments that can be bought from pharmacists; thus every section contains advice on over-the-counter treatments. It is, however, important to realize that such medicines can occasionally have disagreeable side effects, and that they may interact with the medicines a doctor is prescribing. Make a habit of discussing with your doctor whether an over-the-counter treatment is appropriate for you.

Another aim of this book is to help the patient work with the doctor to achieve the best result possible from the treatment given. Each section suggests certain questions to ask a doctor during consultation. These cannot, of course, be comprehensive; but they are intended to be a useful starting point. They are in no way a substitute for questions that concern you particularly. You are not challenging a doctor's competence when you ask such questions: in fact, you will be showing that you are interested in the treatment and want to achieve the best possible result.

These features are of course entirely appropriate to a modern drug handbook; but to them we have added others which, we hope, will give the book added value. Many of the sections go into considerable detail about self-management during ill-ness. This typically includes advice on maximizing the effectiveness of the medicines taken – or of cutting them down so as to achieve results with minimum intake. But they also include many practical suggestions for coping with illness, and indeed preventing it. The aim is to involve the patient as far as possible in *actively* fighting the illness rather than being the passive recipient of medicines. Obviously this is far more relevant to some illnesses than others; but there is usually something the patient can do. Thus *The Patients' Desk Reference* is an all-round approach to drugs and to illness: it sees illness, medicines, doctor, and patient as equally important parts of a whole.

Adverse drug effects

Although all drugs are tested exhaustively before being released on to the market, absolute safety can never be guaranteed. Indeed, no drug is without some side effect(s) which basically need to be taken in the patient's stride. These are listed in each section; the patient is not bound to have them; often they are minimal. By contrast, there will always be the occasional individual who responds adversely to a medicine, and these grave, or potentially grave side effects are also mentioned. In general they are uncommon; don't assume that, because they are mentioned, they are likely to happen. If you are unlucky enough to suffer an adverse effect from any medicine, discuss it with your doctor as soon as possible: in most cases he or she will want to change the treatment. If you feel really awful from your medicine and cannot see a doctor, it *may* be sensible to stop taking it right away. However this is not always the best course because sometimes it is harmful to stop a medicine before the treatment is finished. Therefore, make every effort to get in touch with a doctor to ask if it is all right to stop a medicine. Doctors will be interested in adverse effects and may want to report these to the Food and Drug Administration (FDA).

Drugs today

The words "drug" or "drugs" have acquired a tarnished reputation over the last decade and this is primarily because of the problems of drug abuse and addiction. In this context ''drugs'' usually means heroin, cocaine or amphetamine in its various forms. In medical practice the word ''drugs'' is used interchangeably with ''medicines'' and only a tiny fraction of the medicines in use today produce addiction. There are currently some 2,500 different drugs available for prescription in the USA alone and when the various combination preparations are included this number increases substantially.

Modern medicines are, in large part, the end result of years of patient research. The original idea for a drug has to undergo extensive laboratory testing before being tried out in humans. If all goes well, the government's watchdog committee on drugs (the FDA) will grant a license for investigation of a new drug (IND). Then, extensive trials will take place in humans before the drug is given a product license (new drug application or NDA). Only then may the new drug be prescribed by doctors.

The majority of new drugs are developed by the pharmaceutical companies and it is estimated that it takes at least 10 years and costs $70 million to develop a new drug. It is not unknown for a drug to pass all the clinical trials, only to manifest a rare toxic effect when, for the first time, many thousands of people take it. Inevitably the drug would then have to be abandoned and all the development costs will go to waste.

To allow the company to recoup its development costs the new drug is initially protected by a patent which lasts for about 17 years. When the product license is finally granted, the drug will be sold under a trade name, although it will also have a chemical or generic name. The generic name, for example cimetidine, tells doctors and other professionals what type of drug it is. The trade name (in this case Tagamet) is chosen as a catchy label and may also, but often does not, tell the doctor something about the type of drug it is. In this book, the NAMES YOU WILL HEAR section gives a selection of both generic names and the commonest trade names of most of the drugs likely to be prescribed. The list is *not* exhaustive.

Once a patent has expired, companies other than the original developer may decide to sell the drug and thus it may acquire more than one trade name. However, much prescribing today is done using the generic name only.

We hope that by giving a range of names, including the main variants in English-speaking markets worldwide, you will usually find the one that is applicable to your case. But with the vast array of drugs and different drug names that are now used it is not possible to provide a complete listing.

The future

Research goes on continuously into all areas of drug treatment to find substances that are more effective or have fewer side effects. In certain areas where drugs are not as yet very useful (for example drugs to prevent premature ageing, and to treat obesity or AIDS) there is real promise of better treatments to come. Against this must be balanced the fact that medicine will never provide a drug which can be guaranteed 100 per cent safe and 100 per cent effective.

Prevention of illness and disease

The main focus of modern medicine is still on correcting the disease process once disaster has struck; the shortcomings of this approach are well-illustrated in the patient who suffers a major stroke: once brain cells have died, the only recourse is to re-train other parts of the brain to take over from the damaged parts while trying to prevent further strokes. It would be much more effective to try to prevent the stroke in the first place and increasingly people in the health care professions are directing their attention to the prevention of illness.

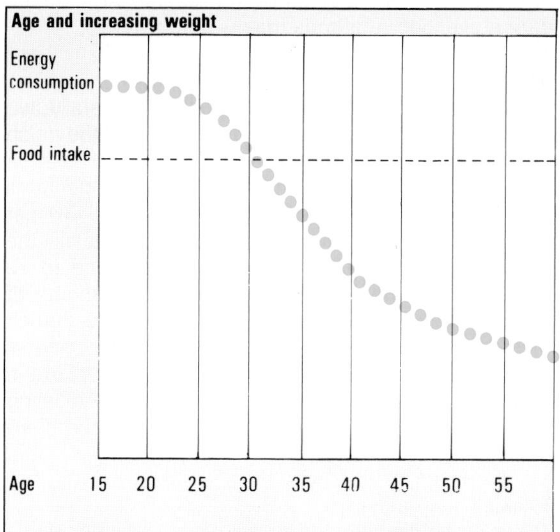

Healthy diet
The source of daily energy supply

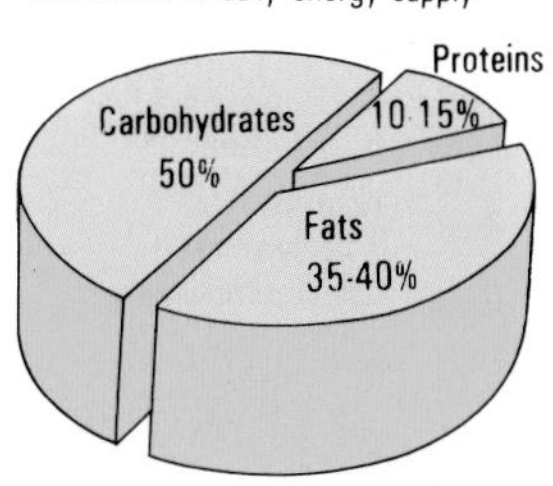

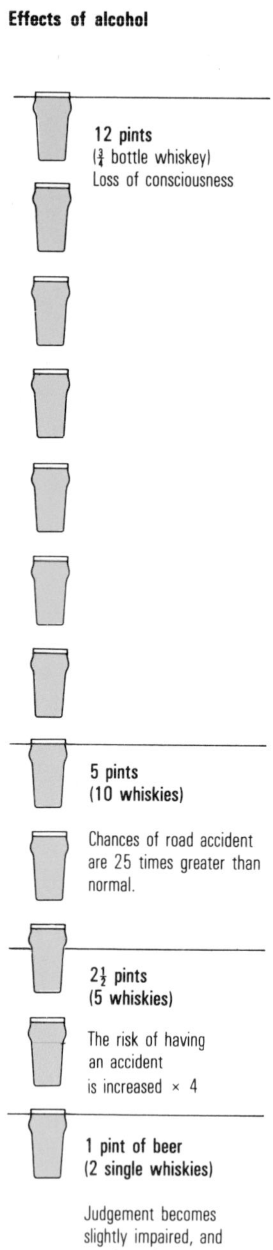
Effects of alcohol
12 pints
(¾ bottle whiskey)
Loss of consciousness
5 pints
(10 whiskies)
Chances of road accident are 25 times greater than normal.
2½ pints
(5 whiskies)
The risk of having an accident is increased × 4
1 pint of beer
(2 single whiskies)
Judgement becomes slightly impaired, and reactions slower

In some cases, the causes of disease are in the environment and the ability of the individual to control these factors is limited. Federal and state governments have a clear responsibility: pollutants in the air, radioactivity and indeed noise are, or should be, controlled by a public body in every country. However, there are ways in which the individual can take action, and they tend to boil down to awareness, and respect for, the risk factors for certain diseases. Thus for heart attack (***myocardial infarction*** – *see page 52)* the main risk factors are cigarette smoking, obesity, high blood pressure and high serum cholesterol. The first two factors are for the individual to control; the second two are, strictly speaking, jointly the concern of the doctor and the patient. Going for health checks regularly is the only certain way to alert the professional to the need for action.

Primary and secondary prevention

These terms have recently crept into the medical vocabulary. In the case of a heart attack, primary prevention means taking steps to prevent a heart attack ever happening. If an individual has already had one heart attack, secondary prevention aims to prevent a further one happening. Between primary and secondary prevention, methods may widely differ.

Diet

The average Western diet is not healthy. Generally, we all eat too much salt, too much animal fat and too much sugar as sucrose (ordinary refined white sugar). Fat, in particular, supplies 40 per cent of the average person's energy needs and this should be reduced to 30 per cent. Protein intake is about right and this is usually the expensive part of our diet. We generally need to increase the amount of fiber we eat and the amount of fruit and vegetables. Convenience foods like French fries, hamburgers and so on often contain much animal fat and salt. They are not necessarily bad foods; but in excess they do not provide a healthy diet. Adjusting diet in this way will help to prevent obesity and heart disease.

Smoking

This is probably the biggest single cause of preventable disease. Smoking is strongly linked with chest disease, heart disease, arterial disease, stomach disease and cancer to name but a few. In the last few years in the US, lung cancer has overtaken breast cancer as the commonest cancer in women, all due to smoking. Un-

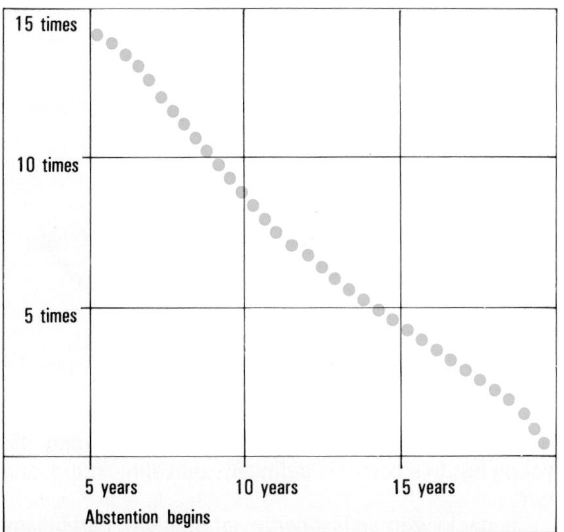

Chances of smokers' dying from lung cancer compared to non-smokers

fortunately, many people who smoke feel that disasters only happen to other people and it is always possible to point to an individual who has smoked all his life and who is fit and well in his eighties. He is the exception that proves the rule. The fewer cigarettes you smoke (preferably none), the more likely you are to remain healthy.

Alcohol

People in most Western countries drink alcohol to excess. Alcohol is strongly linked with liver disease, heart disease and intestinal disease – amongst others. However it is not necessary to stop consuming alcohol completely. Small amounts of alcohol seem to be actually beneficial to long-term health. Women should not exceed 14 units of alcohol per week and men should not exceed 21 units per week (a unit is half a pint of beer, a $4\frac{1}{2}$ ounce glass of wine or a single standard measure of spirits).

Cancer

There is no doubt that many cancers are preventable. For some, this depends on central control to reduce radioactivity or chemical contamination of the environment. Stopping smoking will reduce the risk of lung cancer. Excessive sunlight can cause skin cancer and this is a particular problem for light-skinned people in sunny parts of the world. Unfortunately, having a

Alcoholic content of drinks

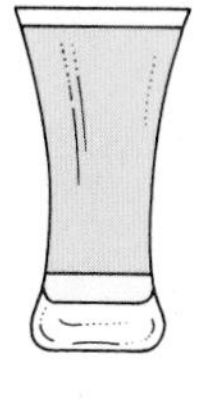

Beer 5% by volume

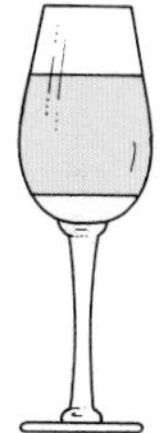

Wine 10% by volume

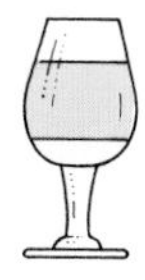

Fortified wine 20% by volume

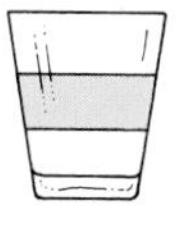

Spirits 40% by volume

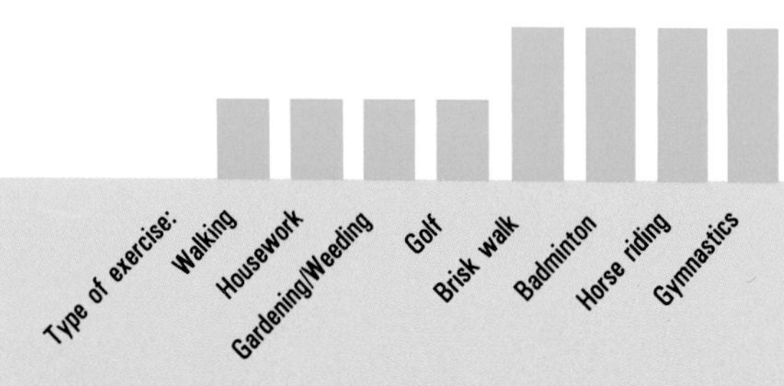

bronzed skin is regarded as fashionable among the young but this vogue is definitely unhealthy in the long run.

Cancer in women is a particular problem, particularly cancers of the breast, the neck of the womb (cervical cancer) and of the body of the womb itself. Screening systems now exist to look at all these problem areas. Women should be encouraged to examine their own breasts for unusual lumps and should have a mammogram and a cervical smear at least every one to two years. Many centers are setting up "well women" clinics for just these purposes. It is hoped that mammography, a simple X-ray examination of the breasts, will improve matters further.

Exercise

In general we all take too little exercise and this contributes to being overweight. This does not mean compulsory jogging for life, but everyone should try to take *some* exercise *each* day. Choose the form of exercise you enjoy most: it should be sufficiently strenuous to increase the heart rate. Recent studies have shown that the standard advice about the need to push for a maximal increase in heart rate (adjusted for age) is unnecessarily rigorous.

Infectious diseases

The big improvement in community health has come from the reduction in infectious diseases following the provision of clean water and effective sewers. It follows that general habits of cleanliness are important to health and everyone should, for example, wash their hands before preparing food before eating.

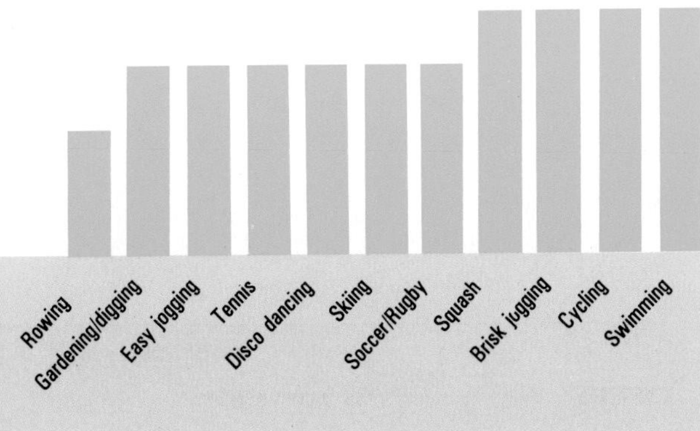

Immunization has done much to reduce the problems of infectious disease in childhood. Children should certainly be immunized against diptheria, tetanus and poliomyelitis and girls against rubella (German measles) if they have not had the natural disease by the age of 12. The whooping cough vaccine has brought immunization into poor repute, but there is little doubt that the risks of this vaccine have been over-stated and the benefits outweigh the risks in the majority of children. Whooping cough in children can be fatal, even with modern drugs.

If you are going abroad, particularly to the tropics, you will need to take special advice on preventing illness. It is, for example, essential to take drugs to prevent malaria, which probably kills more people throughout the world than any other disease. The problem of AIDS is now a real one: the AIDS virus is not easily spread, but is present in the vaginal secretions of women and the semen of men. The contraceptive sheath seems to give some protection against infection during sexual intercourse, though it does not guarantee ''safe sex''. Only a life-long monogamous relationship with an uninfected partner can do that.

All this amounts to only a brief summary of the possibilities of preventive medicine. One of the best ways to discover more is to contact one of the many local or national self-help groups. There is one for almost every disease though the more common, long-term disabling conditions such as diabetes and multiple sclerosis are represented by especially active groups. The chance to discuss problems with someone who has faced them too is reassuring and often prevents those same problems arising.

USING THE BOOK

Principal drug "families" relevant to the illness/disease.

Definition of illness/disease, including selective list of symptoms.

The book's scope is essentially drug treatment of illness. Medical problems never tackled with drugs are generally not included.

*A selection (*not *an exhaustive list) of the common chemical (generic) names of drugs plus some of their most familiar trade names. The list begins with US names, then moves on to give some of the commoner overseas names in English-speaking countries such as Australia, New Zealand, Canada and South Africa.*

Prescription drugs for the illness/disease; how they are given, and, in simple terms, how they work.

A selection of remedies generally available from pharmacists, with comments on their usefulness.

Usual (generally tolerated) and adverse side effects. These are not *exhaustive lists, and reactions in individuals vary widely.*

CYSTITIS

Antibiotics, sodium bicarbonate

NAMES YOU WILL HEAR
Antibiotics
Generic name: sulphamethizole; **trade names:** Microsul, Urolucosil, Urolex, Uroz, Thiosulfil, S-Methizole, Thiosulfil. **Generic name:** ampicillin; **trade names:** Omnipen, Polycillin, Principen, Ampifen, Penbritin, Pentrexyl, Vidopen, Austrapen, Bristin, Amcill, Ampicin, Ampilean, Biosan, Ampil, Famicilin, Pentrex, Petercillin, Synthecillin. **Generic name:** co-trimoxazole; **trade names:** Septra, Bactrim, Fectrim, Nodilon, Septrin. **Generic name:** nalidixic acid; **trade names:** NegGram, Mictral, Uriben. **Generic name:** nitrofuroantoin; **trade names:** Furadantin, Macrodantin.

WHAT IS CYSTITIS?
– An inflammation of the bladder. It may be accompanied by, or mimicked by urethritis, an inflammation of the tube by which urine passes from the bladder out of the body. Typical symptoms are painful and frequent urination, lower abdominal pain, blood in the urine and a high temperature.

CAUSES The root cause is either infection or bruising. The infection may be present in the kidneys or bloodstream and descend to the bladder, but more commonly it ascends from the urethra.

PRESCRIPTION DRUGS
Antibiotics: the common remedy. Many types are available; those listed here are particularly suited to treating cystitis; typically taken in pill form.
How they work: By killing bacteria responsible for infection. However, some bacteria can become resistant to some antibiotics; the antibiotic becomes ineffective, and a different one has to be prescribed. Antibiotics also have a tendency to kill not only the 'target' bacteria, but others as well; as some bacteria are naturally helpful in fighting harmful bacteria, a course of antibiotics can leave you without natural defenses.
Sodium bicarbonate helps relieve discomfort of cystitis.
How it works: by neutralizing acid in the urine.

OVER-THE-COUNTER TREATMENTS
Potassium citrate used to be a commonly recommended treatment but is no longer advised because if the kidneys are damaged a dangerous build-up of potassium could occur.

QUESTIONS TO ASK THE DOCTOR
- How long should I take the antibiotics?
- How soon will the symptoms go?
- How will I know whether they are working?
- What happens if I am allergic to the antibiotics?

SIDE EFFECTS
Antibiotics are usually prescribed for less than one week, but for recurrent cystitis you may take them for several weeks. Antibiotics can make you feel under-the-weather and lethargic; some people are allergic to them, and may develop a rash. Report this to a doctor immediately.
Potassium citrate: A helpful treatment, but it tastes awful, and could make you vomit.

142

The self-management/self-help sub-sections are, where appropriate, sub-divided to include measures for chronic (on-going) illness and acute episodes (sudden attacks).

SELF-MANAGEMENT

If you have had cystitis once, work against future infection – and the need to take antibiotics:

■ After using lavatory paper in the usual way, soap hands and gently clean anus; rinse hands, then pour a bottle of warm water over anus away from vagina.

■ Wear cotton underpants and change them daily. Avoid wearing panty hose. Rinse underwear well and do not use strong detergents or bleach.

■ Always pass urine within 15 minutes of sexual intercourse and then wash the uro-genital area with cool water. Rest – if possible.

■ Drink as little alcohol as possible, and if you do, try to have long drinks, and some bland liquid afterwards.

■ Drink 1-2 quarts of bland liquid or water daily.

SELF-HELP IN AN ATTACK

As soon as the attack begins:

1 Get a couple of heating pads. **2** Drink one pint of cold water and let your stomach settle. **3** Take one teaspoon of bicarbonate of soda mixed in water or jelly. **4** Take two strong painkillers. **5** Fill a pitcher and glass with bland liquid; keep them by you and drink often. **6** Once each hour drink strong coffee. **7** Try to put your feet up, or go to bed. Take your jug and glass, but before resting, drink another half pint of fluid. **8** Put one heating pad on your back and the other high up between your legs, resting against the uretheral opening. **9** Every time you pass water, wash the surrounding area and gently pat it dry. **10** Continue to drink half a pint of liquid every 20 minutes.

The key to self-help is to drink large amounts of fluid, and to take sodium bicarbonate to make the urine less acid. However, if your kidneys do not function normally, this could be dangerous. Before attempting to manage subsequent attacks, get your doctor to measure your kidney function.

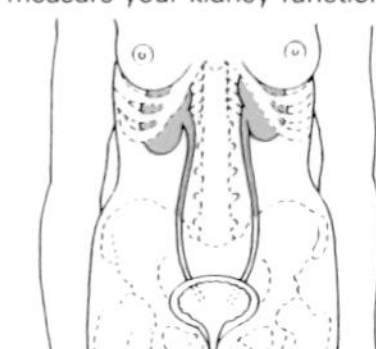

***The kidneys** produce and excrete urine. Waste materials in the blood are extracted in the kidneys and transformed into urine. This passes via the ureter tubes to the bladder where it is stored until the bladder fills up. It then passes through a valve to the urethra, down which it passes to be expelled from the body.*

PATIENT'S EXPERIENCE

"My first treatment for cystitis was a month's course of antibiotics which made me really sick. A few weeks later, back came the cystitis, and more antibiotics were prescribed. Over the next few months I had to take 14 different types of pills. After a variety of investigations, including cauterizing of my urethra, I was prescribed yet more antibiotics. In the end, it was my doctor who said 'try passing water after intercourse'. After all that fruitless medication, it was this simple advice which worked."

The case histories do not relate to actual individuals; they are amalgamations of the typical accounts of illness and disease heard by doctors during consultation. Similarity to any individual's circumstances is purely coincidental. No confidential patient information is disclosed.

143

STANDARD SAFETY PRECAUTIONS WITH MEDICINES

1

Keep medicines out of the reach of children.

2

Keep medicines in the containers in which you receive them – never transfer medicines from one container to another.

3

Your medicines have been prescribed especially for you. Never allow other people to take them. Do not accept medicines which have been prescribed for anyone else.

4

If you have difficulty in opening your medicine container please ask your pharmacist for alternative packaging.

5

If you find the instructions on the label difficult to read, please tell your pharmacist.

6

Always follow the instructions carefully when taking or using medicines. If you have not been given instructions, or if you do not understand them, ask your pharmacist for advice.

The contributors to *The Patients' Desk Reference* are not the only people to believe that a better understanding of medicines allows them to be used to better effect. In the US, and other countries throughout the world, government health departments, pharmaceutical companies and medical faculties of univer-

7

Keep medicines in a cool, dry place unless otherwise directed: some medicines may need to be kept in a refrigerator.

8

Some medicines have an expiry or 'use before' date. Do not use them after this date.

9

Dispose of unwanted medicines carefully. If in doubt, return them to your pharmacist who will dispose of them for you.

10

When buying medicines, please tell the pharmacist about any medicines your doctor has prescribed for you.

11

Some medicines take several days to achieve their intended benefit.

12

If you experience side effects with a medicine, please tell your doctor or pharmacist.

sities are starting to tackle the task of ensuring that patients receive information about their medicines in an easily understandable form.

In the UK, for instance, drugs manufacturers are including (from mid-1988) descriptive leaflets with most medicines.

Gastro-intestinal problems

The gastro-intestinal system includes the esophagus (or gullet), the stomach, and the intestines – both small and large bowel. Food is partly digested in the stomach and then, in the small intestine, further digestion and absorption of nutrients take place. In the large bowel (or colon) water is removed from the contents to form feces (stools) which are discharged through the anus via the rectum. The liver, with the gall bladder, is included in the gastro-intestinal system because this is primarily where all the nutrients absorbed into the body are put to use and ''metabolised''

See also: *Obesity, page 154; organ transplants, page 216; blood and nutritional, pages 218-231; food intolerance, page 230.*

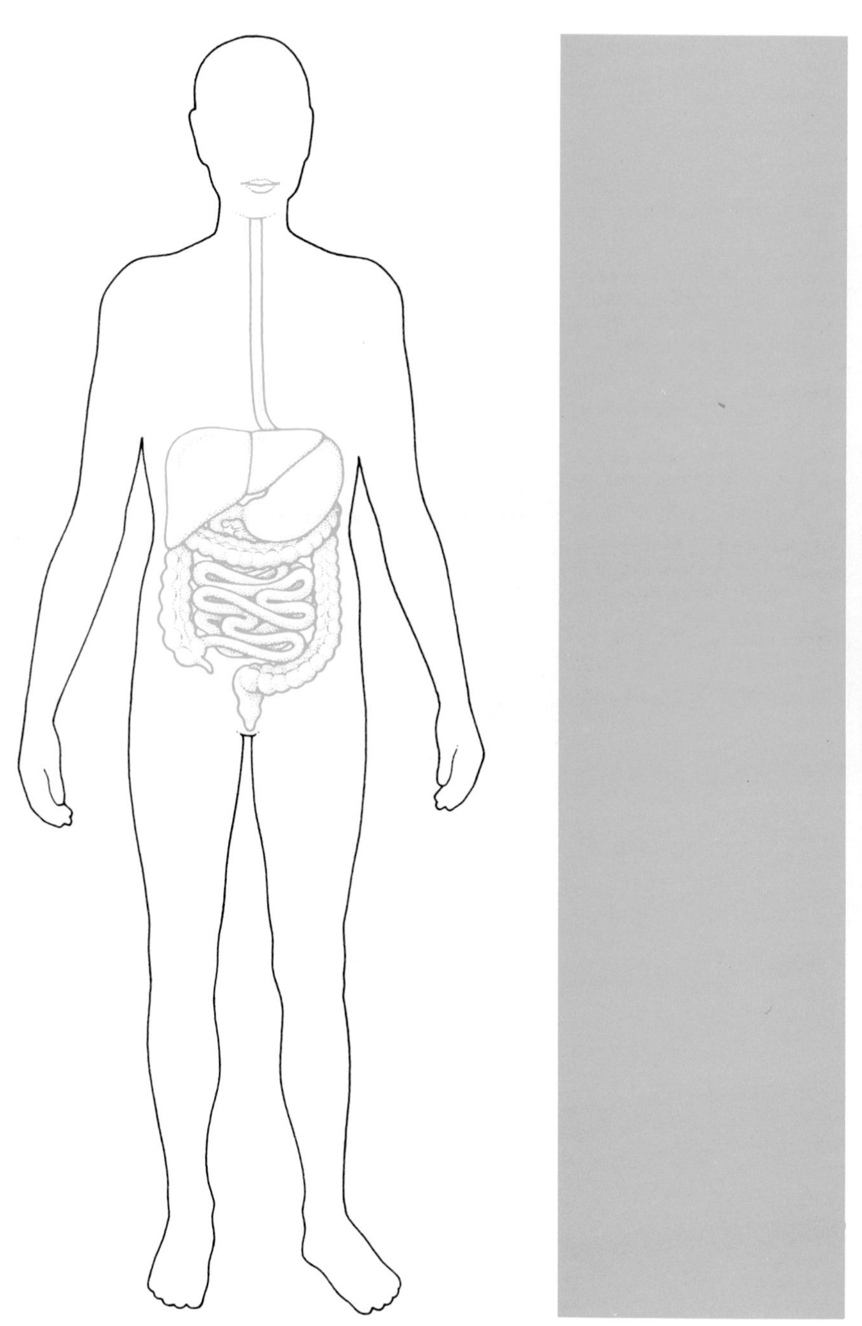

Antacids

NAMES YOU WILL HEAR

Antacids

Generic name: aluminum hydroxide; **trade names:** AlternaGEL, Maalox, DiGel, Mylanta, Gaviscon, Aludrox, Gastrocote, Amphojel, Hasaljel, Alumag. **Generic name:** alexitol; **trade name:** Actal. **Generic name:** hydrotalcite; **trade name:** Altacite. **Generic name:** magnesium hydroxide; **trade names:** Magnesium Hydroxide Mixture, Milk of Magnesia. **Generic name:** magnesium trisilicate; **trade names:** Gaviscon, Gelusil, Trisil.

Anti-emetics

Generic name: metoclopramide; **trade names:** Reglan, Parmid, Primperan, Maxeran, Metramid, Maxolon. **Generic name:** domperidone; **trade name:** Motilium.

H2 antagonists

Generic name: cimetidine; **trade name:** Tagamet. **Generic name:** ranitidine; **trade name:** Zantac. **Generic name:** famotidine; **trade name:** Pepcid.

WHAT IS INDIGESTION?

Pain – typically the aching variety – in the upper abdomen, just under the ribs, in the midriff line. It can be associated with heartburn, a burning pain in the center of the chest, sometimes extending up to the throat, with an acid taste in the mouth; also with waterbrash, when fluid floods into the mouth, often accompanied by nausea. Another meaning of indigestion, used by some people, is belching or burping.

"Hiatal hernia" is a condition in which the stomach bulges up through the diaphragm into the chest, and is often, but not always, accompanied by the symptoms described above.

Esophagitis is inflammation of the gullet, and this causes similar pain, especially after drinking hot liquids. It is caused by stomach acid leaking up into the gullet, particularly when there is a hiatal hernia.

CAUSES Anything which irritates or inflames the stomach can cause these symptoms: too much food or drink, especially alcohol, stress, or spicy foods, and smoking. These all cause inflammation of the stomach lining, or gastritis. Ulcers represent a more severe form of inflammation, when lining is completely lost over a small area – *see* ***peptic ulcer,*** *page 26*.

(If you are male and drink more than 16 units of alcohol per week, you could be over the limit which is safe for you – *see* ***alcoholism,*** *page 94;* in women the limit is less.)

PRESCRIPTION DRUGS

Antacids: available either as pills to be chewed or as liquid.

How they work: absorbing, or neutralizing acid produced by the stomach. It is a common misconception that stomach acid actually causes the condition. In fact its role is to aggravate already existing inflammation. Some preparations also contain alginic acid, which helps the antacid to coat the lining of the stomach or gullet.

Antiemetics lessen the symptoms of indigestion, nausea and heartburn.

How they work: Either by reducing the time food and acid remain in the stomach by stimulating stomach emptying, or by acting on the brain to reduce nausea.

H2 antagonists are expensive, but are highly effective for ulcer healing, both gastric and duodenal, and also for esophagitis, for which higher doses are used. They are less useful for other forms of indigestion and are not normally used unless the diagnosis has been proved by tests.

How they work: The output of acid by the stomach is almost completely stopped by these drugs. *See* ***peptic ulcer,*** *page 26.*

QUESTIONS TO ASK THE DOCTOR

- When should I take the antacids?
- Should I change my diet?
- Have I got an ulcer?

SIDE EFFECTS

Antacids are relatively free from serious side effects, unless taken in gross excess. Bicarbonate of soda, which is often used as a home remedy, will cause serious disturbance to the body's chemical balance if taken regularly. Aluminum-based antacids tend to cause constipation, while magnesium-based preparations lead to diarrhea: this is why most are a mixture of the two.

Antiemetics may, rarely, cause unpleasant involuntary movements of the limbs, especially in the young and the old. They usually stop as the drug wears off.

H2 antagonists have no serious side effects, although cimetidine may interfere with other drugs, and occasionally causes diarrhea. *See* ***peptic ulcer,*** *page 26.*

OVER-THE-COUNTER TREATMENTS

A wide range of antacids is available without prescription, such as Rolaids, Tums, Maalox, Peptobismol or Milk of Magnesia, but if you need to take them continually you should consult your doctor. Expensive preparations are unlikely to be any more effective than simple magnesium hydroxide or aluminum hydroxide (either pills or liquid). Magnesium containing preparations should be avoided by patients with kidney diesase.

SELF-MANAGEMENT

- If you smoke, give up. All forms of tobacco stimulate the stomach to produce acid, the main cause of pain and ulcers.
- If you are overweight, lose weight. Fat in and around the abdomen presses on the stomach, leading to acid regurgitation and heartburn.
- Avoid large meals late at night. Avoid fatty food, as fat delays stomach emptying, encouraging acid regurgitation.
- Avoid foods you know will provoke trouble.

PATIENT'S EXPERIENCE

"I began to suffer from indigestion – a gnawing pain under the ribs – ten years ago. I was working long hours as a foreman printer, and lived on beer and sandwiches, and a roll of antacids per day. After two years I saw my doctor, thinking I had an ulcer. He arranged a gastroscopy, a tube down the throat to look inside the stomach. The specialist said there was no ulcer, but it was very inflamed. I was advised to stop smoking and cut down on the beer. To my surprise I lost 30 lb (12 kg) and the pains went. I still take antacids from time to time, but I know the reason: either missing a meal, stress, or eating something spicy."

SELF-HELP IN AN ATTACK

Once pain starts, a proprietary antacid will probably help; bicarbonate of soda can be used in an emergency, but not regularly. If food relieves your pain, and the symptoms occur frequently, it is quite likely you have an ulcer: see your doctor.

NAUSEA AND VOMITING

Antiemetics, betahistine, glucose-salt solutions

NAMES YOU WILL HEAR

General anti-emetics

Generic name: prochlorperazine; **trade names:** Compazine, Stemetil, Anti-Naus, Mitil, Vertigon. **Generic name:** trifluoperazine; **trade name:** Stelazine. **Generic name:** cyclizine; **trade names:** Marzine, Valoid. **Generic name:** cinnarizine; **trade name:** Stugeron. **Generic name:** metoclopramide; **trade names:** Reglan, Maxolon, Metox, Metramid, Parmin, Primperan, Gastrobid. **Generic name:** domperidone; **trade names:** Evoxin, Motilium. **Generic name:** promethazine; **trade names:** Phenergan, Avomine, Progan, Prothazine, Histantil, Lenazine, Prohist, Profan. **Generic name:** meclizine; **trade names:** Ancoloxin, Antivert, Ancolan, Bonamine, Navicalm.

Meniére's Disease

Generic name: betahistine; **trade name:** Serc.

Glucose-salt solutions

Generic name: sodium chloride: **trade names:** Dioralyte, Rehidrat.

CAUSES

Gastroenteritis or general infection (for example tonsillitis, ear infection, meningitis, kidney infection, appendicitis); obstructions in the bowel, scars from previous operations, or tumors; hormonal changes as in pregnancy and diabetes; disorders of balance, including motion sickness, Menière's Disease and certain viral infections of the ear; brain disease causing pressure on the brain or migraine; certain drugs (digitalis, opiate analgesics, some drugs used in the treatment of cancer and the estrogen component of the contraceptive pill); poisons (iron, lead), alcohol, radiotherapy; psychogenic factors such as anxiety or bulimia *(see pages 84 and 220).*

WHAT ARE NAUSEA AND VOMITING?

Vomiting is a reflex action caused by a stimulus from the vomiting center in the base of the brain. It is usually preceded by nausea – the inclination to vomit – accompanied by sweating, pallor, excessive salivation and dizziness *(see page 96).* Profuse or prolonged vomiting can result in dehydration.

CAUSES See list in margin. All those listed can stimulate the vomiting center in the brain, either via substances in the bloodstream, or by stimulation of nerves.

PRESCRIPTION DRUGS

The choice of drug depends partly on the cause:
Antiemetic drugs can be used to treat vomiting generally, but the side effects are significant. They should not be used if the cause can be rapidly treated and they are only appropriate for cases of persistent vomiting, not for nausea. This applies especially to children and old people, in whom side effects are commonest. They can be given by mouth, or by injection or suppository if the patient is vomiting continuously.
How they work: by acting on the brain, suppressing the stimulus to vomit. Duration of action and the degree of drowsiness caused vary widely. Test different varieties to find which suits you best.

After vomiting, one should drink clear fluid to replace what has been lost. A glucose-salt solution may be a useful alternative to clear fluid, particularly in young children. *See **diarrhea,** page 26.*

Promethazine and **meclizine** have been used for many years to treat vomiting in early pregnancy, with no reports of adverse effects. However, drugs should *only* be used if vomiting is really severe, not for nausea: there is always the potential for drug-induced abnormalities in the fetus. *See **pregnancy,** page 184.*

Severe nausea and vomiting associated with Menière's Disease and vertigo can be difficult to treat. *See **dizziness,** page 96.* **Betahistine** is said to have a specific effect; if it does not work, any of the general antiemetics could be tried.
How it works: not fully understood, but it is thought to improve circulation to the brain. Metoclopramide antagonises dopamine in the brain and thus calms the vomiting centre *(see **migraine,** page 100).*

OVER-THE-COUNTER TREATMENTS

Oral rehydration fluids are useful for maintaining adequate hydration in children; they may be used as soon as vomiting starts. Some motion sickness drugs can be bought without a prescription; self-treatment is appropriate, but it is worth experimenting to find the one that suits best.

QUESTIONS TO ASK THE DOCTOR

■ When can I start on solid foods again?
■ Should I avoid any foods?
■ How long is the vomiting likely to last?
■ Are drugs necessary?
■ How often can I take the treatment?

SIDE EFFECTS

Antiemetics are often antihistamines and tend to have similar side effects. However, the frequency and severity vary as much between people as between drugs. They all cause drowsiness and should not be taken while driving or working in a potentially dangerous environment. This drowsiness is made worse by alcohol. Other side effects include dry mouth, headache and irritability. Muscle stiffness and spasms can occur, usually associated with high doses, but children and some individuals are more sensitive. The effect is reversible with an appropriate drug.

These drugs should not be used in children under 25 lb (10 kg), in people who are dehydrated, nor in people with glaucoma.

Betahistine (not an antihistamine) causes headache and must not be used in people with asthma or peptic ulcer.

SELF-MANAGEMENT

■ Some normal babies regurgitate their feeds. This is no cause for worry if the baby is gaining weight, and it can be at least partially improved by frequent winding, thickening feeds and propping up after feeds. It usually resolves once the baby is on a mixed diet. ■ Any patient who has vomited should be given clear fluids to drink. The most suitable are sugar-salt solution, water, diluted pure apple juice or soda water. ■ Milk and other dairy products should be avoided, as should all fatty foods. Digesting fat causes extra strain on an already irritated stomach. ■ Small amounts of fluid, taken frequently, are easiest to absorb. ■ Fever can cause or aggravate vomiting, particularly in young children, so get the patient's temperature down: *see* ***common cold, page 134.*** ■ Aspirin should not be used when there is nausea or vomiting. ■ Vomiting during pregnancy: Have something to eat BEFORE getting up in the morning. Eat small, frequent meals during the day.

PATIENT'S EXPERIENCE

"My four-year-old daughter suddenly started vomiting in the middle of the night. She did not seem particularly ill, and she didn't have a fever. I had some sugar-salt solution powder, which I made up for her. She wouldn't drink it because she didn't like the taste; so I mixed it with apple juice. She seemed happy to sip it, and it put my mind at rest; however she vomited once more before sleeping for a few hours.

Next morning, she had a slight fever and vomited again, so I phoned the doctor. He told me to give her two teaspoonsful of acetaminophen. When he saw her, he said he thought gastroenteritis, caused by a virus, was the most likely cause. He suggested keeping her on clear fluids during the day and to give the acetaminophen every four hours if she had a fever. By evening she was much better. I kept her on a bland diet next day, but she was fine by then."

WHEN TO SEE A DOCTOR

■ If vomiting persists for more than 24 hours. ■ If a child under six years has diarrhea or fever as well as vomiting: there is a danger of dehydration. ■ If there is vomiting after a head injury. ■ If the patient is not only vomiting but generally ill.

TREATMENT OF MOTION SICKNESS

■ Take the medication about half an hour before starting the journey. ■ Avoid heavy, fatty meals before or during the journey. ■ If in a car or train, face forwards and look out of the window. ■ If on a boat, lie flat, or if you wish to be up and about, try to keep your gaze on the horizon. ■ Have small frequent meals. ■ Don't read or write while in motion.

PEPTIC ULCER

Antacids, H_2 antagonists, mucosal strengtheners, anticholinergics

NAMES YOU WILL HEAR
Antacids
Generic name: aluminum hydroxide/magnesium trisilicate mixtures; **trade names:** Gaviscon, Aludrox, Gastrocote, Alusorb, Adagel, Amphojel, Basaljel, Alumag, Amphojel. **Generic name:** aluminum hydroxide/megnesium hydroxide mixtures; **trade names:** Maalox, Mucaine. **Generic name:** aluminum hydroxide/magnesium carbonate mixtures; **trade names:** Gastalar, Gastrils, Dijene. **Generic name:** calcium carbonate mixtures; **trade names:** Tums, Titralac, Cal-tab.

Histamine (H2) antagonists
Generic name: cimetidine; **trade name:** Tagamet. **Generic name:** ranitidine; **trade name:** Zantac.

Mucosal strengtheners
Generic name: carbenoxolone; **trade names:** Pyrogastrone, Biogastrone, Duogastrone, Bioral Gel. **Generic name:** chelated bismuth suspension; **trade name:** De-Nol. **Generic name:** sucralfate; **trade names:** Corafate, Antepsin, Sulcrate, Ulsanic.

Anticholinergic
Generic name: pirenzipine; **trade name:** Gastrozepin.

WHAT IS A PEPTIC ULCER?

A defect, or a hole, in the lining of the gut – the mucosa. They can occur in the gullet (oesophageal ulcer), stomach (gastric ulcer), duodenum (duodenal ulcer) or rarely in other parts of the gut. Pain in the upper abdomen, or sometimes the chest and back, is the most common symptom. The pain, especially from a duodenal ulcer, is commonly related to meals, often being relieved by food or milk. Most cases are treated with drugs, but surgery may be needed for complications such as bleeding.

CAUSES Although this is a common disease, the mechanism of ulcer formation is not understood. Smoking and heavy alcohol consumption are thought to increase the risk; drugs such as aspirin and indeed various drugs used to treat arthritis can cause ulcers.

PRESCRIPTION DRUGS

Antacids: taken as liquid, or tablets; often taste 'chalky' or 'minty'. (Also widely available over the counter.)
How they work: as the name suggests, antacids work by neutralizing the acid secreted by the stomach; although the volume of acid the average dose neutralizes is small.
Histamine H_2 antagonists: powerful, ulcer-healing drugs, given as tablets, but can be injected into the bloodstream in hospital. They relieve the symptoms of indigestion.
How they work: Stimulation of the H_2 receptors of the stomach promotes the production of acid to help digest food. It is this acid which also causes the pain, and enlarges the ulcer. H_2 blockers specifically block this process.
Mucosal strengtheners: These are also powerful ulcer-healing drugs. Depending on type, they may be taken in liquid form or as capsules or tablets.
How they work: normally, the gut lining (mucosa) defends itself against the acid within the stomach by covering itself with thick slime (mucus). Some of the mucosal strengtheners work by increasing the rate of production of the protective mucus. Others bind to the ulcer itself, protecting it against further erosion by acid.
Anticholinergics: also ulcer-healing drugs.
How they work: by blocking nervous impulses which produce stomach acid.

OVER-THE-COUNTER TREATMENTS

There are many antacids available without prescription;

even if they help with the pain, see your doctor – ULCERS CAN BE HAZARDOUS.

QUESTIONS TO ASK THE DOCTOR

- For how long should I take the medication?
- Are there any foods or drinks I should avoid?

SIDE EFFECTS

Antacids: Tell the doctor about other drugs that you are taking because antacids may interfere with their absorption from the gut. Some antacids (those containing calcium or aluminium) tend to constipate, while others (containing magnesium) may cause diarrhea; otherwise side effects are uncommon.

Histamine H_2 antagonists: may be given for some months until the ulcer heals; sometimes continued indefinitely to prevent recurrence. Side effects are unusual, but in men, impotence and enlargement of the breasts have been occasionally reported, and these drugs can cause confusion in the elderly. Ranitidine is better than cimetidine in this respect. H_2 antagonists can interfere with other drugs taken simultaneously; discuss with your doctor.

Mucosal strengtheners: In the USA, only sucralfate is available. Follow the directions carefully. It has almost no side effects other than constipation and a dry mouth.

Anticholinergics: Several anticholinergics used in the past often produced adverse effects, including dry mouth, constipation, blurred vision and difficulty passing urine. Patients with glaucoma should not take anticholinergics.

SELF-MANAGEMENT

Four steps towards helping an ulcer heal quickly:

- If you smoke, stop. This will speed healing.
- Avoid drinking large amounts of alcohol.
- Eat regular meals. Obviously you should avoid foods which upset you, but there are no hard rules about diet.
- Don't take aspirin-like painkillers *(see page 106)* without consulting your doctor.

SELF-HELP IN AN ATTACK

1 You can relieve the ulcer pain quickly by drinking milk, or taking an antacid.

2 If you have ulcer-healing drugs left from a previous attack, **don't take them without consulting a doctor.**

3 See a doctor, soon. If you vomit blood, pass black faeces, or feel faint, call your doctor or go to hospital.

PATIENT'S EXPERIENCE

"I had a nasty gnawing pain high up in my stomach, which only went away when I ate; it often used to wake me up at night. The doctor gave me some white medicine which helped the pain a lot, and sent me for a telescope test to look for ulcers. I was given an injection which made me drowsy, and the doctor passed a thin tube down my throat – it wasn't bad at all. I was told that I had an ulcer, and started on some special tablets. I haven't had any trouble since."

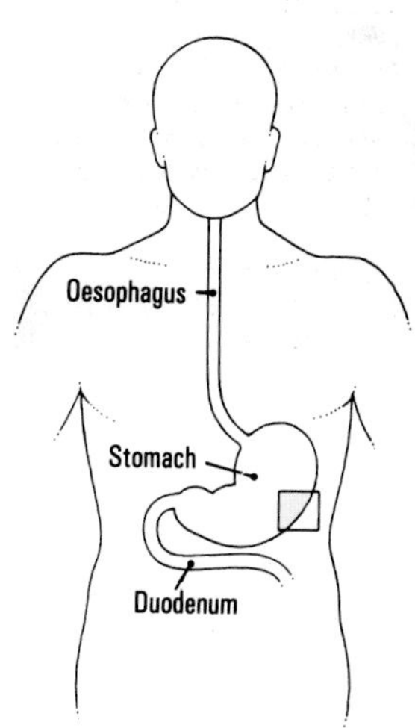

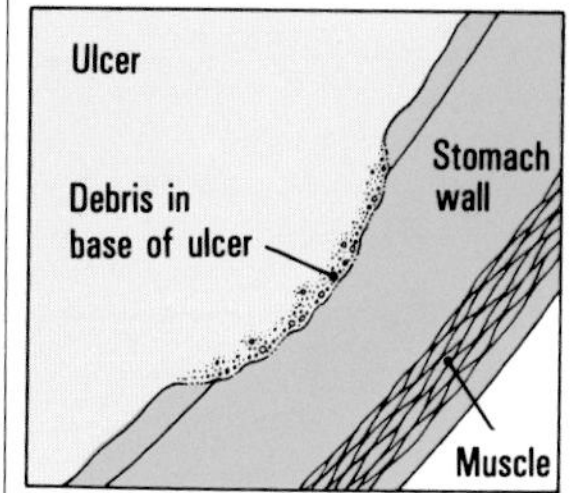

DIARRHEA

Fluid replacements, anti-diarrheal drugs, antibiotics

NAMES YOU WILL HEAR

Glucose-salt solutions
Generic name: sodium chloride; **trade names:** usually precribed by generic name in US, elswhere Dioralyte, Rehidrat.

Anti-diarrhoeal drugs
Generic name: codeine phosphate; **trade names:** usually prescribed by generic name in US, elsewhere Codlin, Diarrest, Kaodene, Paveral. **Generic name:** diphenoxylate hydrochloride; **trade name:** Lomotil. **Generic name:** loperamide; **trade name:** Imodium. **Generic name:** kaolin and morphine; **trade name:** Donnagel; usually prescribed by generic name.

Antibiotics
Generic name: erythromycin; **trade names:** Benzamycin, Erymax, Ilotycin, Pediamycin, Pediazole, Arpimycin, Erycen, Erythroped, Retcin, Erythrocin, Erythromid, EpMycin, Erostin, Emu-V, Ethryn, Eromel, Ilocap, Ilosone, Rythrocaps. **Generic name:** co-trimoxazole; **trade names:** Septra, Septra DS, Bactrim, Fectrim, Nodilon, Septrim.

Non specific agents
Generic name: bismuth subsalcylate; **trade name:** Pepto-Bismol. **Generic name:** kaolin and pectin; **trade name:** Kaopectate. **Generic name:** attapulgite and pectin; **trade name:** Polymagma.

WHAT IS DIARRHEA?

– The frequent passage of loose or liquid feces. Normally the large bowel absorbs most of the water in the digestive system, leaving a semi-solid residue – the feces. When excess fluid passes down the bowel, or when the bowel is unable to absorb fluid, the normally solid feces become liquid, and are passed more frequently. Excessive loss of fluid causes dehydration, which can be fatal.

CAUSES The infection known as gastroenteritis is responsible for most attacks of diarrhea in babies and young children, but can affect people of any age. It is usually caused by rotaviruses, but many other organisms can be involved. All are infectious.

In adults the commonest cause is food poisoning. One type, caused by poisons produced by bacteria in food, starts two to four hours after eating. The other is caused by bacteria (often *salmonella*) themselves multiplying in food; it starts 12-24 hours after eating. Both types may be accompanied by vomiting; the first is less prolonged and is not contagious.

Travelers' diarrhea is a form of gastroenteritis suffered by people newly arrived in a foreign, usually hot, country. It is caused by the local strains of various bacteria or viruses, such as *E.coli*, against which the body has no immunity.

In old or ill people 'false diarrhea' can result from constipation: an overflow of liquid feces by passing the hard, impacted constipated stool, giving the appearance of diarrhea. Medical advice is needed here.

PRESCRIPTION DRUGS

Glucose-salt solution: for infants and young children, or whenever diarrhea is severe. This solution, containing glucose and various salts in the correct proportions, is by far the most important form of treatment, and will prevent dehydration if started early.
How it works: It replaces the sodium, potassium and bicarbonate lost with water in the feces.
Anti-diarrheal drugs: These relieve the painful spasms, and reduce the frequency of diarrhea. They DO NOT prevent dehydration.
How they work: By reducing activity of the bowel. They cause severe constipation if used for too long. They should never be used in children under four, and only with caution in older children and the elderly.
Antibiotics are only used in certain forms of diarrhea.
How they work: by killing the bacteria responsible.

OVER-THE-COUNTER TREATMENT

Both glucose-salt solutions and anti-diarrheal drugs are available from pharmacists. If you feel confident in using them, and take care to follow the guidelines on the package, you will save unnecessary visits to the doctor. BUT for babies under two years, or anyone with severe pain or vomiting, medical advice is essential.

QUESTIONS TO ASK THE DOCTOR

- How can I prevent it spreading to other people?
- Should I drink milk, or avoid it?
- When should I start solid food again?

SIDE EFFECTS

Glucose-salt solution may cause nausea: try one of the flavored varieties, or add a little fruit juice. **Anti-diarrheal drugs** readily cause constipation if continued too long. Some, including Lomotil, can cause drowsiness. These drugs should NOT be used to treat the diarrhea of inflammatory bowel disease *(see page 30).*

SELF-MANAGEMENT

■ Prevention: Food poisoning results from unhygienic food preparation, and inadequate cooking or reheating. Always wash your hands before preparing food, use clean utensils, refrigerate food quickly and reheat thoroughly. ■ When traveling: Avoid eating unwashed, unpeeled fruit, or drinking tap water unless you are sure it has been boiled, or chemically sterilized. Avoid ice cubes in drinks, unless prepared from clean water. ■ For short trips (less than one week), an antibiotic such as doxycycline may be taken as a preventive measure.

SELF-HELP IN AN ATTACK

■ Young children with diarrhea require immediate fluid replacement. Use glucose-salt solution if possible, but any fluid will help. ■ For adults, the discomfort and embarrassment of diarrhea can be reduced by taking anti-diarrheal drugs, but remember also to take plenty of fluids. ■ Solid food should be stopped for 24 hours, but as soon as you feel able, start again with dry bread or toast and small amounts of vegetables. Avoid fatty food and milk products, which can aggravate the symptoms. ■ Be aware of the signs of dehydration: Dehydration results in thirst, dry mouth, fast breathing, and sometimes fever. An early sign is reduction in the amount and frequency of urine passed. Drink enough to keep up normal output.

PATIENT'S EXPERIENCE

"I developed diarrhea after a business trip to the Middle East. The cramping pains started as the plane landed in New York, and I began to feel very ill. My doctor gave me some loperamide which eased the pain and diarrhea."

HOME-MADE GLUCOSE-SALT SOLUTION

A safe substitute for commercial glucose-salt solution can be made up from 1/10 oz (3.5 grams) of salt and 1½ oz (40 grams) of sugar (or half the amount of glucose) in 1 3/4 pints (1 litre) of water. Too much salt is dangerous: 3.5 grams is slightly less than one small level teaspoon. The solution should not be more salty than tears. Fruit juice or squash can be added for taste.

Laxatives

NAMES YOU WILL HEAR

Bulking agents

Generic name: methylcellulose; **trade names:** Cologel, Celevac, Cellucon, BFL, Cellulon, Nilstim. **Generic name:** psyllium; **trade names:** Metamucil, Konsyl, Naturacil, Agiolax, Fybogel, Isogel, Regulan. **Generic name:** sterculia; **trade names:** Normacol, Inotaxine, Karagum, Prefil. **Generic name:** bran; **trade names:** Fybranta, Proctofibre, Trifyba.

Osmotic laxatives

Generic name: lactulose; **trade names:** Cephulac, Chronulac, Duphalac, Lactalose Solution. **Generic name:** magnesium hydroxide; **trade name:** Milk of Magnesia.

Lubricant

Generic name: liquid paraffin; **trade name:** Petrolagar. **Generic name:** mineral oil; **trade name:** prescribed by generic name in USA.

Stimulant laxatives

Generic name: bisacodyl; **trade names:** Evac Q Kwik, Dulcolax, Dulcodos, Toilex, Bisacolax, Laco, Perilax. **Generic name:** senna; **trade names:** Senna Tablets, Senokot. **Generic name:** docusate sodium; **trade names:** Dialose, Kasot, Dioctyl-Medo, Normax, Constiban, Regulex.

WHAT IS CONSTIPATION?

– Failure to pass normal feces (''stools''). What constitutes ''normal'' is open to a wide range of interpretations, but constipation implies the infrequent passage of hard feces, which may be accompanied by pain or discomfort. By contrast, the normal feces passed by people living in rural Africa are bulky and semi-liquid, due to their high-fiber diet of unrefined grain, fruit, and vegetables.

CAUSES By far the commonest cause of constipation is a diet lacking sufficient fiber or roughage. This is a hazard of modern life, with its convenience foods, which are highly processed, removing most of the natural fiber.

Many drugs and medicines can interfere with the normal working of the bowel, causing constipation. The most significant of these are antidepressants and painkillers such as codeine. Lack of thyroid hormone (myxedema) is a rare but important cause of severe constipation, as are many diseases of the nervous system, especially dementia and depression in the elderly. Irritable bowel syndrome *(page 30)* is another cause of constipation.

Constipation in young children is often a result of anxiety about emptying the bowel (fear of pain, embarrassment); or part of a more complex psychological disturbance. This can become a severe problem; treatment often involves the whole family, and is directed at behaviour and feelings rather than at the constipation itself. *See also* ***hemorrhoids,*** *page 34.*

PRESCRIPTION DRUGS

Bulking agents: When prescribed, these are supplements to the diet, and should only be necessary if the patient really finds a high-fiber diet – at least 1 oz (30 grams) – of coarse bran per day too unpleasant (see SIDE EFFECTS).

All bulking agents should be taken with plenty of fluid: at least 3½ pints (1.5 litres) per day.

How they work: by increasing the water in the feces.

Osmotic laxatives also increase the water content of the stool, leading to a larger, softer stool.

How they work: The laxative contains sugars and/or salts which the body does not absorb and these attract (by osmosis) water into the bowel.

Stimulant laxatives may be necessary in the initial treatment of constipation, provided intestinal obstruction has been excluded.

How they work: by acting on the muscle wall of the large bowel, making it propel the contents forward. In excess, they readily cause diarrhea.
Suppositories: Glycerine suppositories stimulate defecation without any risk of side effects. They are best avoided in young children, who find them frightening or painful.
How they work: uncertain, but lubrication plays a part.
Enemas, usually administered by a nurse, are sometimes necessary in the initial management of severe constipation, especially in the elderly.
How they work: by softening hard, dry feces; they also stimulate the bowel muscle by increasing the volume of the feces.

QUESTIONS TO ASK THE DOCTOR

- Why am I constipated?
- How can I improve my diet?
- How long should I use the medicines?
- Have I got hemorrhoids?

SIDE EFFECTS

Bulking agents (including bran) can lead to bloating, increased wind (flatus), and to discomfort. Reducing the quantity, and then building it up gradually, with plenty of fluids, should solve this. **Stimulant laxatives** cause colicky pains as a direct result of their action on the bowel. This is probably inevitable, and acceptable, if the laxative is used for a short period only. **Osmotic laxatives** and **suppositories** have no significant side effects.

OVER-THE-COUNTER TREATMENTS

All the preparations discussed here are available without prescription. Buy them from a pharmacist who is prepared to advise on their use.

SELF-MANAGEMENT

- In addition to bran, many foods are high in fiber, and prevent constipation: wholemeal bread, whole grain cereals, fruits (oranges, grapefruits tangerines, and other citrus fruits), nuts, vegetables (especially peas, beans and carrots).
- A high-fiber diet has other beneficial effects: it lowers blood cholesterol, helps weight reduction, and may deter hemorrhoids. It may also reduce the risk of developing a bowel cancer.
- You should consult your doctor about any change in your normal bowel habits: this is, on rare occasions, a sign of serious disease.

PATIENT'S EXPERIENCE

"I had always tended towards constipation, but after the birth of my third child it got really bad. I developed hemorrhoids, and had to have enemas for several days. My doctor persuaded me to persist with a really high-fiber diet, much more bran and vegetables than I had been eating before. After three or four weeks my motions began to be quite soft: I went regularly – twice a day."

IRRITABLE BOWEL SYNDROME

Anticholinergics, antispasmodics, bulk-forming agents, tranquillizers, antidiarrheal drugs

NAMES YOU WILL HEAR

Anticholinergics
Generic name: dicyclomine hydrochloride; **trade names:** Bantyl, Merbentyl, Procyclomin, Wyovin, Clomin. **Generic name:** propantheline; **trade names:** Pro-Banthine, Propanthel. **Generic name:** methanthiline; **trade name:** Banthine.

Antispasmodics
Generic name: peppermint oil; **trade name:** Colpermin. **Generic name:** mebeverine hydrochloride; **trade names:** Colofac, Duspatalin. **Generic name:** alverine citrate; **trade names:** Spasmonal, Profenil Faible.

Bulking agents
Common name: bran; **trade names:** Fybranta, Proctofibe, Trifyba. **Common name:** psyllium; **trade names:** Metamucil, Citrocel, Hydrocil, Perdium, Mucilosa, Agiolax, Fybogel, Isogel, Regulan. **Common name:** sterculia; **trade names:** Normacol, Inolaxine, Karagum, Prefil.

Antidiarrheal drugs
Generic name: codeine phosphate; **trade names:** Codlin, Diarrest, Kaodene, Paveral, Todlin. **Generic name:** loperamide; **trade name:** Imodium. **Generic name:** diphenoxylate hydrochloride; **trade name:** Lomotil. **Generic name:** kaolin pectin; **trade name:** Kaspectate. **Generic name:** bismuth sulfate; **trade name:** Pepto Bismol.

WHAT IS IRRITABLE BOWEL SYNDROME (IBS)?

The common symptoms include: alternating constipation and diarrhea, sometimes with mucus; pain – dull or gripping – usually in the lower abdomen, but sometimes spreading all over the abdomen, and followed by diarrhea; wind, nausea, flatulence and feeling bloated; suddenly needing to empty the bowel. All these may be intermittent or continuous.

Symptoms *not* due to IBS are: loss of weight; *sudden* change in bowel habit; passing blood in feces. If you have these you *must* seek medical help – your doctor may order hospital tests.

CAUSES Uncertain. The symptoms are thought to be due to abnormal bowel contractions, uncoordinated bowel movements and distension of the bowel. These may be due to lack of fiber in the diet, food intolerance or allergy, or stress. IBS can be triggered off by an attack of gastroenteritis, or bowel infection. In women, symptoms may be worse before periods.

PRESCRIPTION DRUGS

Anticholinergics theoretically lessen bowel activity. Effect may be delayed – see antispasmodics.
How they work: *see* ***peptic ulcer,*** *page 26.*
Antispasmodics can relax the bowel. Both these and anticholinergics may take a couple of weeks to show an effect: in many people they are unhelpful.
How they work: by acting directly on the bowel muscle, causing it to relax.
Bulk-forming agents add bulk to the feces which makes bowel action more regular and co-ordinated. Bran may be taken as natural bran or as bran tablets. Other fiber, for example psyllium, comes as powder – dissolve in plenty of water and drink after meals.
Tranquillizers (and antidepressants) may be prescribed on the basis that IBS is associated with and worsened by stress. However they are not very helpful and tranquillizers can be addictive – *see* ***anxiety,*** *page 84.* It is better to deal with the causes of stress than to take tranquilizers.
How they work: *see* ***anxiety,*** *page 84.*
Antidiarrheal drugs are mainly useful if IBS is accompanied by extremely frequent bowel action.
How they work: *see* ***diarrhea,*** *page 28.*

OVER-THE-COUNTER TREATMENTS

Bulk-forming agents and anti-diarrheal drugs are widely available from pharmacists. *See* ***constipation*** *page 30* and ***diarrhea,*** *page 28,* for details.

QUESTIONS TO ASK THE DOCTOR

■ Do I really need a prescription, or is it best to try natural remedies and self-help first?
■ Will the medicine work, and how soon?
■ How long should I take the medicine/keep up the special diet/high roughage intake?
■ Will the medicine have any side effects?
■ Am I likely to have IBS for life?

SIDE EFFECTS

Anticholinergics can cause a dry mouth, and, rarely, blurring of vision, glaucoma, or inability to pass urine.
Antispasmodics have few side effects, although peppermint oil may cause heartburn.
Bulk-forming agents should be introduced slowly; if introduced too fast, they worsen flatulence. Start with one tablespoon a day of bran or one tablespoon of psyllium and increase over a few days until feces are soft and not too frequent.
Tranquillizers: *see* ***anxiety,*** *page 84.*
Antidiarrheal drugs: *see* ***diarrhea,*** *page 28.*

SELF-MANAGEMENT

■ **Diet:** Eat plenty of vegetables and roughage. Bran can be bought in supermarkets or health food stores, and added to cereal, stews and soups. Eat wholemeal bread and use brown rice.
■ **Certain foods may trigger IBS.** Common culprits include: milk products, wheat, coffee, tea, nuts, peas, beans and even, occasionally, meat. Certain food flavorings and dyes may cause problems too, particularly yellow or red. If you want to find out whether a food affects you, you must exclude it completely from your diet for at least three weeks: if symptoms do not improve, think again. Consult your doctor if in doubt.
■ **Stress:** If you suffer from IBS it is important to find time to relax regularly. Try going swimming or doing aerobics and find a regular time *each day for relaxing your body completely*. Identify causes of stress in your life and change them if possible. Try the relaxation technique described on page 86.

SELF-HELP IN AN ATTACK

■ Rest, and avoid stressful situations.
■ A heating pad often helps.
■ Continue to eat regular small amounts, maintaining the roughage in your diet.

PATIENT'S EXPERIENCE

"I had four years of nausea and feeling bloated. My GP said it was all psychological; but eventually I had severe pains and was going to the bathroom every couple of hours. A specialist diagnosed irritable bowel and advised me to take more roughage and try reducing dairy products. I've given up milk, tea and coffee; I eat quantities of vegetables, take regular bran and go swimming three times a week, and hardly have any problems now . . . maybe just a couple of bad days every six months if I eat something I shouldn't."

HEMORRHOIDS (PILES)

Local anesthetics, astringents

NAMES YOU WILL HEAR
(All are available both as suppositories and ointment)

Local anaesthetics
Steroid also present in those with a letter in brackets:
(B) = betamethasone
(HC) - hydrocortisone
(F) - fluocortolone
(P) - methyl prednisolone
(Other ingredients are present in all these preparations)
Generic name: benzocaine with benzethonium chloride; **trade name:** Corticaine. **Generic name:benzocaine, 8-hydroxyquinoline, menthol zinc oxide, Peruvian balsam in cocoa butter; trade name:** Rectal Medicone. **Generic name:** pramoxine hydrochloride; **trade name:** Tronolane. **Generic name:** lignocaine, lidocaine; **trade names:** Xyloproct(H), Betnovate Rectal(B). **Generic name:** cinchocaine; **trade names:** Proctosedyl(HC), Scheriproct(P), Ultraproct(F), Uniroid(HC). **Generic name:** pramoxine; **trade names:** Anugesic-HC(HC), Proctofoam (HC).

Astringents
Generic name: bismuth subgallate; **trade names:** Anusol, Anusol-HC(HC), Anugesic-HC(HC). **Generic name:** Bismuth subgallate, bismuth resorcin, benzyl benzoate, Peruvian balsam and zinc oxide; **trade name:** Anusol. **Generic name:** as above plus hydrocortisone; **trade name:** Anusol-HC. **Generic name:** belladonna, ephedrine, zinc oxide, boric acid, bismuth oxyiodide, bismuth subcarbonate and Peruvian balsam in cocoa butter and beeswax; **trade name:** Wyanoids.

See also ***constipation,*** *page 30.*

WHAT ARE HEMORRHOIDS?

There are two distinct sorts of hemorrhoids: internal and external. Either can cause pain in the rectum, bleeding, or swellings at the anus called piles.

External hemorrhoids are sometimes extremely painful swellings at the margin of the anus, which appear suddenly, sometimes after straining. They may bleed, but not profusely. They look purplish, measure about $\frac{1}{4}$-$\frac{1}{2}$ in (0.5-1 cm) in diameter, and subside in 3-4 days.

Internal hemorrhoids originate deep inside the anal canal, where the normal mechanism for holding the bowel closed consists of three cushions – pads formed from the bowel lining and containing large veins. A hemorrhoid forms when one or more of these cushions bulges down towards the anal canal. They may then appear as red swellings at the anus. Because of the large veins inside them, internal hemorrhoids bleed readily, indeed they are the most common cause of bleeding from the rectum. They are painful only when they extend down beyond the anal margin, and become ulcerated or congested.

CAUSES With external hemorrhoids, a blood clot forms in one of the veins lying just under the skin of the anus, leading to congestion, swelling and pain.

Internal hemorrhoids are often associated with constipation and straining. In pregnant women they arise from pressure of the enlarging womb on veins in the lower abdomen. Occasionally hemorrhoids may be associated with rectal cancer.

PRESCRIPTION DRUGS

Drugs have only a small part to play. External hemorrhoids are often treated by cooling with ice packs. In acute cases, a doctor, using a local anesthetic, can cut open the 'thrombosed' vein and release the blood clot. The skin heals up quickly, and no other treatment is needed. One of the **local anesthetic ointments** or **suppositories** listed may be used for a few days without harm (see SIDE EFFECTS) if soreness persists, or if incision is thought unnecessary.

How they work: By blocking the nerves to the area.

Internal hemorrhoids must be examined by a doctor in order to exclude other more dangerous causes of bleeding from the rectum. Most internal hemorrhoids will subside in a few days, and local anesthetic preparations may be used to relieve pain during this time, as well as a cooling lotion, regular salt baths and, more important, diet and/or laxatives to promote the easy passage of soft stools. *See **constipation**, page 30.*

Persistently bleeding hemorrhoids, or those internal hemorrhoids which protrude outside the anus, will be referred to a specialist. Several treatments are used: injection of the base of the hemorrhoids, causing them to shrink; stretching the anal canal under anesthetic; removing them by tying them off; surgery.

Astringents protect raw surfaces and may aid healing.
How they work: by sealing exposed tissue. The steroid content of many of these preparations (see drugs list in margin) reduces inflammation and itching, but increases the risk of infection in the skin.
How they work: by suppressing the body's reaction to infection and allergy.

PATIENT'S EXPERIENCE
"When I suddenly developed pain while going to the lavatory and noticed some blood in the pan, I was scared I had cancer. My mother said it was piles, and recommended a tube of cream from her pharmacist. Because of my fear, and the pain, I saw my doctor, who examined me and said it was a fissure: a crack in the skin at the anus. He prescribed lidocaine ointment, and told me to eat bran and also to take a laxative. (I had been rather constipated.) After two days the pain and bleeding stopped."

QUESTIONS TO ASK THE DOCTOR

■ Can I prevent them happening again?
■ Is there any risk that it could be cancer?

OVER-THE-COUNTER TREATMENT

Piles are a common complaint, and many creams, ointments and suppositories are available without prescription. The same risk of sensitization applies to these, and they should be used with caution, not for more than two weeks at a time.

SIDE EFFECTS

There is a risk with all the preparations that the skin will develop sensitivity (allergy) to one or more of the components of the ointment or suppository. Sensitivity is manifested in further irritation and soreness.

SELF-MANAGEMENT

If you have bleeding from the rectum, whether or not it is painful, you MUST consult a doctor. However, local soreness, itching, or small swellings which subside, can be treated by simple home remedies.

■ The simplest solution is to sit in a bath or basin of warm salty water, several times a day if possible. Frequent washing of the anal skin in this way helps prevent the cycle of irritation, soiling, rubbing, leading to more irritation. After washing, the skin must be dried thoroughly, by dabbing, not rubbing, with a towel. A pad of cotton wool helps to keep the skin of the buttocks apart and promotes healing. Small pads containing glycerine and with hazel (Tucks) often give good local relief.

■ To prevent recurrence of these problems, increase the fiber in your diet – *see **constipation**, page 30.*

Pancreatic enzymes, vitamins, minerals, antibiotics

NAMES YOU WILL HEAR

Pancreatic enzymes
Generic name: protease, amylase, lipase combination; **trade names:** Arco-Lase, Pancrease, Donnazyme, Kanulase, Phazyme, Prevenzyme, Viokase, Zypan, Cotazyme, Digepepsin, Pancreatin, Nutrizym, Paneric.

Vitamins
*See **vitamin deficiency,** page 228.*

Minerals
Generic name: ferrous sulfate; **trade names:** Feosol, Feospan, Ferro-Grad C, Ferro-Gradumet, Fentard, Fespan, Ferro-Gradumet, Fer-in-sol, Fesotor, Ferroson, Fesofor. **Generic name:** calcium gluconate; **trade name:** Calcium Gluconate Tablets. **Generic name:** zinc sulfate; **trade names:** ACE & Z Tablets, Eldercaps, Vicon C, Vicon Plus, Vi Zac, Zinc 220, Solvazinc, Zincomed, Z Span, Zincaps.

Antibiotics
Generic name: metronidazole; **trade names:** Flagyl, Trichozole, Neo-Tric. **Generic name:** ampicillin; **trade names:** Omnipen, Polycillin, Ampifen, Penbritin, Pentrexyl, Vidopen, Austrapen, Bristin, Amcill, Ampicin, Ampilean, Biosan, Ampil, Famicilin, Pentrex, Petercillin, Synthecillin. **Generic name:** amoxicillin sodium; **trade names:** Augmentin, Polymox, Triniox, Amoxil, Moxacin, Moxilean, Novamoxin, Penamox. **Generic name:** co-trimoxaxole; **trade names:** Septra, Bactrim, Fectrim, Nodilon, Septrim. **Generic name:** erythromycin: **trade names:** Erythrocin, Ilotycin, Arpimycin, Erycen, Erymax, Erythroped, Retcin, Erythrocin, Erythromid, EpMycin, Erostin, Emu-V, Ethryn, Eromel, Ilocap, Ilosone, Rythrocaps. **Generic name:** tetracycline; **trade names:** Achromycin, Tetracycline Capsules, Chymocyclar, Economycin, Oustramycin, Bio-Tetra, Cyclabid.

WHAT IS MALABSORPTION?

– A term covering a group of conditions in which there is failure to absorb one or more nutrients from the diet. It can take the form of an isolated defect, such as failure to absorb lactose; this results in diarrhea after drinking milk, but few other symptoms. Or, at the other extreme, there may be total gut failure and inability to absorb all nutrients. This occurs typically after surgical removal of the small bowel and results in gross malnutrition and emaciation.

CAUSES These may be divided into two main groups.

First, failure to digest the food. This may occur if pancreatic juices are reduced by chronic inflammation (pancreatitis) or by cancer, or if the bile flow is impaired through liver disease or blockage of the bile ducts. It may also happen if food rushes through the intestine without time to mix with digestive juices, as happens after gastric operations.

Second, failure to absorb digested food. This happens in disease of, or removal of, the small intestine itself. Important examples include celiac disease, an allergy to a constituent of wheat, and Crohn's disease (regional enteritis) in which there is chronic inflammation of the small intestine. Some infections may be responsible too, especially giardiasis.

The consequences of malabsorption are:

Weight loss: the simple result of loss of calories. Fat is particularly rich in calories (twice that of protein and carbohydrate per gram) and so fat malabsorption, prominent in chronic pancreatitis, gives early weight loss.

Diarrhea: undigested food reaching the colon or large bowel is broken down by bacteria, resulting in a laxative effect. In the case of fat, malabsorption causes pale, fatty liquid and offensive feces.

Anemia – see page 224. When the upper small intestine is diseased, there is failure to absorb folic acid and iron. Vitamin B12 is absorbed specifically from the last foot of the small intestine with the help of a chemical produced in the stomach. Disease or surgical removal of either of these segments of the intestine may cause anemia related to B12-deficiency.

Skin rashes: These often follow failure to absorb certain vitamins and minerals.

Osteoporosis (or thin bones) – resulting from failure to absorb calcium and vitamin D.

PRESCRIPTION DRUGS

Pancreatic enzymes, extracted from animal pancreas, are

the mainstay treatments, along with dietary measures, of treating chronic pancreatitis.
How they work: by replacing the body's own pancreatic digestive enzymes in the small intestine. Unfortunately they are inactivated by stomach acid, and so have to be well mixed with food (often making food unpalatable) or given in capsules that dissolve in the duodenum. Alternatively, drugs such as cimetidine or ranitidine may be given to reduce stomach acid *(see **peptic ulcer,** page 26)*. They are not totally effective, and must be combined with a low-fat diet to prevent fatty diarrhea.
Vitamins and **minerals** are prescribed to replace potential deficiencies. Needs will vary from patient to patient. More commonly needed are vitamins B, C, D and folic acid; iron, calcium and zinc.
Antibiotics: metronidazole is usually effective in giardiasis. It is important not to take alcohol at the same time. For further information on antibiotics, *see pages 78-9 and 134-7.*

OVER-THE-COUNTER TREATMENTS

Although vitamins and minerals are widely available, self-treatment should not be attempted.

DIET

Those with celiac disease must, of course, avoid wheat entirely. The diet, in fact, needs to be obsessively strict: eating out can be a real problem. For instance, gravy thickened with flour is enough to damage the small intestine. Other causes of malabsorption, such as chronic pancreatitis and bowel resection, are more generalized in their effect and the diet may thus be just as awkward to maintain. Fat, because it is often poorly absorbed, usually has to be restricted. Sometimes calories can be supplemented by MCT (medium chain triglycerides), a liquid form of fat which is relatively easy to absorb.

SELF-MANAGEMENT

■ It is worth following any prescribed diet carefully. Look at the labels of foodstuffs and become familiar with the constitutents of food. Eating at home is easiest. Try to maintain a varied diet with the necessary vitamins and minerals.
■ You are susceptible to gastroenteritis, and foreign travel is therefore risky.
■ Join any appropriate club or society: discuss your day-to-day problems with others who share the same experience.

PATIENT'S EXPERIENCE

"I have chronic pancreatitis; for ages I couldn't find a pancreatic enzyme preparation that would stop the foul, fatty diarrhea which plagued me constantly.

Eventually I recognized that even on this treatment I could not eat what I liked and went on a strict low-fat diet. The results were dramatic: I now supplement my calories with liquid MCT, and this helps keep up my weight without causing terrible diarrhea."

ULCERATIVE COLITIS

Steroids, sulfasalazine, antidiarrheal drugs

NAMES YOU WILL HEAR

Steroids
Generic name: betamethasone valerate; **trade names:** Betnelan, Betnesol. **Generic name:** methyl prednisolone; **trade names:** Solumedrol, Deltacortef, Codelsol, Delta Phorical, Deltacortril, Deltalone, Deltastab, Precortisyl, Prednesol, Sintisone, Nisolone, Delta-Cortef, Deltasolone, Prelone, Lenisolone, Meticortilone, Predeltilone.

Sulfasalazine
Generic name: sulfasalazine; **trade name:** Azulfidine, Salazopyrin.

Antidiarrheal drugs
Generic name: codeine phosphate; **trade names:** Galcodine, Uniflu, Codlin, Diarrest, Kaodene, Paveral, Codeine Linctus, Codeine Syrup. **Generic name:** diphenoxylate hydrochloride; **trade name:** Lomotil. **Generic name:** loperamide; **trade name:** Imodium. **Generic name:** kaolin and morphine; **trade name:** usually prescribed by generic name. **Generic name:** codeine sulfate; **trade name:** prescribed by generic name in USA. **Generic name:** opium tincture; **trade name:** prescribed by generic name in USA. *See also* ***diarrhea,*** *page 28.*

WHAT IS ULCERATIVE COLITIS?

– An inflammatory condition affecting the colon (large bowel) which is usually chronic. Common symptoms are diarrhea, blood and mucus in the feces and abdominal pain. Symptoms vary from patient to patient according to the amount of colon affected: if the inflammation is confined to the rectum, the stools may be solid but mixed with fresh blood and jelly-like mucus and there will be great urgency to open the bowel; more extensive colitis produces copious liquid stools and may cause chronic ill-health. Occasionally the illness starts acutely: emergency surgery may be needed to remove the colon before it bursts.

CAUSE Unknown. Dietary factors and infective triggers have been suggested. Crohn's disease is a closely allied condition which may produce an identical colitis, managed the same way, but can affect other parts of the intestines as well.

Bleeding from the bowel and diarrhea are serious symptoms that can be caused by other conditions such as dysentery and cancer of the colon, and so investigation before treatment is mandatory.

PRESCRIPTION DRUGS

Steroids are used in tablet or injection form during severe and extensive attacks. They work by suppressing the body's inflammation response and are useful when applied locally to the lining of the colon.
How they work: by reducing inflammation.
Sulfasalazine: This is the mainstay of treatment of ulcerative colitis in remission and relapse, taken as pills. In the colon it is split into two parts, the active one being called 5-ASA. There are recent developments where the 5-ASA itself can be given by mouth in a form which is released in the colon but these are not yet available in the USA.
How they work: by settling inflammation.
Antidiarrheal drugs: Agents such as codeine phosphate, loperamide and kaolin + morphine mixture may slow down the gut and hence reduce diarrhea but have no effect on the underlying inflammation.
How they work: *see* ***diarrhea,*** *page 28.*

OVER-THE-COUNTER TREATMENTS

Some of these antidiarrheal drugs may be available without prescription, but there are risks attached to using "chemical stoppers" for this condition: don't take them without medical advice.

QUESTIONS TO ASK THE DOCTOR

■ How soon should I see an improvement?
■ Will I need long-term treatment?
■ Are there alternatives if this treatment fails?
■ What are the warning signs that I need medical help?
■ What should I do about diet?

SIDE EFFECTS

Steroids: These are very effective in controlling a severe attack but have no place in preventing a relapse while the patient is well and in remission. When taken by mouth or injection, particularly in high dosage, they may cause weight gain, a "moon" face, easy bruising and acne, but your doctor will be aware of these problems and do everything possible to minimize them. *See also **anemia**, page 224*. Steroids must not be stopped abruptly or their dose varied at will by the patient. Side effects are minimal when steroids are given topically as enemas or suppositories, although small amounts will be absorbed into the bloodstream.
Sulfasalazine: This pill, and its newer forms, is effective not only in treating an acute attack but also as prevention. It may therefore be prescribed for months or even years, with appropriate blood count checks. It may induce a certain amount of indigestion, and this can be reduced by building up to the prescribed dose over a few days. Some people may be allergic to the sulfa-component and get a skin rash, in which case the still-experimental 5-ASA preparations may be the answer. It is used with caution in pregnancy. **Antidiarrheal drugs:** *see **diarrhea**, page 28*.

SELF-MANAGEMENT

■ A few patients with ulcerative colitis seem to be sensitive to milk; trying a milk-free diet is worthwhile.
■ When only the lower colon (rectum and sigmoid) are affected, the stool may be paradoxically hard and difficult to pass. Such constipation makes the colitis worse and may prevent the sulfasalazine getting to where it is needed. A high fiber diet is the best way to avoid this problem.
■ It is tempting to stop sulfasalazine once the attack of colitis settles, but you must continue a maintenance dose to prevent relapse unless otherwise advised.
■ Time the use of a steroid enema so that it is kept in for as long as possible. This is usually last thing at night. If used twice a day, lie down for an hour after inserting it in the morning. Many patients find the foam enemas easier to put in and keep in than the fluid ones.

PATIENT'S EXPERIENCE

"I was going to the lavatory every few minutes but passing only a teaspoon of blood and jelly each time. I hardly ever saw any actual motion, and then it was only hard pellets. Once the doctor recommended a high fiber diet, including bran, which I had been specifically avoiding till then, I started to have a decent soft stool each day and the bleeding, frequency and urgency all seemed to settle."

Viral hepatitis vaccine, gamma globulin injections

NAMES YOU WILL HEAR
Viral hepatitis vaccine; gamma globulin injection. No specific drug treatments except these preventive injections. *See also* ***alcholism,*** *page 94 and* ***cirrhosis,*** *page 42.*

WHAT IS JAUNDICE?

– Yellow discoloration of the skin and of the whites of the eyes. It occurs when the amount of bilirubin pigment in the blood is raised. It often causes no symptoms, and may first be noticed by a friend or relative. Sometimes, when jaundice is severe, there is itching, the urine may be dark and the feces paler than usual.

CAUSES Normally, bilirubin pigment, which is produced by the regular turn-over of red blood cells, is secreted by the liver as a waste product in bile. When the flow of bile is blocked or slowed due to a liver problem, jaundice results. Bile flow may be blocked within the liver or outside it. In adults, common problems *within* the liver are: viral hepatitis, alcoholic hepatitis and primary biliary cirrhosis. Certain drugs may also be responsible. Causes of jaundice *outside* the liver are: gallstones blocking the main bile duct; inflammation of the pancreas, and cancer of the pancreas or bile ducts. An infection within the bile ducts may cause jaundice.

Gilbert's Syndrome, a mild, hereditary form of jaundice, affects about 5 per cent of the population. The jaundice becomes more prominent during illness or when dieting or fasting. It does not require treatment.

PRESCRIPTION DRUGS

There are no specific prescription drugs either for jaundice or for viral hepatitis.

However, a **vaccine** is available against one of the four different hepatitis viruses (B). A doctor may advise it for close contacts.

Other regular social and business contacts may in addition be well advised to have an injection of **gamma globulin** to boost their immunity against hepatitis. *See also* ***alcoholism,*** *page 94.*

Because jaundice is caused by so many different diseases, quick, accurate diagnosis is essential.

QUESTIONS TO ASK THE DOCTOR

- What is the cause of my jaundice?
- Do I need special tests?
- If viral hepatitis is suspected, and there is a delay in getting test results, should I take any precautions?

OVER-THE-COUNTER TREATMENTS

None.

SELF-MANAGEMENT

Without the help of special blood tests, and sometimes

a needle biopsy of the liver, it is virtually impossible to decide whether the jaundice is caused by one of many viruses, alcohol, a bacterial infection in the bile ducts, gall stones, or a reaction to medication being taken as treatment for another condition.

There are at least four different viruses which cause hepatitis (labelled, A, B, D and non-A non-B). Apart from jaundice, the early symptoms resemble a 'flu-like illness: fatigue, mild fever, muscle and joint aches and pains, loss of appetite, nausea, vomiting and vague abdominal pain. These symptoms often lessen when the jaundice appears. Also, viral hepatitis may occur without jaundice ever developing.

If you suspect you have viral hepatitis, consult your doctor. If the diagnosis is confirmed (or while you await the results of tests):

- Avoid excessive exercise, though rest in bed is not necessary unless you feel weak.
- Avoid physical contact with other people (including kissing). This includes those living with you, and visitors. Sexual activity does not affect recovery from hepatitis, but you may pass on the infection.
- Avoid alcohol during the acute phase.
- Since hepatitis viruses are passed on by blood, body fluids and secretions, do not share items such as razor blades, scissors, toothbrushes and needles. Carefully cover any cuts.
- A well-balanced diet is usually sufficient during the illness: vitamin supplements are not normally necessary. If there is nausea, it is best to have a large breakfast because nausea is generally least troublesome in the morning, but increases during the day.
- Avoid preparing meals for others, especially if you have hepatitis A. However, by the time the hepatitis is diagnosed, you will have already passed the most infectious phase and infection of close contacts may have already occurred. *See also* ***AIDS,*** *page 214.*
- Symptoms should clear up within a couple of months, but some people require about six months to recover fully.
- In a very few cases, hepatitis may become chronic, causing liver damage and cirrhosis.

Only viral hepatitis requires these precautions. Bacterial infection within the bile ducts and jaundice due to gall stones usually have a more sudden onset with high fever, sweating, upper abdominal pain, nausea and vomiting (cholecystitis). Immediate attention from a doctor is necessary. Admission to a hospital is required for intensive treatment.

PATIENT'S EXPERIENCE

"I had had a cold for about two weeks, and couldn't shake it off. It was my neighbor who noticed that my eyes had turned yellow; the next day I could see that my skin had gone a similar color.

My arthritis, which began some years ago, had also seemed more active. So for a week I took a few extra arthritis tablets. They were the new ones my doctor had recently given me.

After the jaundice appeared, I saw my doctor who arranged some blood tests; he also recommended some precautions at home, and suggested I stay at home until the results came through. Three days later, the results for viral hepatitis were negative, but my jaundice was much worse. My doctor suggested stopping the arthritis tablets. Within a week, the jaundice had cleared and so had the 'flu-like symptoms. We assumed the jaundice was a toxic reaction to the pills."

DRUG-INDUCED LIVER INJURY

This is rare, but has been found with nearly every known drug. Most medicines which damage the liver do so in an unpredictable manner. An allergic type of reaction is found in many people. The diagnosis is often circumstantial: there are no specific tests. Once the offending drug is stopped, recovery usually occurs over a few weeks.

Diuretics, steroids, azathioprine

NAMES YOU WILL HEAR

Diuretics

Generic name: spironolactone; **trade names:** Altex, Aldactone, Diatensec, Laractone, Spiretic, Spiroctan, Spirolone, Spirotone, Sincomen.

Generic name: furosemide; **trade names:** Furoside, Aluzine, Diuresal, Dryptal, Frusetic, Frusid, Lasix, Aquamide, Uremide, Urex, Urex-M, Neu Dural, Novosemide, Uritol, Aquasin.

Steroids

Generic name: methyl prednisolone; **trade names:** Solumedrol, Codelsol, Delta Phorical, Deltracortril, Deltalone, Deltastab, Precortisyl, Prednesol, Sintisone, Nisolone, Delta-Cortef, Deltasolone, Prelone, Lenisolone, Meticortilone, Predeltilone.

Azathioprine

Generic name: azathioprine; **trade names:** Imuran, Azathioprine Tablets.

WHAT IS CIRRHOSIS?

– A chronic liver disease in which damage occurs to normal liver cells, which are then replaced by scar tissue. This process reduces the number of normal liver cells so that liver function becomes less efficient and flow of blood through the liver is partly blocked.

The liver is the single largest organ in the body except for the skin. It is, with justice, called the body's chemical factory, and it has thousands of functions, the important ones being: maintenance of the blood clotting mechanism, production of many blood proteins, blood enzymes, the production of bile, metabolism of fats, maintenance of a normal blood sugar level, the storage of energy, and eliminating drugs and poisons (including alcohol) by converting them into inactive compounds.

Cirrhosis often develops insidiously, but once liver function is impaired, the following may appear: loss of appetite; weight loss; nausea and vomiting; enlargement of the liver; jaundice; itching; abdominal swelling due to fluid accumulation (ascites); vomiting of blood (from an ulcer in the stomach or ruptured veins in the gullet); increased sensitivity to drugs; and mental changes leading to confusion and coma.

CAUSES Excessive alcohol intake is the commonest cause of cirrhosis. Some patients with viral hepatitis may also develop cirrhosis. *See **jaundice,** page 40.* Other rare causes are: inborn abnormalities where excessive iron or copper is deposited in the liver; severe reactions to drugs; some forms of heart disease; disease of the bile ducts (biliary cirrhosis). Alcohol can be readily identified as the cause of cirrhosis, especially if a tiny piece of liver tissue is examined under the microscope. The development of cirrhosis is related to the amount of alcohol consumed, its regularity, and perhaps the individual's state of nutrition. Females are more prone to liver injury from alcohol.

PRESCRIPTION DRUGS

There is no cure and the scarring process cannot be reversed. Treatment is aimed at reducing the extent of liver damage and controlling complications such as accumulation of fluid.

Diuretics such as spironolactone and furosemide taken as tablets once or twice a day may help reduce fluid accumulation.

How they work: by increasing loss of fluid through the kidneys.

Steroids: Prednisolone is the drug most used for reducing inflammation in the liver caused by some forms of chronic hepatitis. For the majority of cases of cirrhosis, however, steroids are unhelpful, and may be harmful, because of fluid retention.
How they work: by blocking inflammatory reaction.
Azathioprine: this is a more powerful suppressant of inflammation than steroids. It is used only under expert guidance in patients with primary biliary cirrhosis.
How it works: *see **organ transplants,** page 216.*

QUESTIONS TO ASK THE DOCTOR

■ What is the cause of my cirrhosis?
■ Do I need special tests?
■ Is specific treatment needed?
■ Will cirrhosis affect my job, diet or activities?
■ Are any special precautions necessary?

OVER-THE-COUNTER TREATMENTS

None.

SIDE EFFECTS

*See **heart failure,** page 54, **anemia** page 224* and ***organ transplants,** page 216.*

SELF-MANAGEMENT

The cause of cirrhosis can only be found by blood tests, and sometimes a "needle biopsy" of the liver. If you suspect you may have cirrhosis, consult your doctor. However, alcohol is by far the commonest cause.

■ Stop drinking alcohol completely.

■ Avoid excessively high protein in your diet. However, a well balanced diet is essential. You may also have to limit the total quantity of fluid you drink. This may in turn lessen the need for diuretics.

■ If viral heptatis is suspected, or found to be the cause of cirrhosis, and you are a carrier of the virus, you may have to follow the same precautions as for viral hepatitis *(see **jaundice,** page 40).*

■ Cirrhosis reduces the body's response to infection, so if a mild infection persists, you should seek the advice of your doctor.

■ Avoid taking any pills or other medicines which are not essential. They may overload an already overworked liver, and the action of most medicines is greatly prolonged in chronic liver disease such as cirrhosis.

■ Aspirin and similar analgesics are best avoided. They can worsen bleeding from the esophagus, or from stomach ulcers.

PATIENT'S EXPERIENCE

"I was managing a textile manufacturing company which began having financial difficulties about five years ago. The pressures mounted up and when it got really bad, I drank. Soon I found myself drinking every day; at the time I didn't think it was excessive – I certainly did not feel ill because of it, and carried on working over 16 hours a day.

Then, a year ago, I began to notice a thinning of my arms and legs and a thickening waistline, together with a decreased appetite. About six months ago, I suddenly woke in the night, vomited large amounts of blood, and passed out. At the hospital I was told I had an enlarged liver due to cirrhosis. This had caused back pressure in the flow of blood through the liver and a distended vein in my esophagus had burst, causing the bleeding. Later tests showed that I had early cirrhosis caused by alcohol.

They told me to give up alcohol completely – advice which was reinforced by my own doctor. With a good deal of nagging from my wife, I've succeeded in not having a drink for six months. My waist and liver have almost returned to normal, and the weakness in my limbs has gone. They say that if I stay off alcohol for good, I have an excellent chance of not dying from cirrhosis."

Cardio-vascular disease

At the center of the cardio-vascular system is the heart which acts as a pump to drive blood around the body. The left ventricle receives oxygenated blood from the lungs via the left atrium and then pumps the blood, under pressure, to the organs of the body through the arteries. From the main arteries the blood passes into a branching network of smaller and smaller blood vessels ending in capillaries which allow the nutrients and oxygen in the blood to reach every cell in the body. The right ventricle receives non-oxygenated blood returning to the heart from the peripheral circulation, via the veins and right atrium, and pumps it at relatively low pressure to the lungs. The heart receives its own circulation of blood via the coronary arteries.
Illustration to show heart and arteries, veins

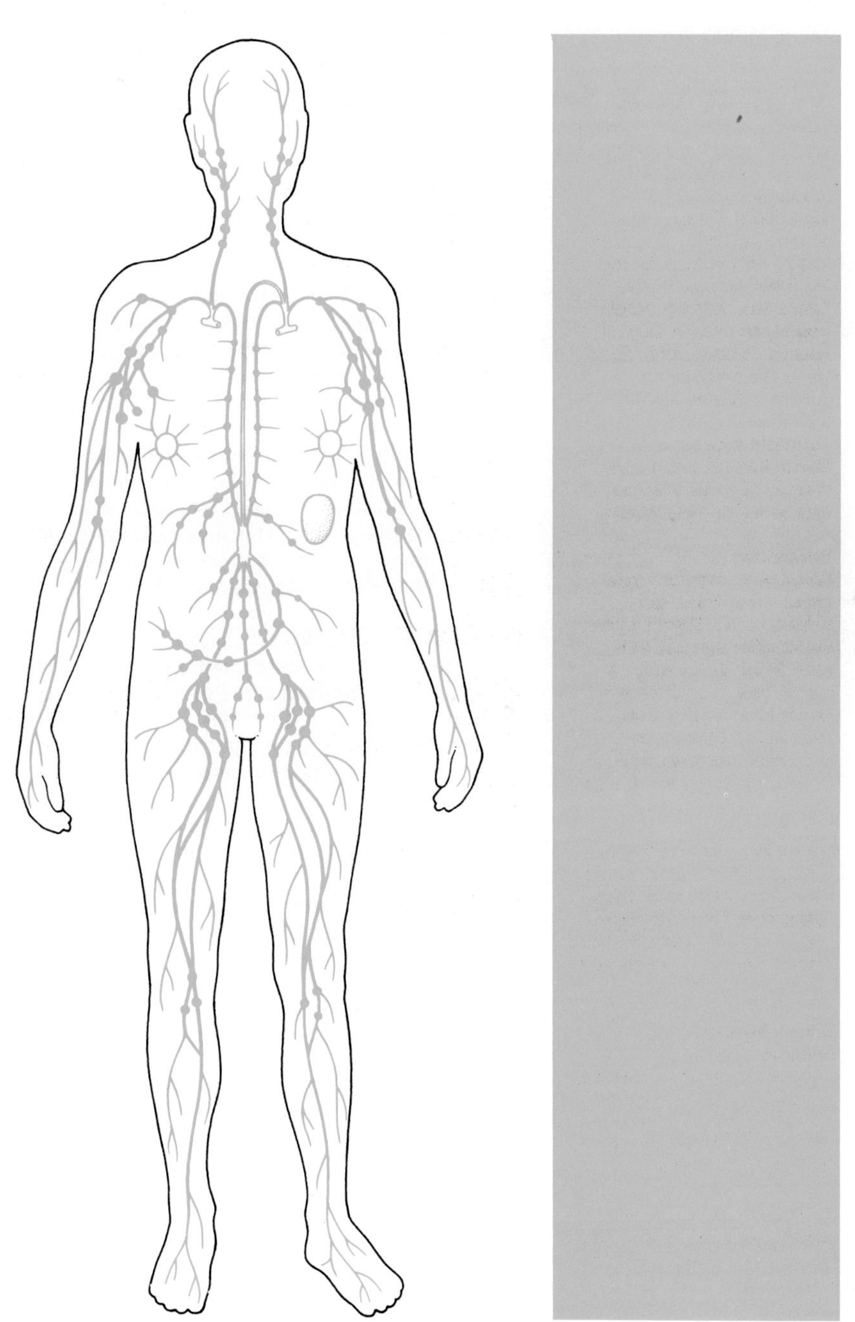

Nitrates, beta-blockers, calcium blockers

NAMES YOU WILL HEAR

Nitrates

Generic name: glyceryl trinitrate (GTN), commonly but incorrectly referred to as nitroglycerin, as tablets, spray or ointment; **trade names:** Coro-nitro spray, Nitrolingual spray, Natirose, Nitrocontin Continus, Suscard Buccal, Sustac, Percutol ointment, Transiderm nitro, deponit (plaster), Nitrolate, Nitrol, Nitrong, Nitrostabilin, Nitrostat, Angised, **Generic name:** isosorbide dinitrate; **trade names:** Caravasin, Cedocard, Vascardin, Sorbichew, Isoket, Sorbid SA, Soni-Slo, Isordil, Isotrate, Novosorbide, Coronex, Apo ISDN. **Generic name:** isosorbide mononitrate; **trade names:** Elantan, Monorit, Mono-Cedocarol. **Generic name:** pentaerythritol tetranitrate; **trade names:** Cardiacap, Mycardol.

Beta-blockers

Generic name: propranolol; **trade names:** Inderal, Angilol, Apsolol, Bedranol, Berkolol, Sloprolol, Cardinol. **Generic name:** acebutolol; **trade name:** Sectral. **Generic name:** atenolol; **trade name:** Tenormin. **Generic name:** betaxolol; **trade name:** Kerlone. **Generic name:** metoprolol tartrate; **trade names:** Lopressor, Betaloc, Lopresor. **Generic name:** nadolol; **trade name:** Corgard. **Generic name:** oxprenolol hydrochloride; **trade names:** Apsolox, Laracor, Slow-Pren, Trasicor. **Generic name:** pindolol; **trade name:** Visken. **Generic name:** sotalol hydrochloride; **trade names:** Beta-Cardone, Sotacor. **Generic name:** timolol maleate; **trade names:** Blocadren, Betim.

Calcium blockers

Generic name: diltiazem hydrochloride; **trade names:** Cardizem, Tildiem, Tilazem. **Generic name:** nifedipine; **trade name:** Adalat. **Generic name:** nicardipine; **trade name:** Cardene. **Generic name:** verapamil hydrochloride; **trade names:** Calan, Berkatens, Securon, Cordilox, Isoptin. **Generic name:** lidoflazine; **trade name:** Clinium. **Generic name:** prenylamine; **trade names:** Synadrin, Segontin.

WHAT IS ANGINA?

Constricting pressure-like pain felt behind the breast bone sometimes spreading to the arms or throat, usually brought on by exertion or emotional upset and relieved after a few minutes by rest.

CAUSES Usually a fixed narrowing of the coronary arteries, caused by cholesterol deposits, which restricts blood flow to the heart muscle. At rest the blood supply to the heart is adequate despite the coronary artery narrowing, but when the heart has to beat faster or more forcefully during exercise or emotional stress, oxygen demand of the heart muscle exceeds the supply and angina results. Resting reduces the heart's rate of beating and hence its need for extra blood. Thus the pain disappears. If an already narrowed artery becomes completely blocked, typically by a blood clot, a heart attack *(page 52)* results.

Angina may also be caused by spasm in an artery of basically normal caliber. This may cause atypical Prinzmetal's angina which may occur at rest. Arterial disease: ultimate causes, *see page 52.*

PRESCRIPTION DRUGS

Three groups of drugs are used. They act in different ways, and may be used alone or in combination.

Nitrates: used to treat an attack as it occurs (a small tablet placed under the tongue or lip – 'sub lingual' – or as an aerosol spray into the mouth. Long-acting nitrates are available as tablets or as an impregnated patch applied to the skin, or a paste held on the skin by tape and are used to reduce the frequency and severity of attacks.

How they work: Nitrates probably widen the coronary arteries and reduce the amount of blood flowing into the heart, allowing the heart to pump more easily.

Beta-blockers: commonly used to reduce the frequency and severity of attacks. Taken as pills, they allow patients to take exercise before the pain comes on.

How they work: by slowing the heart rate and reducing the blood pressure thereby allowing the heart to pump more efficiently.

Calcium blockers: used in same way as beta-blockers.

How they work: by reducing the force at which the heart pumps, by lowering blood pressure and by widening the coronary arteries.

OVER-THE-COUNTER TREATMENTS

Some nitrates may be purchased direct from a pharmacist in an emergency, but only for angina patients under medical care.

QUESTIONS TO ASK THE DOCTOR

- How often can I take nitroglycerin tablets under the tongue?
- How often can I use the spray?
- How quickly will the medication work?
- What should I do if it doesn't work?
- Can I take beta-blockers and calcium blockers just when I need them?
- Can I stop taking beta-blockers and calcium blockers if they upset me?
- Does angina inevitably lead to a heart attack?

SIDE EFFECTS

Nitrates often cause headaches which become less severe as you get used to the medication. Sometimes in older patients, they may cause light-headedness; sit or lie down if this develops. Abrupt cessation of these agents may lead to severe worsening of angina or to a heart attack.

Beta-blockers may cause cold hands and feet, aching muscles, particularly in the legs, feelings of mental and physical slowing and vivid dreams. Occasionally they cause asthma – seek immediate medical advice. **Calcium blockers** may cause headache, flushing of the face, minor ankle swelling and bowel upset (constipation or diarrhea). All these side effects are infrequent and usually minor compared with the consequences of untreated angina.

SELF-MANAGEMENT

Sublingual tablets or spray to relieve an attack can be taken as often as necessary. They should be taken as soon as pain starts, or when you are in a situation in which the pain is likely to occur – prevention is better than cure. These drugs are not painkillers; they help to reverse the cause of the angina. Relief should be obtained within 15 minutes. If the pain does not go away, or your need for tablets or spray increases over a few days, seek medical advice.

The sublingual tablets lose their effect once the bottle has been opened and should be renewed every three months. The spray has a much longer shelf-life; it should NOT be shaken before use.

Smoking is forbidden as it may bring on an attack and is a major cause of coronary artery narrowing. Dieting may be useful: discuss with your doctor.

PATIENT'S EXPERIENCE

"I went to the doctor with what I was sure was bad indigestion and was upset when he told me it was angina. He said I must give up smoking, and once I'd managed it I stopped taking the GTN he'd also given me, as they gave me a headache. Stopping smoking didn't cure the angina, though, which still occurred if I exercised. The doctor presuaded me to carry on with the GTN and also prescribed a beta-blocker. I still have mild headaches and my hands and feet get cold, but at least I'm free of the pain in my chest – in fact, I'm back to the gardening."

WHAT TO AVOID

Try to avoid situations known to bring on angina, for example arguments, walking into a cold wind or walking after a heavy meal. If you cannot avoid a provocative situation, take a sublingual tablet (or spray) immediately beforehand. Try to lead an ordered, regular life. Plan your day to avoid rushing. Sometimes sexual intercourse (emotion and exercise) may bring on an attack; a sublingual tablet or spray before sex may prevent this.

IN AN ATTACK

At the first warning of an attack, sit down and try to relax. Take a sublingual tablet or spray. Do *not* try to manage without your medication.

Antihypertensive drugs, beta-blockers

NAMES YOU WILL HEAR
Beta-blocker
Generic name: labetalol; **trade names:** Normodyne, Trandate, Labrocol. *See also* ***angina****, page* 46 for other beta-blockers.

Diuretics
Generic name: bendroflumethiazide; **trade names:** Naturetin, Aprinox, Berkozide, Centyl, Urizide, Neo-NaClex, Aprinox-M, Pluryl. **Generic name:** chlorothiazide; **trade names:** Diuril, Saluric, Azide, Diubram, Diuret, Diurone, Chlotride. **Generic name:** chlorthalidone; **trade names:** Hygroton, Thalitone, Urid, Uridon, Novothalidone. **Generic name:** clopamide; **trade name:** Brinaldix. **Generic name:** cyclopenthiazide; **trade name:** Navidrex. **Generic name:** hydrochlorothiazide; **trade names:** Esidrex, Direma, Hydro Diuril, Oretic, Hydro Saluric, Dichlotride, Neo-Flumen, Diuchlor-H, Hydro-Aquil, Natrimax, Dichlotride, Urirex. **Generic name:** hydroflumethiazide; **trade names:** Diucardin, Saluron, Hydrenox, Di-Ademil. **Generic name:** indapamide; **trade name:** Natrilix. **Generic name:** mefruside; **trade names:** Baycaron. **Generic name:** methylclothiazide; **trade names:** Aquatensen, Enduron, Duretic. **Generic name:** metolazone; **trade names:** Zaroxolyn, Metenix, Diulo. **Generic name:** polythiazide; **trade names:** Renese, Nephril, Drenusil. **Generic name:** xipamide; **trade name:** Diurexan. **Generic name:** furosemide; **trade names:** Lasix, Aluzine, Diuresal, Dryptal, Frusetic, Frusid, Aquamide, Uremide, Urex, Urex-M, Furoside, Neo-Renal, Novosemide, Uritol, Aquasin. **Generic name:** ethacrynic acid; **trade names:** Edecrin, Edecril. **Generic name:** piretanide; **trade name:** Arelix. **Generic name:** spironolactone; **trade names:** Aldactone, Diatensec, Laractone, Spiretic, Spiroctan, Spirolone, Spirotone, Sincomen.

WHAT IS HYPERTENSION?

Hypertension is abnormally high blood pressure in the arteries, a relatively common condition affecting about one in five of the population, particularly in middle age. (Each time the heart beats it produces a pressure wave consisting of a maximum – systolic – and minimum – diastolic – pressure.)

There is no clear division between normal and raised blood pressure although doctors usually define one for the sake of convenience. Most would regard pressures above 140/95 as hypertensive. Borderline values become important to treat if other factors predisposing to heart attack are present (smoking, high blood cholesterol). Systolic blood pressure often rises with age even when the diastolic does not, but it may still be important to treat it. Blood pressure is not a fixed property but varies depending on activity and time of day. Anxiety and stress (caused, for example, by consulting a doctor) make it rise and allowance must be made for this. Only a persistently elevated blood pressure merits treatment.

Most patients with high blood pressure have NO SYMPTOMS so the condition can go undetected for many years. To identify hypertension you must have your blood pressure measured from time to time.

CAUSES Ninety-five per cent of patients have 'essential hypertension', meaning there is no discernable cause. Rarely it may be due to kidney disease, narrowing of the aorta or the arteries to the kidneys, or abnormal hormone production. Oral contraceptives can occasionally cause hypertension, hence the importance of monitoring blood pressure in women who use them. Hypertension may also develop in pregnancy (pre-eclampsia). Heredity is an important factor; if your parents' blood pressures were high, the chances of your being hypertensive are greater.

Measuring blood pressure: The instrument used is called a sphygmomanometer. An inflatable cuff is wrapped around the upper arm and inflated so no blood can get through. The pressure is slowly decreased while the doctor/nurse listens over the artery at the elbow. When blood starts to flow it creates a thumping noise (systolic pressure). As the pressure continues to fall the sound slowly disappears (diastolic pressure).

Does high blood pressure matter? Emphatically yes. People with untreated hypertension are at increased risk of developing strokes, heart and kidney disease with a consequent reduction in life expectancy. Drugs to lower blood pressure will help to reduce these risks considerably.

PRESCRIPTION DRUGS

Your doctor will aim to lower your blood pressure gradually over a period of weeks. He will start with a low dose of tablets and slowly increase it. If a single agent is not sufficient, another type of drug may be substituted or added.

How they work: Beta-blockers slow the heart and reduce the volume of blood pumped out; **diuretics** cause the kidneys to excrete more salt and water and produce some relaxation in the walls of the smaller arteries; **vasodilators** also relax the walls of smaller arteries. **Converting enzyme inhibitors** prevent the production of Angiotension II, the hormone which raises blood pressure. **Centrally acting drugs** reduce the drive from the brain which raises blood pressure. Sometimes drugs working in different ways are combined into a single pill (see **Combinations** under **NAMES YOU WILL HEAR**).

OVER-THE-COUNTER TREATMENTS

None. Various non-drug treatments (meditation, biofeedback, relaxation exercises) may be helpful in lowering blood pressure, but they involve regular therapy. They are only useful for mild hypertension; their long-term benefit is unproven.

QUESTIONS TO ASK THE DOCTOR

- What tests (if any) do I need?
- Should my family have their blood pressure checked?
- Will raised blood pressure interfere with my job?
- Will I be refused life insurance?
- Will my pregnancy be affected?
- What happens if I forget to take my medication?
- For how long do I have to take mediaction?

SIDE EFFECTS

Treatment for hypertension is usually life-long, so the drugs should be simple to take and as free as possible from side effects. Although no drug is completely free of side effects, modern ones are closer to this ideal.

It is important that you discuss any symptoms you may experience after starting treatment with your doctor. These are not always related to the treatment. Dizziness or light-headedness may occur if blood pressure is lowered suddenly or excessively; **beta-blockers** may

PATIENT'S EXPERIENCE

"My blood pressure was first found to be raised when I was examined for an insurance medical. I was surprised because I felt perfectly well and rather resented the fuss. My own doctor subsequently also found my blood pressure to be high and explained the risks of not having treatment. I've given up smoking and have to take tablets every day."

Combinations
Generic name: amiloride + hydrochlorthiazide; **trade name:** Moduretic. **Generic name:** triamterene + hydrochlorthiazide; **trade names:** Dyazide, Maxide. **Generic name:** amiloride + furosemide; **trade name:** Frumil. **Generic name:** rusemide + spironolactone; **trade name:** Lasilactone.

Vasodilators
Generic name: hydralazine; **trade name:** Apresoline. **Generic name:** minoxidil; **trade name:** Loniten. **Generic name:** prazosin; **trade names:** Minipress, Hypovase. **Generic name:** indoramin; **trade name:** Baratol. **Generic name:** phenoxybenzamine; **trade name:** Dibenzyline.

See also ***angina*** *page 46.*

Converting Enzyme Inhibitors
See heart failure, *page 54.*

Centrally acting drugs
Generic name: clonidine; **trade name:** Catapres. **Generic name:** methyldopa; **trade names:** Aldomet (also contained in Aldochlor, Aldoril-15, 25 and Aldoril D30, D50), Dopamet, Hydromet, Medomet, Alduril, Novomedopa, Alphamex, Hypo-tone.

cause fatigue, cold hands and feet, and impotence in some men. They are not suitable for patients with asthma or bronchitis; **diuretics** can cause excessive loss of potassium and may occasionally cause gout, diabetes and sometimes sexual difficulties. *See also* ***heart failure,*** *page 54.* The majority of people experience relatively few side effects while on these drugs. Many of the drugs can now be given once or twice daily, avoiding a midday dose. Most drugs are best taken prior to breakfast and/or the evening meal. *For side effects of vasodilators see page 55.*

SELF-MANAGEMENT

In order to help control your blood pressure, you should be aware that:

■ There is a relationship between dietary salt intake and hypertension. Although salt restriction may not prevent high blood pressure, it is advisable for patients with hypertension to reduce salt intake by avoiding foods with a high salt content (fast foods, canned foods) and not using salt at the table. Salt substitutes are available.

■ High blood pressure is commoner in people who are overweight. Such patients should loose weight by careful and sensible dieting.

■ Heavy alcohol intake raises blood pressure: hypertensive patients should not exceed two bottles of beer (or the equivalent) per day.

■ As people with hypertension have a higher risk of coronary heart disease and arterial disease of the legs, they should STOP SMOKING. Similarly, a reduction in fat consumption (particularly animal fat) is advisable if the blood cholesterol is high.

■ Don't forget to take your pills regularly. Poor compliance will result in poor blood pressure control. If you do forget them, do *not* take twice the dose next time; resume your normal dose.

■ Regular measurement of blood pressure by a nurse or doctor should be performed every three to four months. It is very useful to obtain a reliable blood pressure measuring device and keep a regular check on your own blood pressure. The new electronic devices which provide a digital read-out, costing $60-100, are quite adequate.

■ There is evidence that regular exercise will also help to lower blood pressure. Dynamic exercise (for example, walking, running, swimming, cycling) is therefore to be recommended; isometric exercise (for example, weightlifting) which produces a surge in blood pressure

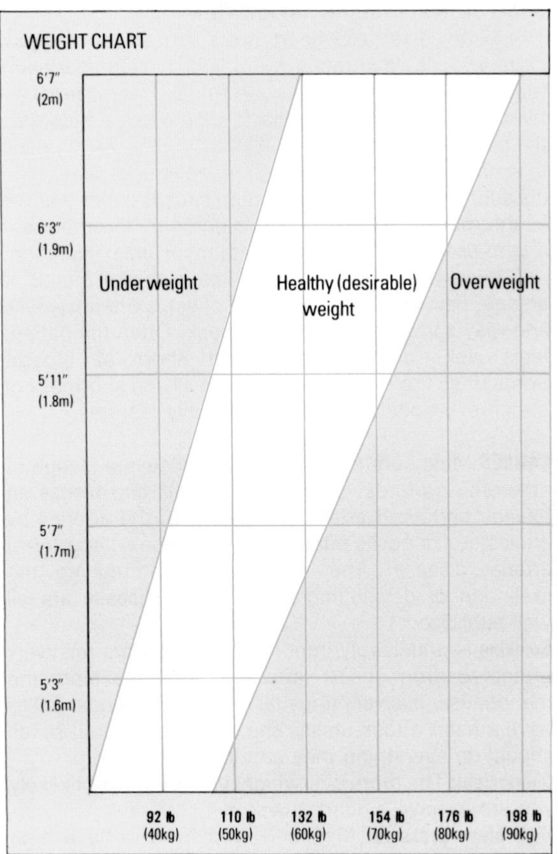

is not a good idea for hypertensive patients. In the long run, most patients with hypertension should be able to lead a perfectly normal life with few restrictions.

SELF-HELP

Hypertension is a long-term problem and you must therefore get repeat prescriptions from your doctor. Be careful not to run out of pills even when your blood pressure is controlled.

It is wise to be cautious when starting additional drugs for other conditions, as they may occasionally interfere with the blood pressure pills. This is particularly true of certain drugs used for treating arthritis. If in doubt, consult your doctor or pharmacist.

MYOCARDIAL INFARCTION

Analgesics, diuretics, antiarrhythmic drugs

NAMES YOU WILL HEAR

Analgesics

Generic name: morphine; **trade names:** Roxanol, Nepenthe, Duromorph. **Generic name:** diamorphine; **common name:** heroin; usually prescribed by chemical name. **Generic name:** pethidine, meperedine; **trade names:** Demerol, Pethilorfan, Pamergan, Pethoid, Demer-Idine; usually prescribed by chemical name. **Generic name:** pentazocine; **trade names:** Fortral, Talwin, Sosegon. *See also* ***pain,*** *page 106.*

Diuretics

Generic name: furosemide; **trade names:** Lasix, Frumil, Dryptal, Aluzine, Aquamide, Uremide, Urex, Lasic, Furoside, Neorenal, Novosemide, Uritol, Aquasin. **Generic name:** bumetanide; **trade name:** Bumex. **Generic name:** ethacrynic acid; **trade names:** Edecrin, Edecril. *See also* ***hypertension,*** *page 48.*

Antiarrhythmic drugs

Generic name: lignocaine hydrochlride, lidocaine hydrochloride; **trade names:** Lidocaine, Xylocaine, Xylocard, Xylocaine, Leostesin, Nurocain, Sarnacaine, Democaine, Leostesin, Peterkaien, Remicane, Remicard. **Generic name:** disopyramide; **trade names:** Norpace, Rythmodan, Dirythmin, Rythmodan. **Generic name:** verapamil; **trade names:** Calan, Cordilox, Securon.

See also drugs used in ***angina,*** *page 46 (for beta-blockers),* ***heart failure,*** *page 54,* ***lipid disorders,*** *page 162,* ***disorders of heart rhythmn,*** *page 56 and* ***hypertension,*** *page 48.*

WHAT IS MYOCARDIAL INFARCTION?

The technical term for heart attack. (An attack of ***angina,*** *page 46,* is by contrast a warning pain from your heart that it may be prone to a heart attack.) Myocardial infarction occurs when the blood supply to the heart (via the coronary arteries) is totally obstructed (as opposed to simply restricted, as in angina): an area of heart muscle actually dies. This obstruction causes a clot (known as thrombosis) to form – hence coronary thrombosis – a term used interchangeably with myocardial infarction.

A heart attack usually feels like a severe attack of angina. Pain in the center of the chest is often vise-like and may spread to the arms or neck. Often the patient feels sick, dizzy, sweaty and short of breath. Sometimes there may be no pain at all and shortness of breath or palpitations may be the only features.

CAUSES Most commonly, possibly because a plague of atheroma ruptures, a blood clot forms and blocks an already narrowed artery. Narrowing of the arteries by cholesterol deposits (atheroma) is a chronic (long-term) arterial disease. The risk factors determining the likelihood of developing such arterial disease are all well-publicized:

Smoking is undeniably important. Women are relatively protected from heart attack before reaching the menopause. It is very unusual for a woman under 50 to have a heart attack unless she smokes. So both sexes should do everything they can to stop smoking.

Overweight: The more overweight you are the more likely you are to have a heart attack.

High blood pressure: Men and women who have high blood pressure are more likely to have a heart attack although the risk is less in women. Attention is now given to measuring blood pressure in young people and to taking action early. *See* ***hypertension,*** *page 48.*

Cholesterol: People with high cholesterol levels are more likely to have heart attacks, as are diabetics.

Family history.

PRESCRIPTION DRUGS

The first thing a doctor will do for the heart attack patient is to give a powerful **analgesic** by injection. This will usually be morphine and will work within ten to 20 minutes. Oxygen is usually given as well. If heart failure develops, digitalis and **diuretics** may also be given – *see page 54.* Sometimes drugs are also given to normalize a disturbed heart rhythm (**antiarrhythmic** drugs). These may be given by injection or by mouth.

In the long term, in order to prevent a further heart attack, particularly in people under the age of 60, beta-blocking drugs are increasingly used. The patient may also need a diet and possibly drugs to reduce cholesterol; drugs to lower the blood pressure may be needed as well – *see* ***lipid disorders*** *and* ***hypertension,*** *pages 162 and 48.*

How they work: ***analgesics,*** *see page 106;* ***diuretics,*** *see page 54;* ***antiarrhythmic drugs,*** *see page 56.*

OVER-THE-COUNTER TREATMENT

None, but some patients may be given a small daily dose of aspirin to try and prevent future heart attacks. Aspirin only works in some individuals and often causes side effects such as indigestion *(page 22).* Ask your doctor before using it regularly.

QUESTIONS TO ASK THE DOCTOR

- What can do to stop this happening again?
- When can I start having sexual intercourse again?
- What is the long-term damage to my heart?
- How likely is another heart attack?
- Can I resume a normal life when I have recovered?

Heart attacks, of course, are serious, but must not be regarded as 'terminal'. On the contrary, the patient's best chance of long-term survival is using the experience as motivation to return to a full life through correct diet and exercise.

SIDE EFFECTS

See ***analgesics,*** *page 106;* ***diuretics,*** *page 54;* ***antiarrhythmic drugs,*** *page 56.*

SELF-MANAGEMENT

- Stop smoking. If you are a regular smoker this is the best thing you can do.
- Exercise in moderation is fine. Usually you should be able to return to full activities within six weeks of leaving hospital. It is a good idea to try to take exercise, such as walking, every day.
- You may be given a diet to lower the fats in your blood. Even if not recommended, it is sensible to reduce the amount of fat in your diet. Most Westerners eat far too much saturated fat from animal sources. Reduce the amount of red meat and bacon you eat, substitute a low-fat spread for butter and use vegetable oil rather than lard for cooking and frying.
- Watch your weight – try to get as close to your ideal weight as possible *(see table, page 51).*

PATIENT'S EXPERIENCE

"When I got the attack of pain in my chest I thought I was going to die. The relief that the injection gave was almost magical. I was rushed to the hospital and stayed in the coronary care unit for two days with various tubes and wires connected to me. After that I was sent to the general ward and was soon up and about. I went home ten days after going into the hospital. I was a bit tired for a few days after going home but within six weeks I was doing everything I did before and within two months I was back at work. I even think my angina is better than it was. That may be because the shock of the heart attack gave me the willpower to stop smoking."

SELF-HELP IN AN ATTACK

At the first warning of chest pain, sit down and try to relax. If you have a supply of nitrate preparation for ***angina*** *(see page 46),* put a tablet under your tongue or use your spray. If the pain is not relieved within 30 minutes, call your doctor, or if he is not available, call an ambulance and go to hospital. If you have never experienced angina before, call a doctor or ambulance earlier.

Diuretics, vasodilators, A.C.E. inhibitors, digoxin

NAMES YOU WILL HEAR

Diuretics

*See **hyptertension, page 48.***

Vasodilators

See hypertension, page 48. Nitrates and calcium blockers have an equivalent function, too – *see **angina,** page 46.*

Ace Inhibitors

Generic name: captopril; **trade names:** Capoten, Acepril. **Generic name:** enalapril; **trade names:** Vasotec, Innovace.

Other drugs

Generic name: digoxin; **trade names:** Lanoxin, Cardiox, Natigoxin, Prodigox, Purgoxin. **Generic name:** digitoxin; **trade names:** Digitaline Nativelle, Digitox. **Generic name:** medigoxin; **trade name:** Lanitop. **Generic name:** lanatoside C; **trade names:** Cedilanid, Lanocide.

WHAT IS HEART FAILURE?

Not to be confused with heart attack, *page 52,* it occurs when the heart cannot pump adequate amounts of blood to the rest of the body, or can only do so by enlarging or by generating abnormally high pressures within the heart cavities during its filling phase. Symptoms are shortness of breath during exercise or even, in severe cases, at rest and when lying flat. Sometimes ankle-swelling and tiredness are symptoms, too.

CAUSE Damage to the heart muscle as a result of coronary artery disease and its outcome, heart attack. Untreated high blood pressure, damaged heart valves and, rarely, primary disease of the heart muscle itself may be responsible.

PRESCRIPTION DRUGS

Diuretics: Two types are commonly used: thiazides long-acting, taken once per day; and loop diuretics, shorter-acting, more potent than thiazides.
How they work: by acting on the kidneys, causing loss of salt and water from the body. By reducing the fluid in the circulation, the pressure in the heart and lungs is also reduced. Diuretics may cause significant loss of potassium from the body, so potassium pills are usually prescribed to make up for the shortage.
Vasodilators: often added if diuretics are inadequate.
How they work: by dilating the arteries they reduce the resistance the heart has to pump against.
A.C.E. inhibitors: a relatively new and promising treatment acting in some ways like diuretics and vasodilators combined.
How they work: Like vasodilators they dilate arteries, but they also have a beneficial effect on hormones (the body's chemical messengers), reducing the body's tendency to retain salt and water.
Digoxin: This is a centuries-old drug derived from the foxglove plant.
How it works: Its key role is in slowing the heart rate in atrial fibrillation *(see page 56).* If this is the cause of heart failure, digoxin is the drug of first choice. It also makes the heart contract more forcefully.

OVER-THE-COUNTER TREATMENTS

None.

QUESTIONS TO ASK THE DOCTOR

■ How much will 'water pills' (diuretics) interfere with my daily activities?

■ Will I need to drink more fluid to replace what is lost by taking diuretics?
■ How long will I have to take the pills?
■ When and how often do I need to take the potassium tablets?

SIDE EFFECTS

Diuretics cause an increase in frequency and volume of urine passed – inconvenient at work, on long journeys or when out of the house. Loop diuretics act within about 30 minutes of ingestion, the effect diminishing four to six hours later. Take the pills at times which suit your daily routine. Thiazides act more gradually throughout the day.

Diuretics do make people thirsty. Counteract this by drinking freely; avoid salty foods, and do not add salt to your food, as this reduces the effectiveness of the treatment. Loss of potassium due to diuretics may jeopardise the proper working of muscles, including the heart; however it is easily replaced by taking potassium tablets. Gout and sexual problems are rare side effects.
Vasodilators may cause flushing of the face, headaches, dizziness and sometimes palpitations.
A.C.E. inhibitors captoril may cause skin rashes, a metallic taste in the mouth and upset of kidney function. Rarely serious depression of the bone marrow has occurred. Ehalapril seems to be less toxic. These drugs are a promising advance in the treatment of heart failure. As with all other treatments for heart failure, medication is usually required indefinitely unless an obvious precipitating factor is removed.

SELF-MANAGEMENT

Only exercise within your limitations, and get adequate rest. Smoking is forbidden. Alcohol can aggravate symptoms in some people by reducing the heart's efficiency. A low-salt diet is helpful in some people and may allow a reduction in medication. Don't attempt it without proper supervision.

SELF-HELP IN AN ATTACK

Attacks of breathlessness sometimes occur at night in bed. **1** Sit up. **2** Put a nitrate tablet under the tongue *(see **angina,** page 46).* **3** Consider taking an extra diuretic tablet, bearing in mind that this will keep you awake passing water. **4** If the attack settles quickly, consult your doctor next day. If the breathing difficulty persists, call your doctor immediately or go to the local emergency room.

PATIENT'S EXPERIENCE

"A few days after discharge from hospital following my second heart attack I noticed I was short of breath after climbing the stairs. Attacks of shortness of breath started to wake me at night and I was only comfortable in bed propped up on four pillows. My doctor gave me some diuretic tablets to take in the morning which made me pass urine very frequently until lunch-time. Frankly, this was nuisance for the first few days, but the effect was less noticeable after a week. My breathing improved enough for me to sleep through the night and this certainly makes it worth putting up with the diuretics. If I want to go out in the morning I can take my tablets at lunch-time."

Antiarhythmic drugs

NAMES YOU WILL HEAR

Class I
Generic name: quinidine; **trade names:** Duraquin, Quinaglute, Quinalan, Kiditard, Kinidin Durules, Quinidoxin, Biquin, Kinidine. **Generic names:** lignocaine hydrochloride, lidocaine hydrochloride; **trade names:** Xylocaine, Xylotox, Lidothesin, Lignostab. **Generic name:** procainamide; **trade names:** Pronestyl, Procainamide Durules. **Generic name:** disopyramide; **trade names:** Norpace, Rythmodan, Dirythmin. **Generic name:** mexiletine; **trade name:** Mexitil. **Generic name:** tocainide; **trade name:** Tonocard.

Class II – Beta-blockers
Generic name: propranolol; **trade names:** Inderal, Angitol, Apsolol, Bedranol, Berkolol, Sloprolol, Cardinol. **Generic name:** acebutolol; **trade name:** Sectral. **Generic name:** alprenolol; **trade name:** Betacard. **Generic name:** atenolol; **trade name:** Tenormin. **Generic name:** metoprolol tartrate; **trade names:** Lopressor, Betaloc. **Generic name:** nadolol; **trade name:** Corgard. **Generic name:** pindolol; **trade name:** Visken. **Generic name:** sotolol hydrochloride; **trade names:** Betacardone, Sotocor. **Generic name:** timolol maleate; **trade names:** Blocadren, Betim.

Class III
Generic name: amiodarone; **trade name:** Cordarone X.

Class IV – Calcium blockers
Generic name: verapamil hydrochloride; **trade names:** Calan, Isoptin, Berkatens, Securon, Cordilox, Berkatens, Securon.

Cardiac glycosides
Generic name: digoxin; **trade names:** Lanoxin, Cardiox, Natigox, Prodigox, Purgoxin. **Generic name:** digitoxin; **trade names:** Crystodigin, Digitaline Nativelle, Digitox.

WHAT IS NORMAL HEART RHYTHM?

The adult heart normally beats at a rate of 70-80 beats per minute (bpm). In young children the rate may exceed 90 bpm and in athletes it may fall to below 60 bpm. The rate of the healthy heart (called sinus rhythm) is automatically controlled from centers within the nervous system which transmit electrical impulses to the heart. In response to exercise or anxiety, the rate increases; during sleep or rest, it decreases. The diagram on page 59 shows how the heart maintains a co-ordinated pumping action by means of its own natural pacemaker which transmits impulses through the heart muscle to the chambers.

WHAT IS ABNORMAL HEART RHYTHM?

There is a wide range of disturbances of heart rhythm from the harmless to the potentially lethal. Paradoxically, the harmless rhythm disturbances – the odd ''missed'' or ''jumped'' beat, also called palpitations – are often the ones which cause the patient most alarm; whereas more serious rhythm disorders, which require medical treatrnent, may be completely unnoticed.

Disorders of rhythm (dysrhythmias) may be subdivided into two main categories depending on whether the heart is beating too slowly (less than 60 bpm) or too quickly (more than 100 bpm). The first, **bradycardias,** do not respond well to drug treatment; if treatment is required, they respond best to a pacemaker which can prevent the heart rate falling too low. The second, **tachycardias,** are more common, and can be due to a number of different types of dysrhythmia.

Diagnosis of a specific type of dysrhythmia depends on examining an electrocardiograph (ECG).

CAUSES A minor disturbance, such as a ''missed'' or ectopic beat, usually has no serious underlying cause and can be considered a simple variation of normality. Even frequent ectopic beats or short-lived palpitations are often harmless; they are sometimes caused by an excessive intake of stimulants such as caffeine, alcohol or nicotine. Clearly, if the heart is diseased or damaged, the whole range of cardiac dysrhythmias can occur, but even the more serious types of dysrhythmia do not always reflect irreversible heart disease or damage.

The diagnosis of a dysrhythmia does not necessarily indicate the need for treatment. The doctor's decision about treatment depends upon the nature of the dysrhythmia, the potential complications and the level of accompanying symptoms.

PRESCRIPTION DRUGS

The following are some of the more common types of dysrhythmia, usually forms of tachycardia, with examples of typical treatments. The terminology used relates to the part of the heart from which the dysrhythmia originates: either from the ventricles (ventricular) or from the atria (atrial or supraventricular). The terminology also describes the nature of the abnormality: if there is a "missed" or "jumped" beat it is called an ectopic beat; if there is rapid but coordinated beating, then the straightforward term *tachycardia* applies; if there is rapid but uncordinated activity of the atria or ventricles, *flutter* or *fibrillation* apply.

Atrial (supraventricular) tachycardia: This dysrhythmia is not usually serious (in most cases the heart is structurally normal), but the heart rate may be sufficiently fast (ranging from 120 to 240 bpm) to cause uncomfortable palpitations and symptoms such as breathlessness, chest tightness and light-headedness. The patient may also produce increased amounts of urine. Paroxysms are often recurrent, but with a variable duration (minutes to hours) and a variable frequency (from several episodes per day to only one or two per year). Occasional paroxysms may respond to the Valsalva Maneuver (see SELF-MANAGEMENT), but if long-term treatment is requred, the calcium antagonist drug, verapamil, or one of the beta-blockers is usually effective. Alternative medications include disopyramide and amiodarone.

Atrial fibrillation or atrial flutter: These have similar symptoms to atrial tachycardia but they are typically seen in patients who have a damaged heart. With both dysrhythmias, but especially atrial fibrillation, the overall heart rate is not only fast (about 160 bpm) but irregular. Conversion to normal sinus rhythm is only occasionally possible and the usual aim of treatment is to keep the heart rate under control at about 80 bpm with one of the cardiac glycosides.

Ventricular ectopic beats: Ectopic beats, both ventricular and supraventricular, occur occasionally in most normal individuals ("My heart missed a beat"). Treatment is not necessary. But ventricular ectopic beats also occur in association with a heart attack *(see **myocardial infarction,** page 52)* in which case some short treatment may be given. Ectopic beats sometimes also occur in long-standing heart disease; long-term drug treatment will be given to suppress them. The drugs in class I are often used for this purpose, with amiodarone as an alternative.

PATIENT'S EXPERIENCE

"My elderly mother had been tired for some time, breathless, too, even when she walked short distances, and her feet began to swell. She complained that she felt her heart beating very fast at times. I am a trained nurse, so I checked her pulse. It was slow. I was taken aback by her doctor's verdict: he told her not to worry – she was just getting old.

My fears were confirmed when she blacked out while shopping. She was fine almost immediately afterwards, but I took her back to the doctor and said I thought she should see a specialist about her heart.

The cardiologist said that she needed a pacemaker and admitted her straight into hospital. She was anxious about having a pacemaker fitted, but the specialist assured her it was a simple operation which, even at her age, shouldn't cause complications. The pacemaker box was put under her skin below the collar bone. The wires led into a vein, then to the heart. She had to have antibiotics for a few days to prevent infection of the operation site.

The improvement was dramatic. She passed an enormous amout of urine, her feet went back to normal, and the dreadful tiredness eased. She has to have the pacemaker checked regularly, but it will probably last a few years."

Antiarhythmic drugs

Ventricular tachycardia: The effects of this dysrhythmia range from minor upset to shock and cardiac arrest. The rate falls in the range 120-250 bpm. Ventricular tachycardia usually reflects an underlying cardiac problem and if the episodes are frequent or associated with severe symptoms, then treatment with a class I or class III drug is usually given.

How the drugs work: There is considerable overlap in function: see below. In general though, they dampen down electrical impulses to the heart, or their transmission from the atria to the ventricles, or their transmission through the heart muscle. See above for reasons underlying the choice of drug. See under NAMES YOU WILL HEAR for drug names.

Class I drugs stabilize the electrical activity within cardiac muscle cells.

Class II – beta-blockers – block the effects of adrenaline on the heart. They are often used to slow the heart, or to prevent the development of rapid heart rhythms arising from the atria. Generally, these drugs are used for the less serious types of dysrhythmia.

Class III – amiodarone – has a similar action to Class I drugs. It tends to be reserved for particular types of dysrhythmia arising from either the atria or the ventricles. It is often used when there has been a poor response to some of the other drugs.

Class IV – calcium antagonists – suppress the excitability of the heart muscle and the transmissions of electrical impulses.

Cardiac glycosides work mainly by interfering with the transmission of electrical impulses from the atria to the ventricles.

OVER-THE-COUNTER TREATMENTS

None.

QUESTIONS TO ASK THE DOCTOR

- Is there a serious underlying heart problem?
- What can I do to prevent an attack coming on?
- Will I need to take pills forever?
- What are the risks if I run out of pills?
- Do the pills have serious side effects?

SIDE EFFECTS

With all these drugs, side effects are common. Forty per cent of patients have to stop taking them because of side effects, but treatment can be continued if the effects are not too troublesome. Alternatively side effects may indicate overdose or a potentially serious adverse effect which should be reported to a doctor so that the dosage can be reduced or the treatment withdrawn.

Common side effects: Minor stomach upsets occur with **quinidine** and **mexiletine;** dry mouth, urinary retention and blurred vision with quinidine and **disopyramide;** tiredness, cold hands and feet, and sometimes breathing difficulties, with **beta-blockers;** skin rashes and skin pigmentation with **amiodarone;** constipation with **verapamil.**

Effects of overdosage (requiring a dosage reduction): **Class I** drugs can cause disturbances of the central nervous system including mental confusion, twitching, tremor, slurred speech and dizziness. **Digoxin** often causes nausea and vomiting. Adverse effects with **procainamide** which may require the drug to be stopped: skin rash, joint stiffness and malaise.

SELF-MANAGEMENT

This is only occasionally possible and worthwhile, and for only one type of dysrhythmia: paroxysmal atrial tachycardia – see PRESCRIPTION DRUGS. If the paroxysms are only occasional, a breathing technique called the Valsalva Maneuver may enable the patient to "switch off" the paroxysm and restore a normal sinus rhythm. Take in a deep breath and then slowly, but forcibly, blow the breath out through tightly pursed lips: rather like blowing up a balloon. Your doctor will rehearse the technique with you.

PATIENT'S EXPERIENCE

"I was under heavy stress at work when I first noticed that my heart was occasionally missing a beat; sometimes it even gave a hard thud. I was very worried: my father had had a coronary thrombosis at 65 and died of a cardiac arrest. I went to my doctor who did an eletrocardiogram. He asked me whether the extra beats increased with exercise. I told him that when playing squash the extra beats disappeared, but returned once my heart rate was normal again. His verdict was better than I had hoped. Apparently extra beats during exercise are an indication of coronary artery disease; my problem was therefore more likely to be a disorder of heart rhythm. He told me to avoid or cut down on coffee and alcohol, and suggested that the stress at work might be aggravating the problem."

THE HEART'S NATURAL PUMPING ACTION

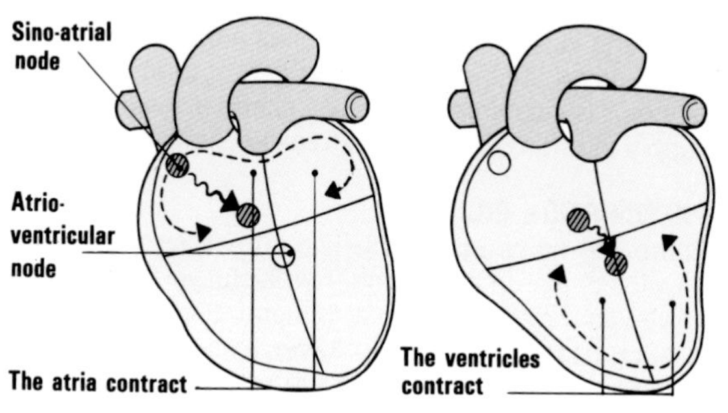

The heart is a muscular pump *which works by contraction and expansion of its muscle fibres. A natural pacemaker, the sino-atrial node, initiates each pumping action by transmitting impulses. These make the atria contract; they also pass through the atrial walls to the atrio-ventricular node, which relays the impulses to the ventricles, causing them to contract in turn.*

Aspirin

NAMES YOU WILL HEAR
Generic name: aspirin; **trade names:** Ascriptin, Ecotrin, Measurin, Aspirin, Bi-Prin; combination products are avoided. See also pain, page 106.
Generic name: heparin; **trade names:** Coumadin, Marevan, Warfilone, Warnerin.

WHAT IS A STROKE?

When the blood supply to any part of the brain is cut off, the brain cells stop working and the area of the body controlled by those brain cells is also unable to function. The right side of the brain controls the left side of the body and vice versa. The most common problem is weakness or paralysis of one side of the body. Speech, vision or balance may also be affected.

If the blood supply to the brain is restored within a short time, then function usually recovers. This type of stroke lasts less than 24 hours and is called a transient ischemic attack. It is sometimes indicative of substantial arterial disease which can be corrected surgically – consult your doctor. If the blood supply is not restored, then the affected part of the brain dies and recovery depends on the ability of other parts of the brain to take over the role of the damaged part. If damage is mild, good recovery occurs over several months. In severe cases, however, there is permanent disability. Some patients may suffer from epilepsy following a stroke *(see page 111)*.

CAUSES Blood supply may be affected by:
Thrombosis: arteries narrow because of atherosclerosis *(see page 44)* and eventually shut off the blood supply completely. Onset of symptoms may be sudden, but is usually graded over several hours or days. Recovery of physical function in major strokes of this type is often poor because other arteries are also diseased, so there is little prospect of blood flow being restored through collateral channels.
Hemorrhage: One of the small arteries bursts and leaks blood into the brain tissue. Damage is caused by the resulting blood clot as well as by a reduction in the blood supply. Onset of symptoms is usually sudden; headache is common.
Embolus: A small blood clot or clump of cells originating in the left side of the heart travels up the arteries to the brain and lodges where the arteries are smaller. This in turn cuts off the blood supply to part of the brain. If the embolus is very small, it breaks up and allows the blood supply to return to normal (a transient ischemic attack).

PRESCRIPTION DRUGS

There are no drugs which will cure a stroke once it develops. Thrombotic and hemorrhagic strokes are more common in patients with high blood pressure and in such cases treatment to lower blood pressure may help to prevent a stroke – *see* ***hypertension,*** *page 46*.

Aspirin or similar drugs in small daily doses (300-600 mg/day) may reduce the frequency of transient ischemic attacks. Clinical trials have not been entirely convincing, especially with women.
How it works: By making platelets (small blood cells) less likely to stick together and therefore less likely to form clumps within the circulation.

OVER-THE-COUNTER TREATMENTS

Aspirin as a treatment for stroke patients should be taken only under medical advice; your doctor may recommend that you buy supplies direct from a pharmacist.

QUESTIONS TO ASK THE DOCTOR

Major stroke:

- Since there are no effective drugs, what can be done to aid recovery?
- How long can I expect to continue to improve?
- How can I prevent another stroke?

Transient ischemic attack:

- How long should I take aspirin?
- How will I know when it is working?
- What happens if I am allergic to aspirin?

SIDE EFFECTS

If **aspirin** is necessary, treatment is for life. The problem is that in substantial, long-term dosage, the drug loses some of its effect, and side effects are more likely. The main side effect is a mild stomach upset such as heartburn. More severe effects such as an ulcer or bleeding from the stomach are rare with small doses. *See also* ***pain,*** *page 106.*

Rarely, severe asthmatic attacks may be precipitated by even a single aspirin tablet – this can be fatal. For patients unable to take aspirin, other drugs such as warfarin may be used.

SELF-MANAGEMENT

Prevention is the key.

- Do not smoke.
- Have your blood pressure checked once a year.
- Reduce your intake of saturated fat and salt.
- Take regular exercise.

SELF-HELP IN AN ATTACK

1 Get medical help as soon as possible. **2** Lie down and keep calm. **3** Accept that you may have to go into hospital for help with your recovery.

PATIENT'S EXPERIENCE

"When I first woke up, unable to move my left side, I thought I would never walk or work again. Progress has been slow, but with physiotherapy I can now walk unaided and have returned to work. I was depressed by the slow rate of progress at the start, but now I do think the effort has been worthwhile."

AFTER A STROKE

Having had a stroke, you will be treated as necessary with physiotherapy, speech therapy and occupational therapy while still in hospital. After you get home it is important to continue exercises you learned from the physiotherapist to maintain maximum functional improvement. Although most improvement occurs in the first six months, function can continue to improve over several years.

Vasodilators

NAMES YOU WILL HEAR
Vasodilators
Generic name: nifedipine; **trade names:** Adalat, Procardia. **Generic name:** prazosin; **trade names:** Minipress, Hypovase. **Generic name:** thymoxamine; **trade name:** Opilon. **Generic name:** isoxsuprine; **trade names:** Vasodilan, Defencin, Duvadilan, Vasotran. **Generic name:** naftidrofuryl; **trade name:** Praxilene. **Generic name:** cyclandelate; **trade names:** Cyclospasmol, Cyclobral. **Generic name:** inositol nicotinate; **trade name:** Hexopal. **Generic name:** oxpentifylline; **trade name:** Trental.

Several important disorders of circulation are featured elsewhere in this book: for example angina *(page 46)* and stroke *(page 60)*. Here are covered circulatory problems affecting the legs and, to a lesser extent, the arms. Three relatively common types are covered.

PERIPHERAL VASCULAR DISEASE

Narrowing of the arteries with reduction of the blood supply to the tissues in the legs. It is most noticeable when exercising. On walking, a cramp-like pain (intermittent claudication) occurs (most often in the calf muscles) after going a certain distance. It ceases a few minutes after stopping. The distance that can be walked before the onset of pain is less when going uphill or walking into the wind. It is worse in overweight patients because of the increased work necessary to move a heavy body. The skin becomes dry, scaly and cold and there is loss of surface hair on the legs. Gangrene may develop in severe cases.

CAUSE Atherosclerosis *(see page 52)*.

PRESCRIPTION DRUGS

There are no effective drugs for this problem. Self-help is therefore essential. Some severe cases require surgery (replacement of a narrowed artery).

QUESTIONS TO ASK THE DOCTOR

- Must I stop smoking?
- What about weight loss and low fat diets?
- Would surgery help?

SELF-MANAGEMENT

Prevention is the key. *See* ***angina,*** *page 46.*

DANGER SIGNS:

- Development of black areas of skin, especially heels and toes.
- Infections in feet.
- Worsening of calf pain.

VARICOSE VEINS

Veins carry blood back to the heart. In the legs this process is helped by the pumping action of the muscles and the valves within the veins which (when healthy) prevent blood flowing backwards. Veins are said to be varicose when they become distended and tortuous because the valves are not working properly. The main problem is often cosmetic, but ankle swelling and aching in the legs may occur. Occasionally ulceration develops around the ankles.

CAUSES A defect in the valves, or obstruction to venous blood flow caused by conditions such as obesity.

PRESCRIPTION DRUGS

Varicose veins are not helped by drug treatment. Some patients require surgery.

QUESTIONS TO ASK THE DOCTOR

- Will any treatment be necessary?
- What can I do to minimize the problem?

SELF-MANAGEMENT

If you are overweight, diet. Avoid long periods of standing and raise your feet on a support when sitting. Wear support hose if advised by your doctor. Avoid tight garments round the abdomen. Get regular exercise. If an ulcer develops, contact your doctor.

RAYNAUD'S PHENOMENON

A disorder of blood vessels in the hands (or occasionally the feet) which results in constriction of small arteries in response to cold or emotion. In most patients this is simply an exaggeration of the normal response to cold. Sometimes it may occur if the arms are exposed to excessive vibrations.

CAUSES Usually unknown. Occasionally a diseased blood vessel, or some other disease elsewhere in the body is implicated. Sometimes an anomalous bone in the neck (cervical rib) may compress the subclavian artery and cause symptoms. Beta-blockers can precipitate the proslem in susceptible subjects.

PRESCRIPTION DRUGS

Vasodilators may help some people. They are often prescribed on a trial-and-error basis: if the first does not work, another is tried. There is no single ideal drug at present. Drugs are only necessary in severe cases.
How they work: by making the small blood vessels increase in diameter and less likely to constrict.

QUESTIONS TO ASK THE DOCTOR

- Is there likely to be an underlying cause?

SIDE EFFECTS

See page 55.

PATIENT'S EXPERIENCE

"I could only walk 100 yards on level ground before I got pains in the back of my legs. I had been smoking for 30 years and was up to 25 a day. My doctor told me to stop smoking; he said treatment would not be much use if I continued to smoke. That was what made me try to give up. It was awful doing without cigarettes at first, but now my health is better than it has been for years; and I can walk at least a mile without stopping."

Anticoagulants

NAMES YOU WILL HEAR
Oral anticoagulants
Generic name: heparin; **trade names:** Coumadin, Panwarfin, Sofarin, Marevan, Warfilone, Warnerin. **Generic name:** phenindione; **trade names:** Dindevan, Haemopan, Danilone. **Generic name:** nicoumalone; **trade names:** Sinthrome, Sintrom.

WHAT IS A BLOOD CLOT?

Usually a normal process essential to stop excessive bleeding from an injury. However, blood clotting can occur where it is unwanted – typically within the deep veins of the legs (deep venous thrombosis). The clot (thrombus) impairs the flow of blood to the heart and fluid builds up in the leg below the site of blockage. The leg becomes swollen, painful and warm. Sometimes part of the clot breaks off and travels in the blood stream, usually to the lungs (pulmonary embolus). This may cause chest pain (which is often worse on taking a deep breath or when coughing). Breathlessness, a fast pulse, coughing up blood and fever may also occur, and if the embolus is large it can be fatal.

CAUSES **1** Obstruction or slowing of blood flow in the legs: this can occur after lying several days in bed, especially with a pillow under the knees, or after a long flight or other journey. **2** Damage to the wall of a vein resulting from an accident, an operation, or inflammation around the vein. **3** Taking oral contraceptives *(see page 179)*. **4** A rare genetic defect in the clotting mechanism.

PRESCRIPTION DRUGS

Heparin is used in most patients as soon as the diagnosis is made. It has to be given by injection and is thus mainly used in a hospital.
How it works: by improving the effect of a natural anticoagulant in the blood, which in turn stops the action of natural blood clotting factors. It is a fast-acting remedy.
Warfarin is usually also started when the diagnosis is made or a few days later: it takes a few days to develop its full effect. It is taken as pills, colored for different strengths, and may constitute life-long treatment if the problem is recurrent.
How it works: by reducing clotting factors.
Phenindione is given in rare cases of a patient being allergic to warfarin. **Nicoumalone** is an increasingly little-used alternative to warfarin.

OVER-THE-COUNTER TREATMENTS

None.

QUESTIONS TO ASK THE DOCTOR

- How long will the treatment take?
- How will treatment be controlled?
- What exercise should I get?
- Do I need to be careful about what I eat?

- Can I take other medication?
- What are the main side effects?

SIDE EFFECTS

Heparin's main side effect is spontaneous bleeding, typically from stomach, bowel or kidney, or into the skin (bruising). This is generally the result of an overdose. Careful dose control is essential to minimize the problem. Occasionally it can cause a severe loss of platelets which are necessary to prevent uncontrolled bleeding. Because the drug is administered under hospital supervision the risk is minimized, and in any case heparin's effect is quickly reversed.

Warfarin: As with heparin, the main side effect is spontaneous bleeding. Thus the dose must be carefully adjusted under hospital supervision for each individual. Blood samples are necessary, daily at the start of treatment but less often when the treatment has stabilized. Long-term warfarin users are at a small but significant risk and must be carefully counselled from the start in recognizing bruising and bleeding into the urine and the bowel, and in reporting such facts immediately. Because warfarin is broken down by the liver, it is subject to some serious drug interactions which may drastically alter its effect. Be sure to check ALL drugs with your doctor. A rare but serious side effect of warfarin is gangrene of skin, fat or other tissues. It usually occurs soon after warfarin is started, and may lead to amputation. Allergic reactions are rare.

SELF-MANAGEMENT

Take your warfarin pills regularly at the same time each day to achieve a uniform effect. Avoid any major dietary changes; don't eat foods rich in vitamin K (for example, cauliflower, spinach, brussel sprouts). Also, if on warfarin, avoid crash diets. These may drastically reduce the amount of vitamin K available and may lead to severe bleeding. Prevent recurrence of deep venous thrombosis by:

- Avoiding prolonged immobility: if you have to lie in bed, wriggle your toes and move your legs at least every 30 minutes while awake. If you are taking a long journey, get up and walk every hour.
- Regular gentle exercise such as walking or cycling.
- Avoiding oral contraceptives, particularly the combined contraceptive pill.
- Wearing support hose if advised to do so.
- Avoiding other drugs, particularly aspirin. You may use acetaminophen for pain relief.

PATIENT'S EXPERIENCE

"I had had two episodes of thrombosis in my leg veins and was not keen on taking pills which, a friend told me, are also used as rat poison. However my doctor explained that the dose of warfarin could be controlled so that it made my blood less likely to clot but without a great risk of bleeding. I am now in the habit of taking my warfarin at the same time each day and the problem seems to be well controlled. I haven't been troubled by thrombosis for the past three years."

SELF-HELP IN AN ATTACK

If your leg swells up, consult your doctor as soon as possible and avoid exercising until your leg has been examined. If you need something for the pain, take acetaminophen. If possible, go to bed, lying with your feet up: elevate the foot of the bed.

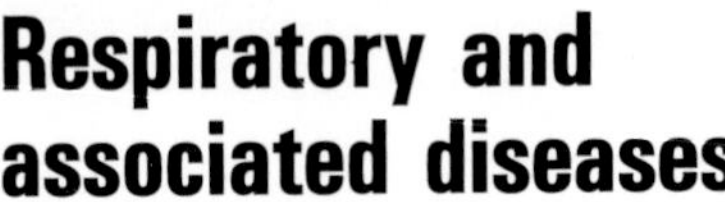

Respiratory and associated diseases

The lungs receive oxygen from air breathed in and this oxygen is transferred to the blood in the spongy tissue of the lungs. In exchange, carbon dioxide is transferred to the lung tissues, and then breathed out. Difficulties in breathing happen when the lung tissue is congested, inflamed, or otherwise damaged or if the air passages are narrowed, as in asthma.

Illustration Lungs and heart with illustrations of possible pathology eg 1) ''shadow on the lung'' – cancer or TB 2) patchy pneumonia – infection 3) narrowed airways – asthma

See also: *Lung cancer, page 202.*

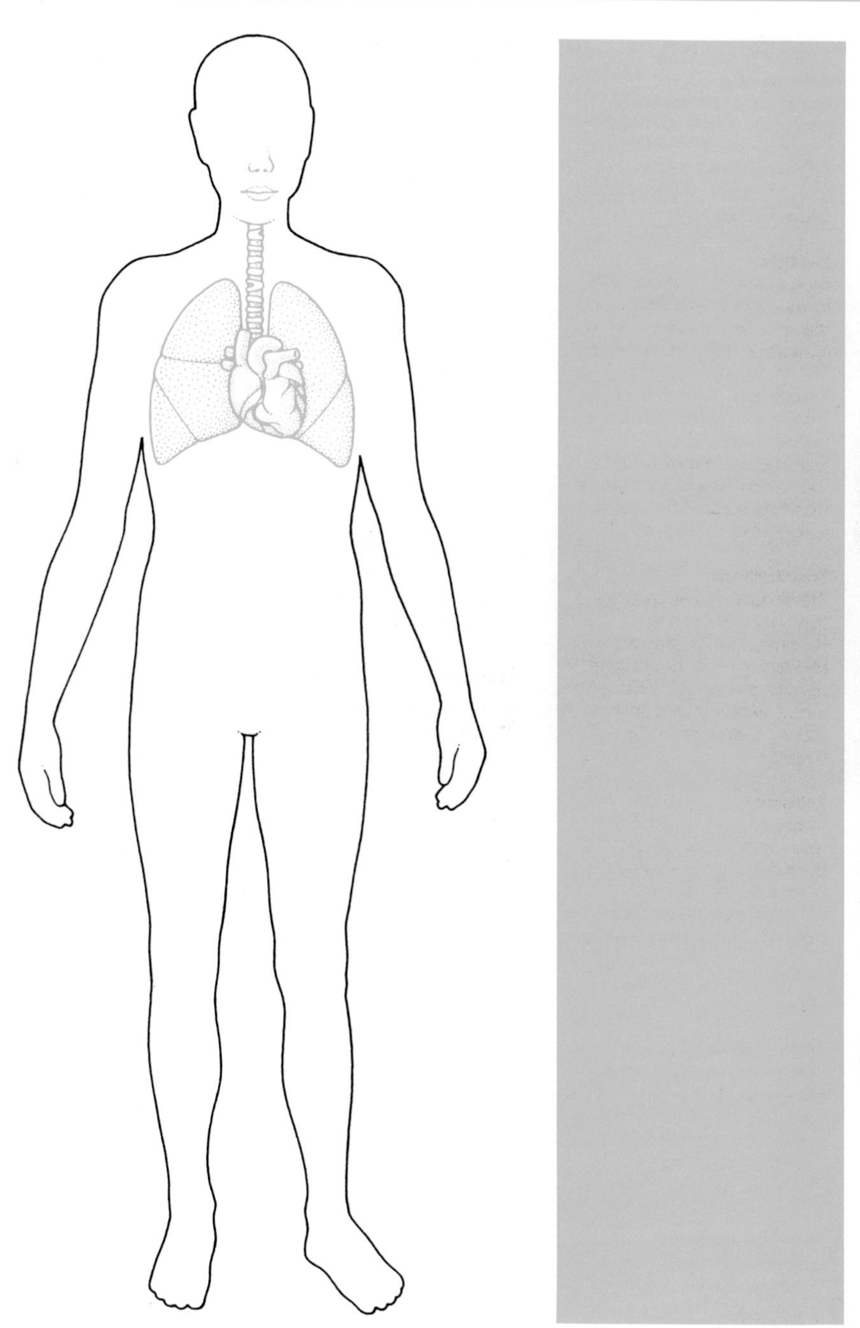

COUGH

Decongestants, mucolytics, expectorants, bronchodilators, antibiotics, cough suppressants

NAMES YOU WILL HEAR

Decongestants
Generic names: pseudoephedrine hydrochloride: Atrohist, Co-Tylenol Cold Medication, Dimetane-DX Cough Syrup, Fedahist, Novahistine, Robitussin, Actifed, Sudafed, Sudilex, Drixora Repetabs, Eltor.

Mucolytics
Generic name: acetylcysteine; **trade names:** Mucomyst, Mucodyne, Mucosirop. **Generic name:** bromhexine hydrochloride; **trade name:** Bisolvin.

Expectorants
There are many expectorants such as guaifenesin, iodide, chlorides, bicarbones, squill and ipecacuanha. These are seldom used alone, but are often found in combination with bronchodilators or mycolytics.

Bronchodilators
Generic name: theophylline hydrate; **trade names:** Neulin, Nuelin, Theocontin, Theo-Dur, Theograd, Iphylline, Elixophyllin. **Generic name:** metaproferenol sulphate; **trade name:** Alupent. **Generic name:** salbutamol, albuterol; **trade name:** Ventolin, Proventil.

Antibiotics
Generic name: amoxycillin sodium; **trade names:** Amoxil, Moxacin, Moxilean, Novamoxin, Penamox, Polymox. **Generic name:** co-trimoxazole; **trade names:** Septra, Septra DS, Bactrim, Fectrim, Nodilon, Septrim. **Generic name:** trimethoprim; **trade names:** Iprol, Monotrim, Syraprim, Trimopan.

Cough suppressants
Generic name: codeine phosphate; **trade names:** Dimetane DC Cough Syrup, Robitussin DC Cough Syrup, Triamine Expectorant with codeine, Codeine Linctus, Codeine Syrup, Dimotane Co, Galcodine, Phensedyl, Tercoda, Terpoin, Unifly, Codlin, Diarrest, Kaodene, Paveral, Todlin. **Generic name:** pholcodine tartrate; **trade names:** Dia-Tuss, Duro-Tuss, Pholtex, Copholco, Copholcoids.

WHAT IS A COUGH?

Muscular contraction of the diaphragm whose function is to expel mucus or foreign bodies from the respiratory tract. A cough is usually useful and does not always require treatment. If a dry cough is due to thick secretions, these can be "loosened" so that they can be coughed up; a dry cough which is disturbing sleep can be "suppressed". Coughing at night may be an early sign of asthma *(see page 74)*.

CAUSES Mucus, produced by the respiratory tract as a response to infection or inflammation. It may be produced in the chest, or may arise in the nose and throat as in a common cold or hay fever. Smoking irritates the lungs and gives rise to cough, hoarseness, reduced lung function, bronchitis, heart disease and lung cancer. Cough may signify serious lung disease. On the other hand, respiratory infections may be followed by a cough which can persist for several weeks, without there necessarily being major disease present.

PRESCRIPTION DRUGS

Decongestants will suppress mucus production in the nose in cases of infection or allergy.
Mucolytics are supposed to make mucus in the chest less thick and easier to cough up.
Expectorants stimulate coughing in order to clear mucus.
Bronchodilators will dilate constricted airways and also make mucus easier to cough up.
Antibiotics will kill bacteria if present.
Cough suppressants will act on the "cough center" in the brain and suppress the cough.

OVER-THE-COUNTER TREATMENTS

Simple decongestants, expectorants, bronchodilators and cough suppressants can all be bought from a pharmacist. Decongestants are often used when the upper airways are congested, and expectorants and bronchodilators when mucus is being coughed up from the chest.

Cough suppressants should only be used if there is no thick mucus or the patient needs rest. Bronchodilators are useful for wheeze and night cough in asthma sufferers *(see **asthma,** page 74)*.

It is better to choose medicines with only one active ingredient. *See **common cold,** page 134.*

QUESTIONS TO ASK THE DOCTOR

■ Which of these drugs do I really need?

■ How long will they take to work?
■ What will happen if I stop them too soon?
■ Have I got asthma?

SIDE EFFECTS

Antihistamines, which are usually found in **decongestants,** cause drowsiness in many people and should not be taken when driving or working in a potentially dangerous environment. They potentiate the depressant effect of alcohol. For more information on the side effects of decongestants, *see* ***middle ear infections,*** *page 256* and ***hay fever,*** *page 260.* **Mucolytics** cause gastric irritation and should not be used by patients with a history of indigestion or peptic ulcer. Some **Bronchodilators** can cause tremor and palpitations, especially if the recommended dose is exceeded, or in sensitive individuals. *See* ***asthma,*** *page 74.* Antibiotics can cause nausea and lethargy; they may also give rise to an allergic reaction, usually a rash. Report it to a doctor immediately. *See also* ***pneumonia and pleurisy,*** *page 78.* **Cough suppressants** cause constipation.

SELF-MANAGEMENT

It is important to differentiate between **1** a cough caused by a post-nasal drip (from mucus production in the nose): this is best treated with a decongestant; **2** a cough caused by mucus production in the chest or asthma for which mucolytics or bronchodilators are the best treatment **3** a dry, useless cough, for which a cough suppressant may be used. Inhalation of steam *(see* ***sinusitis,*** *page 262)* is often useful for patients with sticky mucus in the chest. **4** Cough caused by serious lung disease (asthma, cancer) and **5** cough caused by cardiac failure.

■ Encourage children to blow their noses and cough up any mucus.
■ Stop smoking – if smoker's cough is already a problem, you need to give it up now.
■ Drink plenty of fluids, especially water.
■ Patients with recurrent attacks of wheezy bronchitis or asthma should seek advice on starting treatment with bronchodilators as soon as a cough starts.

Consult a doctor if:

■ Mucus coughed up is green or yellow ■ Mucus contains blood ■ There is pain in the chest with coughing ■ A cough is accompanied by a high temperature ■ A cough is associated with shortness of breath or wheeze ■ A cough continues for more than ten days.

PATIENT'S EXPERIENCE

"My little boy of three had a cough and cold. I gave him some cough medicine to stop him coughing at night, but although it helped a little, the cough continued. After a week I took him to the doctor. The doctor explained that it was wrong to suppress the cough and that it would have been better to dry up the runny nose that was causing it, and prescribed a decongestant. He didn't need antibiotics and his cough cleared after about a week."

DOCTORS' EXPERIENCE

"Most coughs will clear spontaneously and treatment just tends to ease the symptoms and hasten recovery. Bronchodilators are useful if there is mild asthma associated with the cough. Antibiotics are not necessary unless the secretions have become infected."

"It is amazing how many smokers want antibiotics to clear up their smoker's cough. They don't seem to realize how much damage is done to the lungs by smoking; I often test their lung function with a peak flow meter, and show them how it progressively improves over a few months when they stop smoking."

BRONCHITIS AND EMPHYSEMA/1

Antibiotics, bronchodilators, steroids, mucolytics, antitussives, inhalants

NAMES YOU WILL HEAR

Antibiotics

Generic name: ampicillin; **trade names:** Omnipen, Polycillin, Principen, Ampifen, Penbritin, Pentrexyl, Vidopen, Austrapen, Bristin, Amcill, Ampicin, Ampilean, Biosan, Ampil, Famicilin, Pentrex, Petercillin, Synthecillin. **Generic name:** amoxycillin; **trade names:** Amoxil, Augmentin, Polymox, Trimox, Moxacin, Moxilean, Novamoxin, Penamox. **Generic name:** co-trimoxazole; **trade names:** Septra, Bactrim, Fectrim, Nodilon, Septrim. **Generic name:** trimethoprim; **trade names:** Proloprim, Monotrim, Syraprim, Trimopan. **Generic name:** erythromycin; **trade names:** Benzamycin, Erymax, Ilotycin, Peidazole, Arpimycin, Erycen, Erythroped, Retcin, Erythrocin, Erythromid, EpMycin, Erostin, Emu-V, Ethryn, Eromel, Ilocap, Ilosone, Rythrocaps.

Bronchodilators

Generic names: salbutamol, albuterol; **trade names:** Ventolin, Proventil. **Generic name:** terbutaline; **trade names:** Brethine, Bricanyl, Feevone. **Generic name:** fenoterol; **trade names:** Berotec, Partusisten. **Generic name:** metaproferenol; **trade name:** Alupent. **Generic name:** isoetharine; **trade names:** Bronkosol, Numotac, Bronchilator. **Generic name:** aminophylline; **trade names:** Phyllocontin, Theodrox, Anodrophylline, Carophyllin, Euphyllin, Retard, Peterphyllin. **Generic name:** theophylline hydrate; **trade names:** Neulin, Nuelin, Theoconton, Theo-Dur, Theograd, Iphylline, Elixophyllin. **Generic name:** ipratropium bromide; **trade name:** Atrovent.

WHAT ARE BRONCHITIS AND EMPHYSEMA?

Acute bronchitis is characterized by cough, production of yellow or green phlegm and fever resulting from infection of the lower air passages (the bronchi). The infection usually spreads from the upper airways and in fit individuals is commonly a self-limiting viral infection which requires symptomatic treatment only. In patients with pre-existing lung disease, acute bronchitis is more serious, requiring antibiotic therapy and even hospital admission.

Chronic bronchitis and emphysema is an extremely common condition in industrialized countries, though cigarette smoking far outweighs occupational and environmental exposure as a causative factor. Although separate pathological entities, chronic bronchitis and emphysema frequently develop together and can be impossible to distinguish; indeed they are here considered as one. The severity of the disease varies from a simple smoker's cough and morning phlegm to total breathless incapacitation.

Chronic bronchitis is characterized by long-term coughing and excess phlegm production due to damage to the airway.

Emphysema is enlargement of the air spaces in the lung tissue beyond the smallest airways (the bronchioles). A major feature of chronic bronchitis and emphysema is limitation of airflow which may produce wheezing, though the airflow obstruction is not usually as variable or as reversible as in asthma.

The term chronic obstructive airways disease, COAD (or chronic obstructive pulmonary disease, COPD) is used to describe the picture of chronic bronchitis and emphysema with airflow obstruction. Chronic bronchitis develops insidiously, starting usually in winter with a chronic cough and morning sputum, but eventually continuing year-long. The sufferer may be breathless on exertion, or when at rest. Wheezing may be prominent. In advanced cases there is a lack of oxygen reaching the tissues which become blue (cyanosed). Eventually respiratory failure can develop and the resulting strain on the heart can produce heart failure.

The progress of the disease is very variable. Some patients never have more than cough and phlegm; but there is usually a gradual deterioration in respiratory function with increasing breathlessness. In patients whose lungs are already damaged with chronic bronchitis and emphysema, acute infection should be treated seriously: resistance is lowered and lung function can rapidly deteriorate.

Although chronic bronchitis and emphysema is a progressive disease, it can be slowed or halted by removal of the factors which cause it.

CAUSES The major factor is cigarette smoking, though other forms of atmospheric pollution are also implicated and in some people there may be an inherited predisposition to damage from inhaled pollutants.

Tobacco smoke causes swelling of the bronchial walls with enlargement of the mucous glands and damage to the fine hair cells which clear secretions from the lungs. Smoke also inhibits the action of certain enzymes which normally protect the lungs from damage.

PRESCRIPTION DRUGS

Antibiotics: those listed are most commonly used for acute exacerbations of chronic bronchitis. Some patients with persistent or repeated infection require continuous antibiotics, particularly during winter.

How they work: by killing bacteria responsible for infection. Bacteria can become resistant to the action of some antibiotics and the choice of antibiotic from the large number available will depend on local resistance patterns.

Bronchodilators are widely used to alleviate chronic bronchitis and emphysema. However, they are only effective if there is reversible airways narrowing. There are three types: sympathomimetics, anticholinergics, and methylxanthines, and they are taken as pills or by inhalation.

How they work: the three groups act on different receptors to open up the airways and can be used in combination for additive effect. *See **asthma,** page 72.*

Sympathomimetics are chemically related to adrenaline and are best inhaled directly into the lungs since they act faster, with fewer side effects, by this route. They are usually prescribed as an aerosol inhaler. The modern sympathomimetics listed are selective in their action on the lungs rather than the heart. Many are now available but all act similarly and none has a particular advantage. After inhalation the effect is usually seen within 30 minutes.

Anticholinergics: Ipratropium bromide is the only anticholinergic drug usually available for this condition, although others are being developed. It can only be taken by inhalation and takes longer to work than the sympathomimetics. While both types have an immediate effect on airway narrowing, in COAD they are

PATIENT'S EXPERIENCE

"I had a smoker's cough for years and thought nothing of it. My first cigarettes of the day used to help get the phlegm up. In my 40s I became breathless going upstairs and put it down to middle age, but by the time I was 50 I had to stop half-way up. I was rushed into hospital when an attack of 'flu went to my chest and I was barely able to breathe. I now use two inhalers and theophylline tablets and after 35 years have finally stopped smoking. I still get breathless climbing stairs and a smokey atmosphere makes me cough and wheeze. I have to take antibiotics at the first sign of infection, but I do feel better for having stopped smoking."

DOCTOR'S EXPERIENCE

"Robert was 63 and had been a professional footballer in the years after the war; now he works on the ground staff of the local team. He had always prided himself on his fitness and he indeed looked fit. However, he was getting increasingly breathless. He couldn't run, and was fighting for breath after climbing the steps at the club. He had always smoked, and had a morning cough and phlegm. His lungs were over-inflated and wheezing. Testing revealed lung function only 50 per cent of normal. I explained the problem: chronic wheezy bronchitis due to cigarette smoking. The damage had been done; he found it hard to accept that even a natural athlete has no guaranteed immunity to the effects of cigarettes. He was helped considerably by inhaler therapy and by stopping smoking; but he remained yet another member of my vast team of chronic bronchitics."

Steroids
Generic name: beclomethasone dipropionate; **trade names:** Becotide, Vanceril. **Generic name:** betamethasone valerate; **trade name:** Bextasol. **Generic name:** methyl prednisolone; **trade names:** Solumedrol, Codelsol, Delta Phorical, Deltacortril, Deltalone, Deltastab, Precortisyl, Prednesol, Sintisone, Nisolone, Delta-Cortef, Deltasolone, Prelone, Lenisolone, Meticortilone, Predeltilone. **Generic name:** betamethasone; **trade names:** Betnelan, Betnesol.

Mucolytic
Generic name: acetylcysteine; **trade names:** Mucomyst, Mucodyne, Mucosirop.

Cough supressants
Generic name: codeine phosphate; **trade names:** Ambinyl Cough Syrup, Dimetane DC Cough Syrup, Robitussin DC Cough Syrup, Triamine Expectorant with codeine, Codeine Linctus, Codeine Syrup, Dimotane Co, Galcodine, Phensedyl, Tercoda, Terpoin, Uniflu, Codlin, Paveral. **Generic name:** pholcodine tartrate; **trade names:** Dia-Tuss, Duro-Tuss, Pholtex, Copholco, Copholcoids, Davenol, Expulin, Galenphol, Pavacol D, Pholcomed, Rinurel. **Generic name:** dextromethorphan; **trade name:** Cosylan.

Inhalants
Generic name: benzoin tincture compound; **trade name:** Friar's Balsam. **Generic name:** menthol and benzoin inhalation; usually prescribed by generic name.

most effective when taken regularly three or four times a day.

Methylxanthines are chemically related to caffeine and are non-selective in action, with a stimulant effect on the heart as well as the lungs. The modern formulations are oral preparations.

Steroids are related to cortisone produced by the adrenal gland. They are sometimes given, by mouth or by injection, for acute flare-ups of chronic obstructive airways disease and in patients with advanced disease for whom all other therapies have proved ineffective. Since potential side effects are so great it is essential that they are only used when really necessary.

Inhaled steroids *(see also **asthma**, page 74)* are a valuable and safe long-term therapy for wheezy bronchitis, though they will only work if there is at least some degree of reversible airways narrowing. They are not effective during an acute attack since an inadequate amount of the drug reaches the bronchial wall: they must be used regularly to be effective. They are less effective in bronchitis than in asthma. This treatment is not, however, standard in the USA.

How they work: by reducing the inflammation in the bronchial wall which causes airway obstruction.

Expectorants ease removal of bronchial secretions.

How they work: theoretically by increasing the volume and reducing the stickiness of secretions; there is little hard evidence that they are of any value.

Mucolytics contain enzymes which reduce the stickiness of bronchial secretions.

How they work: by breaking down the structure of sticky phlegm. They may be of value in some lung diseases, but in chronic bronchitis their worth is very doubtful.

Antitussives will suppress coughing.

How they work: by acting on the brain to inhibit the cough reflex. Useful for a dry, non-productive cough.

QUESTIONS TO ASK THE DOCTOR

- How often should I use the inhalers?
- Can you check that I am using inhalers correctly?
- Can I take extra puffs of a bronchodilator inhaler if my breathing is bad?
- Should I have influenza vaccine?
- Should I have a supply of antibiotics to start taking as soon as I develop an infection?

SIDE EFFECTS

Antibiotics can cause allergic reactions such as skin rashes. Report them to a doctor immediately. Broad spectrum antibiotics may cause severe rashes. **Bronchodilators;** Sympathomimetics rarely have side effects. *See **asthma,** page 74.* Anticholinergics are usually free from serious side effects, though in high dose they can cause retention of urine, glaucoma *(see page 270)* and a dry mouth. With **methylxanthines** there is little difference between the effective dose and the toxic dose. Nausea, abdominal discomfort and headaches are common side effects. A change in dose, timing of medication or drug formulation may help. The amount of drug in the blood may need to be measured to ensure that the dose is both non-toxic and effective.

Steroids: may cause thinning of bones, bone fractures, peptic ulcer and psychiatric upsets *(see **asthma,** page 74).*

A short treatment with steroid pills is unlikely to be harmful but prolonged therapy (more than a few weeks) does carry the risk of numerous side effects which have to be weighed against the benefits of treatment. Long-term steroids suppress the body's normal secretion of cortisol and it is essential that you do not change (or stop) the dose of steroids without your doctor's advice. *See **anemia,** page 224.*

OVER-THE-COUNTER TREATMENTS

Steam inhalation preparations are widely available. It is the steam which is of value, not the aromatic extras, though these can make the process of inhaling more pleasant.

SELF-MANAGEMENT

■ ***You must stop smoking.*** Even in advanced disease, you may gain benefit. Various techniques such as nicotine chewing gum, hypnotherapy or acupuncture may help, but ultimately it comes down to willpower. Join (or form your own) no smoking group.

■ Avoid smoky atmospheres and sudden changes to extremes of air temperature.

■ Excess weight makes normal people breathless and contributes to breathlessness induced by lung disease. If overweight, diet. *See ideal weight table, page 51.*

■ While exercise will not necessarily improve lung function, regular exercise such as brisk walking can improve exercise tolerance and your feeling of well-being.

■ Vaccination against influenza may be helpful in preventing acute attacks.

■ Long-term oxygen at home may be an option for some patients (see margin) but its use must be regulated.

SELF-HELP IN AN ATTACK

■ As soon as you feel infection starting, with phlegm changing color from white to yellow or green, see your doctor for a course of antibiotics. If these have already been provided, start taking them.

■ Stay indoors: do not try to work through the attack.

■ If phlegm is sticky and difficult to clear, steam inhalations may help. *See sinusitis, page 262.*

OXYGEN

Oxygen is usually given in hospitals for severe acute attacks. In advanced disease, long-term oxygen at home for at least 15 hours a day has been shown to be of value in improving well-being and survival. This can be provided at home by oxygen concentrator, about the size of a small apartment refrigerator. However, only a minority of patients are suitable for this type of treatment and hospital assessment is essential.

Methylxanthines, beta stimulants, mast cell stabilizers, steroids, anticholinergics

NAMES YOU WILL HEAR

Mast cell stabilizers
Generic name: cromolyn sodium; **trade names:** Intal, Nalcrom, Lomudal. **Generic name:** ketotifen; **trade name:** Zaditen.

Beta stimulants
Generic names: salbutamol, albuterol; **trade name:** Ventolin, Proventil. **Generic name:** terbutaline; **trade names:** Brethine, Bricanyl, Feevone. **Generic name:** fenoterol; **trade names:** Berotec, Partusisten. **Generic name:** metaproterenol; **trade name:** Alupent. **Generic name:** isoetharine; **trade names:** Bronkosol, Numotac, Bronchilator.

Methylxanthines
Generic name: aminophylline; **trade names:** Phyllocontin, Theodrox, Androphyllin, Cardophyllin, Somophyllin, Aminophyl, Corophyllin, Euphyllin Retard, Peterphyllin. **Generic name:** theophylline hydrate; **trade names:** Neulin, Nuelin S, Theocontin, Theo-Dur, Theograd, Iphylline,. Elixophyllin.

Anticholinergic
Generic name: ipratropium bromide; **trade names:** Atrovent.

Steroids
Generic name: beclomethasone dipropionate; **trade names:** Vanceril, Becotide, Viarox. **Generic name:** betamethasone valerate; **trade name:** Bextasol. **Generic name:** methyl prednisolone; **trade names:** Solumedrol, Codelsol, Delta Phorical, Deltacortril, Deltalone, Deltastab, Precortisyl, Prednesol, Sintisone, Nisolone, Delta-Cortef, Deltasolone, Prelone, Lenisolone, Meticortilone, Predeltilone. **Generic name:** prednisone; **trade name:** Decortisyl. **Generic name:** Triamcinolone; **trade name:** Azmacort.

WHAT IS ASTHMA?

Narrowing of the small air passages of the lungs (the bronchioles), so that it becomes difficult to move air in and out. In most cases the condition is completely reversible – the bronchioles can recover from the spasm. Asthma varies in severity from the mildly inconvenient to the potentially fatal. Wheeze and shortness of breath are the commonest symptoms, but persistent cough may be the presenting symptom and in young children cough is often a warning sign of an attack. Some asthmatics get infrequent attacks, others may be affected nearly all the time. Asthma often starts in childhood, but it can also start in late adulthood.

CAUSES Asthma often runs in families along with associated conditions such as eczema, hay fever, or other allergies. The mechanism of asthma is not fully understood, but attacks can be triggered by any of the following:

- Allergies: some asthmatics are allergic to such everyday items as house dust (strictly speaking, the house dust mite), pollen, fungal spores, dogs, cats or birds. Usually the allergy is to things *inhaled*, but occasionally asthma can be triggered by allergies to foods.
- Emotion: stress can provoke attacks in some people who already have the diesase.
- Viral respiratory infections: colds or flu commonly precipitate asthmatic attacks, especially in early childhood (typically, before the age of four).
- Sudden exposure to cold air.
- Exercise can occasionally precipitate an attack.
- Smoke (including cigarette smoke).
- Some drugs, including beta-blockers *(see **hypertension**, page 46)* and aspirin.

PRESCRIPTION DRUGS

Beta stimulant bronchodilators: long the mainstay of therapy. Most commonly taken as pressurized aerosol, but also available as tablets or as a solution for a nebulizer. Rarely, in an emergency, they can be given by infusion into a vein. They can be used to maintain relaxation of airways or reverse an attack which has clearly started.

How they work: by directly stimulating the airway muscle, making it relax, just as adrenaline does. Modern drugs like terbutaline, salbutamol and fenoteral act selectively on the airways, having much less effect on the heart. These drugs are also useful in allergic asthma, as they inhibit release of those chemicals which cause the airways to narrow.

Methylxanthines can be useful for prevention and treatment. They are usually given as tablets or by injection.

How they work: probably by acting directly on the muscles in the walls of the air passages, causing them to relax.

Beta stimulants: used to *treat* attacks once in progress, and also to prevent them occurring. Beta stimulants can be given as tablets (or by injection) but are most commonly inhaled by means of an aerosol spray.

How they work: by stimulating the part of the nervous system which causes the muscles in the walls of the air passages to relax. Consequently, the air passage widens, allowing air to pass in and out more freely.

Mast cell stabilizers: Drugs such as cromolyn are useful for the *prevention* of attacks; they are not for the *treatment* of attacks. These drugs are usually only effective if inhaled, and there are several ways of taking them including aerosols, inhalation of fine powder from capsules using a device called a spinhaler, and nebulizers (see illustration).

How they work: possibly by acting on the mast cells which release the chemicals which cause airway narrowing.

Steroids: powerful drugs, used in the treatment of many illnesses; in asthma, they can be used in small doses to prevent attacks, or in large doses to treat severe attacks. Usually steroids are taken in small doses by metered aerosol which avoids the major side effects, or by inhalation of a powder. In bad attacks, a doctor must first give a suitable dose in pill form. If despite being on an inhaled steroid, your asthma flares up, you will be unable to inhale the steroid effectively, and at considerable risk of developing a severe attack. IF YOUR DOCTOR HAS GIVEN YOU STEROID TABLETS, TAKE THEM AT ONCE, AND SEE HIM IMMEDIATELY

How they work: The action of steroids in asthma is complex, but basically they damp down inflammation in air passages and cause the muscle in the walls of the air passages to relax.

Anticholinergics are usually used in addition to a beta stimulant or methylxanthine. The only one in common use in asthma is ipratropium bromide. It is available as an inhaler, and a solution of the drug can be used in a nebulizer.

How they work: by blocking mechanisms which normally cause bronchial muscle to contract, thereby producing relaxation and widening of the bronchioles.

The trachea or windpipe *divides into two in the chest.*

The right and left *main bronchi.*

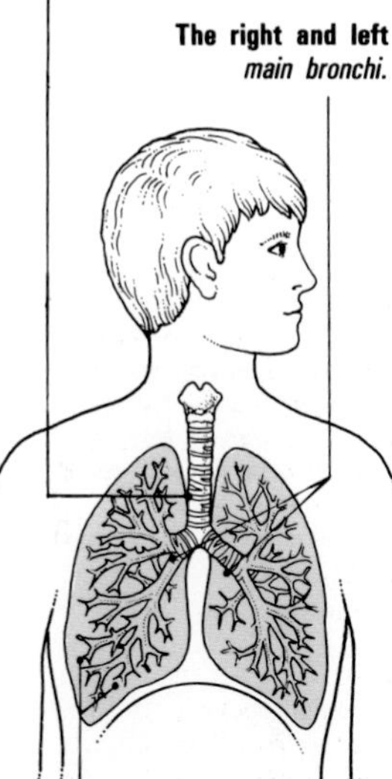

Right and left bronchi *divide into ever-smaller bronchi, and then into bronchioles.*

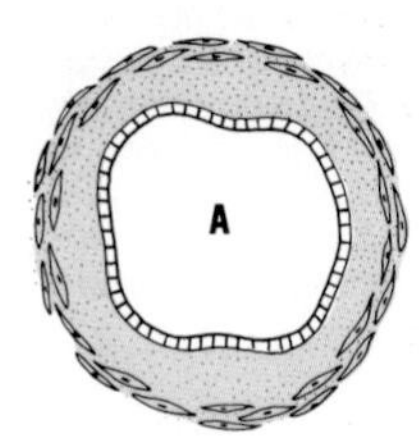

A *shows a (much magnified) normal bronchiole. The muscle is the thin band of surrounding cells. (Actual width may be as little as one mm.)*

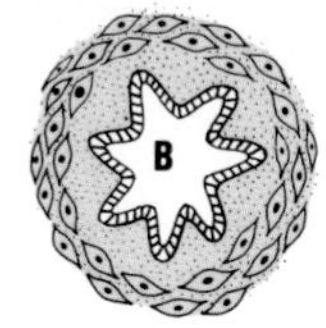

In B *the muscle has contracted, narrowing the air passage. In a really bad attack, the bronchiole may be blocked completely.*

Inhalation devices

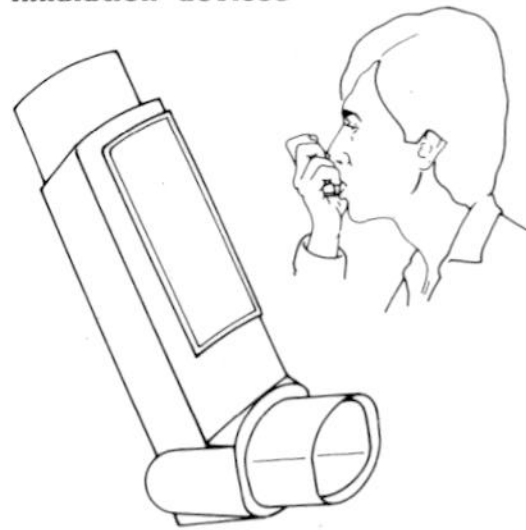

Pressurized inhaler: *effective, convenient to carry. You have to learn to synchronize breathing in with activating the puff; simple for all but the very young or uncoordinated.*

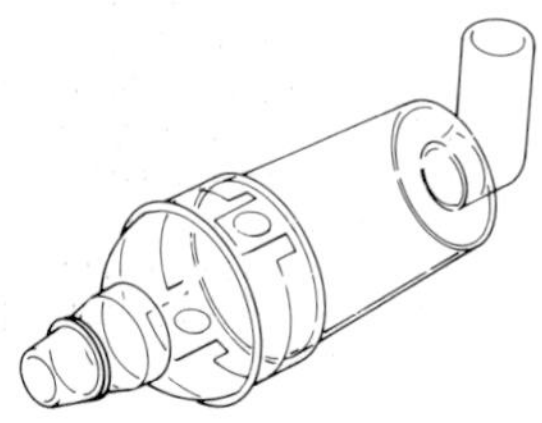

Plastic spacers *like this can be used in conjunction with aerosol inhalers. The drug is puffed into the chamber of a spacing device, from which it is then inhaled. It enables children as young as three years to use an aerosol; the alternative is a nebulizer.*

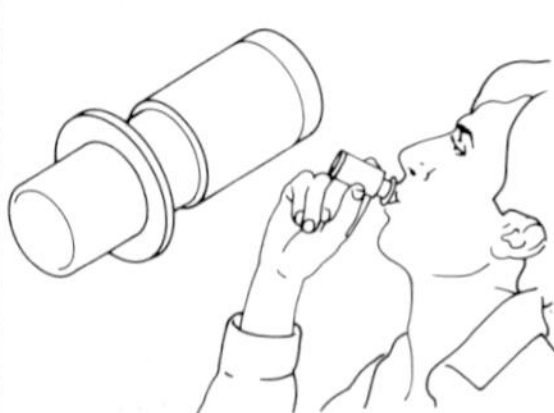

Dry powder inhaler: *Cromolyn comes in small plastic capsules which are impaled on a needle inside the device. When air is inhaled through the device, the drug is dispersed by a tiny propellor.*

OVER-THE-COUNTER TREATMENTS

Don't try to treat yourself. Remember ASTHMA KILLS 2,000 PEOPLE ANNUALLY IN THE US. All attacks should be reported to a doctor.

QUESTIONS TO ASK THE DOCTOR

- Is this drug meant to *prevent* attacks, or help to *treat* an attack once it has started?
- Is there a right and a wrong way to use the aerosol/spinhaler/nebulizer?
- How long should I take the drug?
- If the drug fails, is it safe for me to increase the dose?
- Does it matter in which order I take my inhalers?
- Is it worth having an allergy test?

SIDE EFFECTS

Methylxanthines are usually prescribed in a sustained release formulation, taken once or twice daily. It is often sensible to take the last dose just before going to bed so that the drug is acting while you are asleep. Methylxanthines can be interfered with by other drugs including ulcer healing agents and some antibiotics. If you are on other medication it is important to tell your doctor. In any case he will need to do blood tests from time to time, to make sure you are getting the right amount. It is also very important NOT TO EXCEED THE PRESCRIBED DOSE of these drugs, as adverse side effects are not uncommon, and can be serious. Mild side effects include nausea, stomach pain, loss of appetite, headaches and anxiety; serious side effects include heart rhythm disturbance and fits.

Beta stimulants: much easier to use than previous generations of bronchodilators, modern beta stimulants such as Ventolin (albuterol) have been developed to give insignificant side effects, though mild tremor is not uncommon.

Cromolyn prescribed for *prevention* of attacks, are taken regularly even when free of asthma. Adverse effects are unusual, and rarely serious; cough and mild wheezing are the most common.

Steroids: long-term treatment with steroids worries people who have heard of the side effects of these drugs. But in asthma, the long-term treatment is usually with an inhaler, which delivers a comparatively small dose straight to the lungs. The only significant side effects reported are thrush, a fungal infection causing white spots in the mouth and throat. Steroid pills and injections are another matter: they can cause serious side-effects, such as stunted growth in children, brittle bones, high blood pressure, sugar diabetes, depression and other psychiatric illness being the most common. These take a long time to develop, and since steroid pills and injections are usually a temporary measure, such side effects can usually be avoided. However, the dangers are real and if steroids have to given by mouth they are often given every other day, and always in the lowest possible dose.

Anticholinergic: patients with glaucoma (raised pressure in the eyeball) should not use this drug, nor should men with prostate trouble (usually older men who have difficulty passing water) – a doctor must advise in these cases. Anticholinergic inhaler side effects are not common but include glaucoma, constipation, difficulty passing urine, and heart palpitations.

SELF-MANAGEMENT

■ Get a peak-flow meter, and keep a regular log of the severity of your asthma. If there is any significant or progressive deterioration, SEE YOUR DOCTOR.

■ If you have a child taking drugs by nebulizer (see diagram) heed the warnings given about over-using the apparatus. The very young can succumb to asthma quite quickly; doctors prefer patients to go to the hospital before an attack builds up to a serious level.

■ Resolve to *contest* your asthma *all the time*; don't let it build up. Carry a bronchodilator inhaler with you. Don't miss out on the steroid inhaler dose: long-term asthma can do you more damage than an inhaled steroid. Remember you can use a bronchodilator inhaler to prevent attacks *as well as* treat them. One puff gives relief for up to four hours.

■ If you use both a steroid inhaler and a bronchodilator inhaler, take the bronchodilator *first*: it will make the air passages widen, so allowing the subsequent steroid dose to penetrate better.

■ Discuss the possibility of allergy tests with your doctor. This is a complex area, but worthwhile for many patients with long-term asthma. Once you know your allergies, you can take evasive action.

PATIENT'S EXPERIENCE

"I've had asthma since I was a child – it runs in my family. Provided I make the effort to control it properly, with an albuterol and a steroid inhaler, it is not a nuisance – but I can still remember how unpleasant my childhood attacks were. I can do certain types of exercise – swimming is no problem – but running makes me wheeze."

IN AN ATTACK

■ Shake the inhaler before use. Hold it a few inches in front of your open mouth or use a spacer device.

■ Breathe in slowly and as deeply as possible. Fire the spray as you begin to inhale, and try to hold your breath for ten seconds. If the attack persists, and particularly if you are getting tired or cannot speak, SEEK URGENT MEDICAL HELP. Many asthmatics now have nebulizers at home, and these deliver a larger dose than an inhaler. If it is not effective within the period specified by the doctor/hospital, seek medical help immediately.

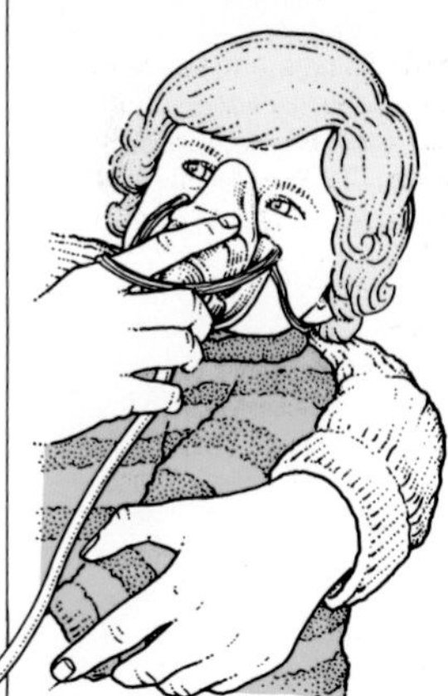

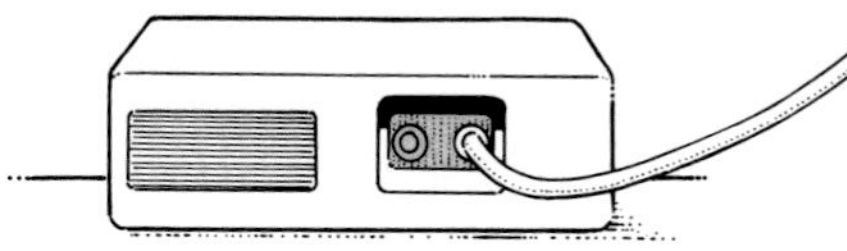

Nebulizer: *These vary in design. The drug, in liquid form, is placed in the small container attached to the mask. When oxygen is passed through, a fine inhalable mist is produced. Portable nebulizer for use at home has air instead of oxygen.*

PNEUMONIA AND PLEURISY

Mucolytics, bronchodilators, cough suppressants, antibiotics, analgesics

NAMES YOU WILL HEAR

Mucolytics
Generic name: acetylcisteine; **trade names:** Mucomyst, Mucodyne, Mucosirop. **Generic name:** bromhexine hydrochloride; **trade name:** Bisolvin.

Bronchodilators
Generic name: theophylline hydrate; **trade names:** Neulin, Theocontin, Accurbron, Elixophylline, Theo-Dur, Somophyllin, Theobid, Theograd, Iphylline. **Generic names:** salbutamol, albuterol; **trade names:** Ventolin, Proventil.

Antibiotics
Generic name: amoxycillin sodium; **trade names:** Amoxil, Augmentin, Polymox, Trimox, Wymox, Moxacin, Moxilean, Novamoxin, Penamox. **Generic name:** co-trimoxazole; **trade names:** Septra, Septra DS, Bactrim, Bactrim DS, Fectrim, Nodilon, Septrim. **Generic name:** erythromycin; **trade names:** Benzamycin, Erymax, Ilotycin, Pediazole, Pediamycin, Arpimycin, Erycen, Erythroped, Retcin, Erythrocin, Erythromid, EpMycin, Erostin, Emu-V, Ethryn, Eromel, Ilocap, Ilosone, Rythrocaps. **Generic name:** tetracycline; **trade names:** Tetracycline Capsules, Achromycin, Mysteclin, Chymocyclar, Sumycin, Economycin, Oustramycin, Bio-Tetra, Cyclabid.

Cough suppressants
Generic name: codeine phosphate; **trade names:** Ambinyl Cough Syrup, Dimetane DC Cough Syrup, Triamine Expectorant with codeine, Robitussin DC Cough Syrup, Codeine Linctus, Codeine Syrup, Galcodine, Phensedyl, Tercoda, Terpoin, Uniflu, Codlin, Diarrest, Kaodene, Paveral, Todlin. **Generic name:** pholcodine tartrate; **trade names:** Dia-Tuss, Duro-Tuss, Pholtex, Copholco, Copholcoids, Davenol, Expulin, Galenphol, Pavacol D, Pholcomed, Rinurel.

Analgesics
see\also ***pain,*** *page 106.*

WHAT ARE PNEUMONIA AND PLEURISY?

Pneumonia is an inflammation of the lungs. It causes fever, shortness of breath and cough with the production of yellow or green sputum; occasionally blood can come up too. Pleurisy is an inflammation of the membrane covering the lungs and this causes pain on breathing and other movements.

CAUSES Of pneumonia, usually a bacterial infection, although viruses, other organisms and even chemicals may occasionally be to blame. Pleurisy usually results from disease within the lung – typically pneumonia.

There are different types of pneumonia: lobar pneumonia is confined to one section or lobe and characteristically develops abruptly in young people; bronchopneumonia is patchy and widespread. This is the type most commonly in children and old people.

PRESCRIPTION DRUGS

Treatment will vary. The main concern is to treat the cause of the inflammation. A secondary aim is to relieve the pain while treating the underlying cause.

Mucolytics, bronchodilators, cough suppressants: *see* ***cough,*** *page 68.*

Antibiotics will only work in cases of bacterial pneumonia; they are ineffective against viruses. The choice of antibiotic will depend on many factors, including: whether the patient has an allergy; whether kidney or liver damage is present; the severity of the illness; whether the patient could be pregant; the type of bacteria most likely to be causing the infection; whether the patient has had an antibiotic recently. If the patient is very ill, more than one antibiotic may be used in combination, and these may be given by injection. Some antibiotics are inactivated by food and have to be taken between meals. The antibiotic may be changed during treatment if the patient does not respond or if sputum cultures show that the organism responsible is resistant to the drug. Treatment typically lasts between five and ten days, but duration depends on the nature of the infection.

How they work: by killing or by stopping the bacteria from multiplying, thus relying on the body's own defenses to complete the elimination. The problem with antibiotics is that bacteria can develop resistance to them, and this happens, typically, when treatment is stopped before all the bacteria have been killed. It may well be worse to take half a course of antibiotics than none at all. This is also why a different antibiotic is likely to be used if the patient is ill again after a short interval – typically less than a month.

Analgesics: aspirin and acetaminophen will ease pain and help reduce fever. *See* ***common cold,*** *page 134.*

In addition to the drug treatment, two other forms of therapy may be useful: oxygen to help patients who are finding breathing difficult; and physiotherapy to help loosen secretions and encourage coughing. Thus cough suppressants are rarely used in the early stages. Oxygen may be needed if the patient's lung function is significantly impaired.

OVER-THE-COUNTER TREATMENTS

Diagnosis of pneumonia and pleurisy are usually made by a doctor after examination of the chest, and with the help of an X-ray. Self-treatment is inappropriate and potentially dangerous.

QUESTIONS TO ASK THE DOCTOR

- How long will the treatment take to work?
- How long should I take the medicine?
- What will happen if I stop taking the medicine?
- Is permanent lung damage likely?

SIDE EFFECTS

Mucolytics, bronchodilators, cough suppressants: *see* ***cough,*** *page 68.*

Antibiotics can cause nausea, vomiting, diarrhea and allergic reactions, which usually present as a rash, and should be reported to the doctor immediately. Some antibiotics can activate thrush in babies, or in the vagina. Tetracyclines cause staining of developing teeth, and should not be given to children under 12 years or to pregnant or breast-feeding women. Some antibiotics, particularly those given by injection for serious infections, may cause further side effects such as loss of hearing or balance: all developments should be discussed with the doctor.

Acetaminophen has no common side effects when taken in the correct dose; *see* ***pain,*** *page 106,* as also for aspirin's side effects.

SELF-MANAGEMENT

Not all patients with pneumonia or pleurisy need to be admitted to hospital. It is important for the patient to drink plenty of fluids as dehydration can make secretions thicker and more difficult to cough up. Pain in the chest should be controlled with analgesics, so that it does not inhibit coughing, which must be encouraged.

PATIENT'S EXPERIENCE

"My baby of six months had a cough with a fever and she was very restless. She seemed to be breathing rather fast. I took her to the doctor, who listened to her chest and then asked me to take her for an X-ray. This showed a patchy pneumonia on both sides of the chest. She was admitted to the hospital where she was given antibiotics by mouth and also physiotherapy to help clear the chest infection. After three days her temperature had settled and she was drinking well again. The doctor said that she could go home but that she must continue the antibiotics. After a week he repeated the X-ray which showed that the infection had cleared. He then stopped the antibiotics; she has been fine ever since."

NAMES YOU WILL HEAR
Generic name: rifampin; **trade names:** Rifadin, Rifamate, or in combination with isoniazid, Rifater, Rifinah and Rimactane. **Generic name:** isoniazid; **trade names:** INH, Laniazid, Rifamate, Nydraxid, Rimifon, Isotinyl, Isotamine. **Generic name:** pyrazinamide; **trade names:** Pyrazinamide, Rifater, Zinamide, Tebrazid, Pyrazide. **Generic name:** ethambutol; **trade names:** Myambutol or, in combination with isoniazid, Mynah. **Generic name:** streptomycin; **trade names:** Streptomycin, Darostrep, Novostrep. **Generic name:** ethionamide; **trade name:** Trecator-SC.

WHAT IS TUBERCULOSIS?

– Infection with the tuberculosis (TB) bacillus. In the great majority of cases it is only the lungs which are involved, but TB may also infect lymph nodes, kidneys, bowel and brain. Early symptoms include lack of energy and loss of appetite. Later a cough develops and yellow phlegm is produced. Weight loss, a slight temperature and severe nocturnal sweating are common. If untreated, symptoms worsen progressively, weight loss becomes very marked and after some months the disease ends in death from 'consumption'. That, at any rate, is how our grandparents saw TB. Though it should be a disease of the past it is all too common among various immigrant groups and alcoholics. Treatment with modern antibiotics is almost always effective, providing it starts at an early stage. The most serious form of tuberculosis affects the membranes around the brain (tuberculous meningitis). This is hard to treat and often ends in coma and death, but is fortunately rare in western countries.

CAUSES Infection occurs most often by inhaling droplets of moisture containing live bacilli coughed into the air by an infected person. Catching TB from infected cow's milk remains, even in developed countries, a real, if rare possibility. Most people who catch TB have been heavily exposed, for example by living with or working closely with an infected person. Others catch it because they have a lowered resistance to infection, which can be caused by cancer, alcoholism, or long-term treatment with steroids.

PRESCRIPTION DRUGS

Anti-tuberculous antibiotics are specific for TB and rarely used for other infections. Often two or more are combined in a single tablet. Rifampin, isoniazid, ethambutol and pyrazinamide are taken as tablets. Streptomycin is given by injection into a muscle.
How they work: by killing the TB bacilli. TB responds only slowly to the drugs and it can be weeks before the symptoms improve. If only one antibiotic is used, the TB bacillus will become resistant. The antibiotic is then ineffective and all the symptoms will return. Thus, two, three or sometimes four antibiotics are used simultaneously. However, although the symptoms may disappear within a month, this does not mean that the disease is cured. There are often a few bacilli left dormant which will grow and cause further disease if the treatment stops too soon. Most treatments last at least

six months; severe cases may need 18 months. **Pyridoxine** (Vitamin B6) may help prevent side effects from izoniazid (see below).

QUESTIONS TO ASK YOUR DOCTOR

- How long should I take the antibiotics?
- How soon will I start to feel better?
- What side effects should I watch out for?
- What happens if I am allergic to the antibiotics?
- Will the drugs react with any other pills?
- When will I be non-infectious?

SIDE EFFECTS

Indigestion is common with these **antibitoics;** it may go away after a few days. If it does not, the antibiotic will be changed. Itchy skin rashes may occur. Rifampin makes the urine appear a reddish-orange color. Sometimes the tears are also colored and soft contact lenses may become stained.

Some side effects are more serious and should be reported to a doctor straight away. Rifampin, isoniazid and pyrazinamide can affect the liver: usually this is only noticed in blood tests, but in a few cases, major liver damage may develop. Isoniazid can cause the hands and feet to tingle and to become numb. Ethambutol can blur the vision, especially when reading, or distort color vision. With all these reactions the doctor will need to decide which drug is responsible; the symptoms will recover if the drug is stopped immediately.

Drug interactions: Rifampin causes the liver to work faster, which means that medicines being taken for many diseases including diabetes, blood clotting and heart problems, and for oral contraception will be less effective and the dose may need adjusting; or the patient may need a change of drugs.

SELF-MANAGEMENT

Apart from the antibiotics, there are no effective treatments for TB. You can help ensure that the treatment is successful by:

1 Taking all tablets as prescribed *each day* for the *whole treatment time.* Don't miss a day's tablets because you are feeling better. The TB might become resistant.

2 Eat a varied diet, including fresh vegetables, to help gain weight. Appetite improves with treatment.

3 Drink as little alcohol as possible. Don't smoke.

4 Report any side effects to your doctor as soon as possible so that he can change the antibiotics.

PATIENT'S EXPERIENCE

"I had always been very fit. Then, some months ago, I seemed to have no energy. My appetite was poor and I lost weight quite dramatically. I started to cough up yellow phlegm most days and noticed that I would wake at night covered in sweat. My doctor sent me to hospital for a chest X-ray and the hospital doctors immediately asked for a specimen of my phlegm. Then they told me I had TB and that I would have to stay in hospital for a few days to start treatment. In fact I stayed two weeks, after which the doctors said I was not infectious and could go home as long as I would continue with the tablets every day for nine months. Later all my family were X-rayed and my father was also found to have TB. I may have caught it from him."

TO AVOID PASSING ON TB

Don't socialize, or go to work until your doctor says it is safe. In particular, avoid close contact with children. These precautions are, however, usually only necessary in the first month of treatment. You can act normally with your own family, but do encourage them to attend hospital for a TB check, and avoid kissing.

Problems of the central nervous system

The brain is the central clearing house for all the messages that come to it, from the eyes, ears and other special sense organs, and from the many nerves which take orders to and receive messages from every part of the body. The way the brain has developed in humans differentiates us in fundamental ways from the rest of the animal kingdom – but brain function is still poorly understood.

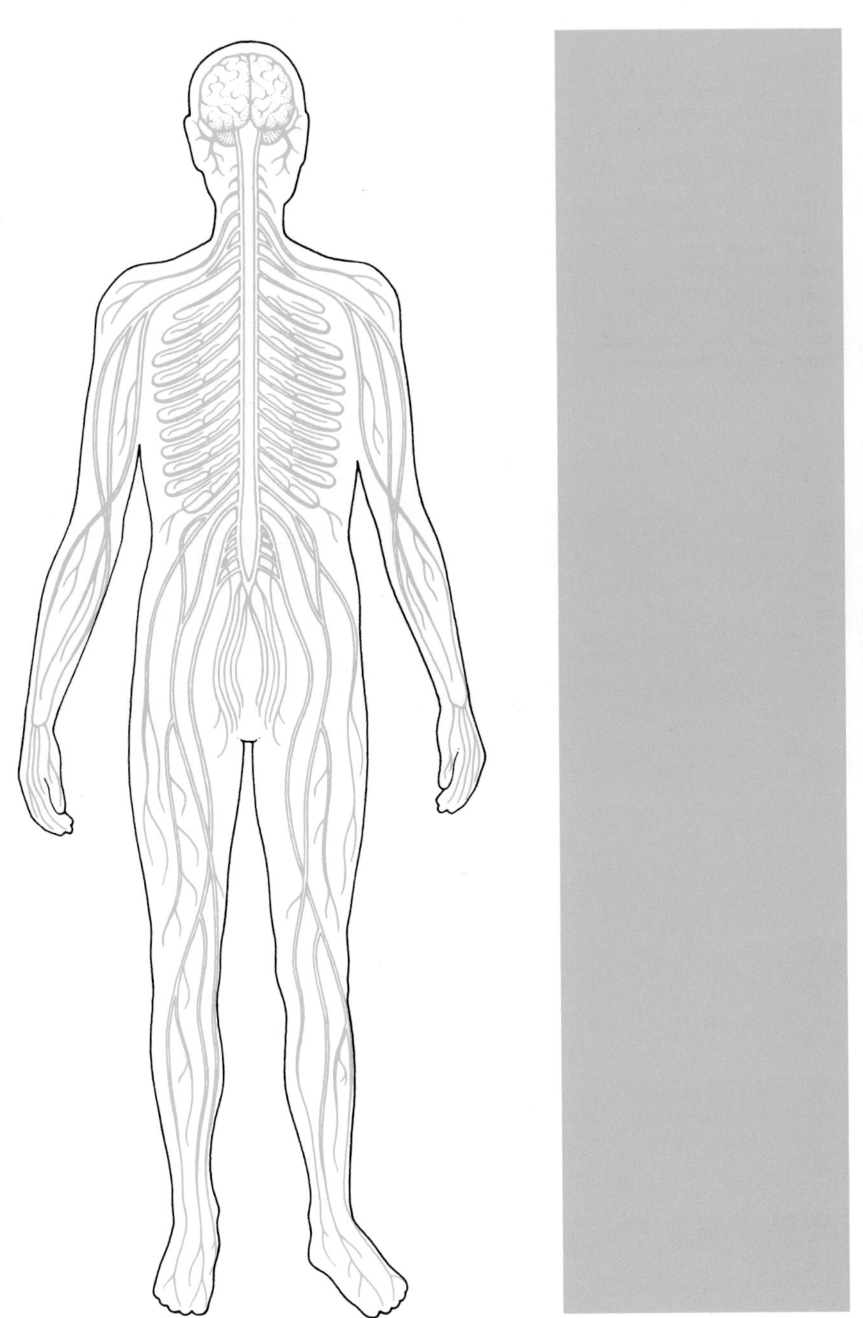

Benzodiazepines, beta-blockers

NAMES YOU WILL HEAR
Generic name: buspirone; **trade name:** Buspar. **Generic name:** alprazolam; **trade name:** Xanax. **Generic name:** bromazepam; **trade name:** Lexotan. **Generic name:** chlordiazepoxide; **trade names:** Librium, Relaxil. **Generic name:** clobazam; **trade names:** Frisium, Urbanol. **Generic name:** clorazepate; **trade name:** Tranxene. **Generic name:** diazepam; **trade names:** Valium, Alupram, Atensine, Evacalm, Solis, Tensium, Valrelease. **Generic name:** lorazepam; **trade names:** Ativan, Almazine.

WHAT IS ANXIETY?

Fear, ranging from a vague sense that something unpleasant might happen, to an overwhelming attack of panic (although the last is distinguished by some experts from anxiety). Patients suffering from anxiety say they feel nervous, tense, uneasy, agitated, edgy and apprehensive; they are often full-time worriers. Their physical symptoms include a dry mouth, choking feelings, tense muscles, a tight or painful chest, rapid pounding of the heart, breathing difficulty, sweating, dizziness, light-headedness, shaking and a strange sensation of distance from the world. Many people with anxiety wrongly attribute these symptoms to a heart attack, or to a brain tumor. This makes them feel even more anxious.

CAUSES The commonest cause of anxiety is stress. One of the most stressful experiences of all is the death of someone close, but problems in marriage, unemployment, poverty, poor housing and growing older can also play havoc. The support of family and friends is crucial for emotional well-being, and those who do not have this are much more likely to become anxious.

PRESCRIPTION DRUGS

Benzodiazepines: commonly called tranquilizers. They offer relief from anxiety in the first six weeks of a course of treatment but after that there will be no marked changes: the drugs will maintain the level of improvement, but will not increase it.

Benzodiazepines have a major role in the treatment of insomnia – *see page 92.*

How they work: by acting on the brain to calm the patient down. Some are fast-acting, some slow-acting. Some are short-acting and some long-acting. Lorazepam takes effect more quickly than diazepam and chlordiazepoxide, and is often prescribed for panic attacks. Another difference between the various tranquilizers is how long they continue to have an effect once they begin to work. Lorazepam is short-acting and disappears from the body fairly quickly.

Buspirone is a newly released non-benzodiazepine with little risk of dependency.

Beta-blockers: These are not tranquilizers, but can reduce the physical symptoms of anxiety such as shaking and palpitations. They are of no value in anxiety except where patients are excessively concerned about tremor or rapid heart beat.

How they work: *see **hypertension**, page 48.*

OVER-THE-COUNTER TREATMENTS

None.

QUESTONS TO ASK THE DOCTOR

- How long should I take them?
- Can I drink alcohol or take other tablets at the same time as the tranquilizers?
- If I become pregnant, will the drugs affect my baby?
- Can I take the tablets only when I feel I need them?

There is a real risk of dependence on tranquilizers: see SIDE EFFECTS.

IS THERE AN ALTERNATIVE TO TRANQUILIZERS?

If you do not take tranquilizers, there is every chance that your anxiety will decrease by itself within a few weeks. You will then attribute your improvement not to the pills, but to your own efforts; the chance of dependence on tranquilizers is put at one remove. If you are too severely anxious to cope unassisted, tranquilizers *can* be useful in breaking the vicious circle long enough for you to change your circumstances.

SIDE EFFECTS

The most common side effects of **benzodiazepines** are drowsiness and lethargy during the first two weeks of taking the pills. Concentration and memory may also be affected, so it is advisable to put off important tasks or decisions, driving, or working with mechanical or dangerous machinery.

The most serious risk is dependence bordering on true addiction. One in every three people who take tranquilizers continuously for more than six months will experience unpleasant withdrawal symptoms when the pills are stopped. These include: anxiety and insomnia – the very symptoms the drugs were prescribed to cure; panic attacks; poor memory and concentration; lack of energy. Often, people going through withdrawal feel as if they have flu. Some lose their appetite, feel nauseous, perhaps actually vomiting; others suffer severe hunger. Constipation, diarrhea, headaches, muscle aches and pains often develop. Muscles can even twitch and jerk quite dramatically. Blurred or double vision, and acute sensitivity or numbness can also play a part in withdrawal. Bright lights and loud noises can become unbearable, and sometimes unusual smells and tastes are noticed. Withdrawal symptoms usually develop a couple of days or even a week after stopping the medication. Symptoms are often at their worst after a week without drugs and can disappear

PATIENTS' EXPERIENCES

'After two or three years on tranquilizers I realized I was not living. I was just existing. I felt as if I was drugged all the time. I didn't notice anything around me – not even the colors of the flowers or the birds singing.'

'I am going through withdrawal at the moment. My whole body aches, I am physically sick and my head feels as if it is in a vise.'

'I had my last tablet one-and-a-half years ago. It took nearly a year to get back to normal. It seemed so very slow, as if I was never going to get better. Only by looking back could I see any improvement.'

DOCTORS' EXPERIENCES

'If you have an office with 30 people in the waiting room, and someone comes in wanting tranquilizers, it is tough to spend 15 minutes explaining why they should not have them. It's much easier to give them.'

'If you take the trouble to reassure patients, explain things to them, but they keep coming back, after a time you feel defeated. The temptation is to say 'Take this.' Sometimes I find myself giving tranquilizers as a sort of admission of failure.'

DO SOMETHING DIFFERENT
Take your mind off your anxiety by doing something active. Here are some suggestions:

- Take decaffeinated tea or coffee.
- Telephone a friend.
- Count backwards from 100 to 1.
- Read a magazine.
- Knit or sew.
- Sing or dance to music.
- Take a walk.
- Go jogging.
- Work in the yard.
- Take a shower.

You may find it difficult to distract yourself at first, but with practice it will become much easier. Try to concentrate on what you are doing, rather than on what you feel.

Once you have completed the sequence one to nine, keep your eyes closed and keep breathing slowly and deeply. Let your whole body become more and more deeply relaxed for a few minutes longer without first tensing your muscles. Count silently to three and open your eyes.

within a month, but they may persist for up to a year.
Beta-blockers: *see* ***hypertension****, page 48.*

SELF-MANAGEMENT

Relaxation techniques really can help. When you feel anxious, sit in a comfortable chair, or lie down, and close your eyes. Begin to breathe slowly and deeply and keep this rhythmic breathing going thoughout the relaxation session. Go through each of the muscle groups below, one at a time. Tense the muscles for five seconds and then relax them for 20 seconds.

1 Curl your toes and press your feet down.
2 Tense your thighs, straighten your knees and make your legs stiff.
3 Make your buttocks tight.
4 Tense your stomach. **5** Clench your fists.
6 Bend your elbows and tense your arms.
7 Hunch your shoulders.
8 Press your head back into a cushion to tense your neck muscles.
9 Clench your jaws, frown and screw up your eyes.

To relax each muscle group effectively you need to talk yourself through both the tension and relaxation phases. Try the following silent self-instructions:

Tense up

- Tense the muscles slightly – don't strain them.
- Hold it.
- Feel the tension in the muscles.
- Notice where the tightness is.
- Keep the muscles tense.
- Concentrate on the tension.

Relax

- Feel the tension leave the muscles.
- Feel them grow more and more relaxed.
- Feel them become heavier and heavier.
- Feel the warmth flow through them.
- Feel the tension drain away.
- Let all the tension go.
- Feel warm and heavy.
- Say words like 'calm' and 'relax' silently.
- Feel more and more relaxed.
- Let the feeling increase.

TRANQUILIZER WITHDRAWAL PROGRAMME

Once you have decided to give the withdrawal program a try, your first step should be to write down your reasons for making that decision. Looking back at these reasons will help you later on. List them in order of importance.

Now write down the order in which you are going to cut down on your pills. Begin with the pill you could most easily do without, and end with the most difficult.

Cutting down in stages

Cut down in stages, beginning with the part of the day during which you need the pills least, and working up to the time when you need them most. If, for example, you take pills four times a day, cut them down in 8 stages:

Stage 1
Cut out half of your least important pill.
Stage 2
Cut out the other half.
Stage 3
Cut out half of your second least important pill.
Stage 4
Cut out the other half.
Stage 5
Cut out half of your second most important pill.
Stage 6
Cut out the other half.
Stage 7
Cut out half of your most important pill.
Stage 8
Cut out the other half.

If you find it impossible to cut down in this way, set yourself a maximum limit of pills that you will take each day and keep to this limit until you feel ready to reduce to a lower limit.

Cutting down at your own pace

The more gradually you reduce your pills, the less chance there is of withdrawal symptoms and the less severe they are likely to be. As withdrawal symptoms can take some time to develop, you should remain at each stage for at least one week. It is likely that you will need to remain at some stages for several weeks before you feel ready to move on, particularly as you near the end. It is not unusual to take several months to come off the pills altogether, and some people need a year or more.

MONITORING YOUR ANXIETY

As soon as you begin to feel anxious, write down in a notebook:

- The time of day.
- Where you are.
- What you are doing.
- Who you are with.
- How you feel.

This record will enable you to pinpoint the circumstances which are likely to make you anxious. Use relaxation exercises to prepare yourself the next time they crop up. You may not be able to get rid of feelings of anxiety altogether; but you may well find you can keep them under some control.

Benzodiazepines, beta-blockers

NAMES YOU WILL HEAR
For benzodiazepines (tranquillizers) *see* ***anxiety,*** *page 84;* for beta-blockers *see* ***angina,*** *page 46.*

WHAT IS STRESS?

''Stress disorder'' is an increasingly common diagnosis in general practice. Stress is used here in the sense of tension, or psychological pressure. People vary in the degree of stress they can tolerate before they develop problems in coping. Sometimes it is difficult to recognize the signs of stress in oneself; for many, coping with stress is a matter of pride and the thought of being labelled as unable to cope is unwelcome. Some families seem to condition people to ''go it alone''; others recognize early stress symptoms and encourage children or adults to seek support. Stress disorders, like tension states *(see* ***anxiety,*** *page 84),* may be present in the form of symptoms which can also be caused by infection – sore throats, diarrhea and cystitis-like symptoms are common examples. This can cause much confusion for the doctor.

CAUSES Stressful lifestyles involving long hours of work in crowded environments at high pressure are associated with many physical diseases or conditions such as high blood pressure, stomach and duodenal ulcers, migraine, eczema and dermatitis, heart attack and cancer. The underlying cause is presumably a continual drive on the body's internal mechanisms. The common stress disorders constitute an early-warning system: your body is telling you to ease off the pressure or suffer the consequences.

PRESCRIPTION DRUGS

Many stress-related symptoms can be helped by medication, but if stress is the cause, then the symptoms will not be completely cured until you have begun to reduce the stress.

Propranolol, a beta-blocker, will reduce tremor (shaking hands or legs) and butterflies in the stomach before an exam, and may, by the same means, ease stage fright.

Stress-induced heartburn or indigestion can be treated in the same way as ordinary heartburn or peptic ulcer (*see pages 22 and 26*), but these will resolve quicker if drug treatment is combined with stress reduction in your lifestyle. The same is true of tension headaches or back pain.

Hypertension, migraine, asthma and eczema will react in the same way, requiring more of the usual medication at times of stress.

Many people with stress-related disorders are doubtful about taking tranquillizers as such; they don't want to be slowed down. This is a reassuring sign the times.

OVER-THE-COUNTER TREATMENTS

Symptomatic treatment can be used, but it will not solve all the problems of stress disorders. Painkillers and antacids are the main over-the-counter remedies. It may be worth trying homeopathic or herbal remedies too as they have no side effects.

QUESTIONS TO ASK THE DOCTOR

- Do you think my symptoms are caused by stress?
- What if I can't see that my lifestyle is stressful?
- Do you think I would benefit from tranquillizers?

SIDE EFFECTS

One major problem with **tranquillizers** is their sedative effect *(see **anxiety,** page 84)*. They are even more sedative when combined with alcohol or antihistamines *(see **hay fever,** page 260)*. In addition, they create dependence: withdrawal symptoms make it difficult to come off them once you are "hooked". Getting hooked is tragically easy and can happen within a matter of a few weeks. Both the medical profession and the lay public are becoming wary of tranquillizers – for good reason.

Propranolol and other beta-blockers are not particularly sedative, nor are they addictive. In general they have few side effects as long as you are not asthmatic or diabetic and there is no tendency to asthma in your family *(see **hypertension,** page 48)*.

SELF-HELP

*(See also **anxiety,** page 84; **irritable bowel syndrome,** page 32; **insomnia,** page 92).*

- Ideally, self-help groups and health workers should collaborate to make non-drug treatments such as yoga, relaxation classes, books and tapes widely available. These, combined with modifying one's lifestyle to give a balance of activity, stimulation, work, exercise, rest and play are sound long-term measures.
- Once you have identified and tackled a stress-related disorder, don't be surprised if it recurs some time later. Get back into your chosen routine and try to eliminate the new source of stress. It takes practice to become a cool calm personality.
- Alcohol and stress: Alcohol is of course the time-honored tranquillizer, and this is what makes it dangerous. Its effect is first to stimulate and then to dull the senses. Stress does not go away because you have drunk yourself under the table – the symptoms are usually worse next day. Above all, alcohol should not be combined with prescribed tranquillizers or antihistamines.

PATIENT'S EXPERIENCE

"I went through a six-month period of having to go to the doctor's office practically every week. If it wasn't my eczema getting worse, it was heartburn, then cystitis, then thrush, then headaches. I had 12 different prescriptions in three months. Finally I had this aching throat – I thought I must have got a chicken bone stuck in my gullet. This time the doctor called me back for a long appointment and pointed out how I kept coming running in with a new symptom. I broke down and cried – I just felt overwhelmed by it all. I began to see how I'd been trying to compensate for my awful marriage by working 24 hours a day – I was living on aspirin and coffee by that time. To cut a long story short, it really helped to see what it was all about. I found I could cope better once I stopped drinking caffeine and started going to a health club after work, doing the relaxation exercises I'd been taught there. I never even contemplated using tranquillizers – that would be a living death to me."

DOCTOR'S EXPERIENCE

"It's relatively easy to help people who come in and say they are under stress and ask what they should do about it. Easy to say, not so easy to do, as I've found myself – it depends on the level of motivation. Often, however, I can spot a stress disorder miles away, but can't get the patient to recognize it for what it is. Stress, they say, what stress? It's as if the workaholic within them really resists making a connection between, say, seven-day working weeks and nervous indigestion. Everyone recognizes "pre-exam diarrhea" but it seems much more difficult to accept that the same mechanism can operate continuously."

NAMES YOU WILL HEAR
Stimulants
Generic name: caffeine; **trade name:** No-doz, Proplus. **Generic name:** dexamphetamine; **trade names:** Dexedrine, Durophet. **Generic name:** cocaine; **trade name:** none. Fecamfamin and prolintane are ingredients of various stimulant preparations available outside the USA and tend not to be sold separately.

WHAT IS FATIGUE?

The sensation of being tired. This is normal, of course, after a hectic day looking after young children or after exercise or a late night. It is when you have the same feeling of being worn out day and night, regardless of how much you are actually doing during the day, that makes you worry about fatigue as a symptom. It may well be associated with other symptoms such as headaches and sore throats, or a general feeling of being run down. It may be difficult to get to sleep, once you are overtired, and this completes a vicious cycle.

CAUSES Normal tiredness apart, fatigue can have a host of medical causes. Viral illnesses such as 'flu or infectious mononucleosis (Epstein Barr virus infection) may be followed by months of general malaise and fatigue – the ''post-viral syndrome''. Bacterial infections such as pneumonia and urinary tract infections can also lead to fatigue which generally resolves once the treatment is over. Tension, anxiety and depression, or just continuing difficulties in your personal life, can easily lead to a feeling of continuing fatigue.

Anemia, pregnancy *and* ***hypothyroidism*** are also common medical causes of fatigue (*see pages 224, 184, 166*).

There are also many drugs which cause fatigue – see margin. Less common conditions in which fatigue is a major symptom include ***tuberculosis*** *(see page 80)*, ***multiple sclerosis*** *(see page 128)*, ***cancers*** *(see pages 200-213)*, myasthenia gravis and narcolepsy.

PRESCRIPTION DRUGS

Tonics used to be a mainstay of prescribing for people suffering from fatigue. It is now recognized that none of the ingredients (*see* **NAMES YOU WILL HEAR**) could possibly have a real chemical effect on tiredness; if they do ''work'' at all, it is through psychological suggestion (the placebo effect) which of course can be a powerful force, but is nothing to do with the medicine itself. Tonics are now prescribed in limited quantities for the older generation who have grown up believing in them.

If tiredness is caused by depression, then the appropriate prescription drug is one of the less sedative antidepressants like imipramine (*see* ***depression,*** *page 116*). This takes several weeks to have optimum effect, but the sleep pattern may improve within a week of starting treatment.

Amphetamine is very rarely prescribed by doctors for fatigue because of the danger of dependence and long-term side effects (*see below*). It is prescribed in cases of narcolepsy, usually under close supervision by a neurologist.

OVER-THE-COUNER TREATMENTS

Tonics: *see* **PRESCRIPTION DRUGS.**

Vitamins are often advertised for their pick-me-up effects and bought by an unsuspecting public. They are unlikely to have any chemical effect unless there is a deficiency which can usually be detected by a medical examination or a blood test. Again, when they do "work" in the absence of evidence of a deficiency state, it is presumably by a placebo effect (*see above*).

Caffeine is widely consumed in tea (40 mg per cup), coffee (100-150 mg per cup) and "cola" drinks (20-30 mg per glass). It certainly has a short-term effect in countering fatigue in most people (not all) and is also sold over the counter as 50 mg pills, useful in long-distance driving.

QUESTIONS TO ASK THE DOCTOR

- Should I have tests for medical causes?
- Is there any point in taking vitamins?
- Would a change of scene help?

SIDE EFFECTS

Caffeine in large quantities produces irritability and interferes with sleep, although some people are more sensitive to it than others. It may increase cholesterol levels in the blood.

Amphetamine use induces dependence to a variable degree. This is one major reason for limiting its use; another is that severe psychotic episodes similar to schizophrenic breakdowns can occur even long after stopping the drug.

SELF-HELP

- Sit down and think about your symptoms. Is your tiredness related to stress, work, bringing up small children, poor sleep? Has it come on gradually or suddenly, out of the blue? Is your body giving you an important message to slow down, or are you in fact ill? Is there anything else wrong – in your body or in your lifestyle? All this information will be useful to your doctor if you do seek medical help.
- Get used to the idea that apart from cups of coffee, there are no magic potions to cure fatigue. If it isn't caused by a medical condition, then the best you can do is to try changing your timetable to give the best combination of rest, mental stimulus and exercise.

PATIENT'S EXPERIENCE

"Five years ago I was working as a barmaid. I got gradually more and more exhausted over a period of several months, and started to lose weight. I thought it was just the night work at first, but I was just as tired once I'd given up the job. Finally someone said I should get a blood test for anemia and I went to the doctor. I mentioned the tiredness and the sweating at night, and she sent me for tuberculin testing. That's how they found out I had TB as well as anemia. They put me on treatment as soon as I'd had the X-rays, and after about six weeks I felt great."

DOCTOR'S EXPERIENCE

"Fatigue can be the earliest sign that someone has a major disease like tuberculosis, multiple sclerosis or even cancer. But for every one of those "small-print" textbook cases, there are ten of the others – parents of young children who are up every night, students working flat out for exams, people in the early stages of depression. I wish tonics did work, but I don't believe in pretending they're going to solve anyone's problems. We have started a relaxation class in the health center now and I hope many people will use that instead of drugs. I see it as a training program for learning how to cope without medication."

DRUGS WHICH CAN CAUSE FATUGUE

Antihistamines *(see* ***hay fever,*** *page 260);* ***sedatives*** and ***tranquillisers*** *(see* ***anxiety,*** *page 84);* ***antidepressants*** *(see* ***depression,*** *page 116);* ***anticonvulsants*** *(see* ***epilepsy,*** *page 110)* and even some antibiotics.

NAMES YOU WILL HEAR

Benzodiazepines
Generic name: flunitrazepam; **trade name:** Rohynpol. **Generic name:** flurazepam; **trade name:** Dalmane. **Generic name:** nitrazepam; **trade names:** Mogadon, Nitrados, Noctesed, Remnos, Somnite, Surem, Unisomnia, Arem, Hypnotin, Noctene, Dormicum. **Generic name:** temazepam. **trade names:** Restoril, Euhypnos, Normison, Levanxol. **Generic name:** triazolam; **trade name:** Halcion.

Antihistamines
Generic name: promethazine; **trade names:** Phenergan, Avomine, Progan, Prothazine, Histantil, Lenazine, Prohist, Profan. **Generic name:** trimeprazine; **trade names:** Temaril, Vallergan, Panectyl.

Chloral derivatives
Generic name: chloral hydrate; **trade names:** Noctec, Chloralex, Chloradorm, Chloralix, Dormel, Elix-Nocte. **Generic name:** dichloralphenazone; **trade name:** Welldorm.

Chlormethiazole
Generic name: chlormethiazole; **trade name:** Heminevrin.

WHAT IS INSOMNIA?

Probably the most reliable definition is persistent sleeplessness. It really is a common problem: in any one year up to 30 per cent of the population of a developed country will seek help for insomnia. Sleep needs vary a great deal; older people need less.

CAUSES are numerous, indeed more than one factor may be involved at any given time. The most important causes are: anxiety; depression; medical conditions causing pain, indigestion, constipation, cough, breathlessness, itching, fever; environmental factors including bedroom comfort and neighborhood noise; daytime naps – not a true cause as the person who sleeps during the day will need less sleep at night; certain drinks including tea and coffee (which are stimulants), alcohol (which helps put you to sleep, but tends to disrupt sleep later in the night); excessive food or fluid intake before bedtime; menopausal symptoms such as hot flashes and excessive sweating.

PRESCRIPTION DRUGS

Sleeping pills – hypnotics – are only really useful for short-term relief of insomnia. The cause or causes of the sleeplessness should always be sought and the thrust of attention brought to bear on these.

Benzodiazepines, also called minor tranquillizers, constitute the bulk of sleeping pills. A number of types are available, the essential differences between them being their duration of action: nitrazepam, for example, is long-acting (16 hours) whereas triazolam is short-acting (4 hours). They should only be prescribed for short-term treatment – no more than a few weeks.
How they work: In low dosage these drugs have a calming effect, and in high dosage a sleep-inducing effect. In common with all hypnotics, they affect the part of the brain controlling wakefulness. How exactly this is achieved is not fully understood.

A number of **antihistamines** have marked sedative properties and are used to exploit this effect, especially in children. Results vary from child to child.
How they work: by acting on the brain.
Chloral derivatives, principally chloral hydrate, are sometimes used to treat insomnia in children and the elderly. They are also a relatively safe and effective alternative to benzodiazepines.
How they work: by acting on the part of the brain which controls wakefulness.

Chlormethiazole is occasionally used, primarily in some elderly people.
How it works: by acting on the brain.
Antidepressants are genuinely helpful for insomnia if depression is the cause. Many have useful sedative properties and can prevent early waking (at 4 am or so), which is characteristic of depressive illness.
How they work: *see* ***depression,*** *page 116.*

QUESTIONS TO ASK THE DOCTOR

- Do I really need sleeping pills?
- Will the sleeping pills leave me "hung over"?
- If I wake in the middle of the night, is it all right to take another pill?
- Can I increase the dose if the first is ineffective?
- Will the sleeping pills interact with any other pills I am taking?
- How long before bed should I take them?
- Should I take them for less than a week?

SIDE EFFECTS

Benzodiazepines' sedative effect diminishes with continued use and they are addictive, and users will become dependent on them. They may produce withdrawal effects characterized by insomnia, anxiety, loss of appetite and tremor. The outcome could be worse, in terms of insomnia, than the original problem. *See* ***anxiety,*** *page 84.*
Chloral derivatives may bring about a tolerance-reduced response to the same dose – as can all hypnotics.

All **hypnotics** can impair judgement and increase reaction time, thereby interfering with ability to drive or operate machines. Alcohol should be avoided with all hypnotics because together they can cause a dangerous level of sedation, and coma.

SELF-HELP

■ Avoid daytime naps. ■ Go to bed only when tired. ■ A warm milky drink half an hour before bedtime often helps. ■ Physical exercise during the day often aids relaxation. ■ Try to avoid thinking about getting to sleep or worrying about the day's events. Try to think about pleasant places and memories instead. ■ Avoid stimulant drinks – tea, coffee and so on. If you are unable to fall asleep within half an hour, get up and do something else such as reading. Return to bed only when sleepy. ■ Get up at the same time every day, irrespective of how much sleep you had during the night. ■ Try relaxation techniques – *see* ***anxiety,*** *page 84.*

PATIENT'S EXPERIENCE

"I developed insomnia after my mother died and my doctor willingly gave me sleeping pills. After a while I became so dependent on them that the prospect of a night without them was terrifying. For years I took them until I moved house and had to change my doctor. The new doctor explained the hazards of taking sleeping pills long-term and together we worked out a plan to stop them. She was very sympathetic and taught me about relaxation and gave me simple instructions about bedtime routine and getting up at the same time every morning. In the beginning it was a struggle, but I succeeded and I sleep more soundly now than I ever did."

INSOMNIA IN CHILDREN

If you have long-lasting problems with your child's sleep pattern, it is well worth asking your doctor to refer you to a child psychologist.

BARBITURATES

At one time popular, these are rarely used now because overdose can kill, because they have significant interactions with drugs like warfarin, and because stopping them quickly can cause severe withdrawal symptoms.

NAMES YOU WILL HEAR
Generic name: disulfiram; **trade name:** Antabuse.

COMMON PROBLEMS ARISING FROM ALCOHOLISM

Liver disease: The liver can be damaged without there being any symptoms or obvious signs, indeed problems may only be picked up by blood tests or liver biopsy. Many forms occur: The mildest, such as fatty liver, can be reversed if the patient stops drinking. Others, such as ***cirrhosis,*** *page 42,* causes permanent scarring. The damage is permanent, but the liver may improve in function if the patient stops drinking completely.

Stomach disease: Alcohol directly damages the stomach lining, causing inflammation and sometimes bleeding. The patient may retch or vomit, often in the mornings, or vomit blood.

Damage to the pancreas: Either an acute attack of inflammation of the pancreas (pancreatitis) can occur, or the pancreas can be permanently scarred, producing chronic abdominal pain, diabetes and malabsorbtion.

Nervous system damage: Nerve damage may give rise to tingling or numbness in the hands and feet and unsteadiness, even when not drunk. Periods of forgetfulness can signify brain damage or vitamin deficiency.

Bowel damage: gives rise to diarrhea, and malabsorbtion.

Heart damage: There may be palpitations. Breathlessness and swelling of the feet can be caused by alcoholism giving rise to heart failure.

DO YOU HAVE A DRINKING PROBLEM?

The following questions are used by some doctors to find out if there is a drink problem:

- Have you ever felt you should cut down your drinking?
- Have people ever annoyed you by

WHAT IS ALCOHOLISM?

The rough-and-ready definition is addiction to alcohol which may affect any aspect of an individual's well-being, mental health or social life. Being an alcoholic does not imply that someone has gross physical damage, or is continually drunk.

There is no absolute level of drinking that always produces damage, just as there is no absolutely safe level of drinking below which damage never results. Typical current recommended levels of safe drinking (SA) are 15 units of alcohol per week for men, and ten per week for women. These levels are set so that it is *unlikely* that below them physical harm will result. They demonstrate that women are more at risk from alcohol than men. A unit of alcohol consumption is equivalent to one half pint of normal strength beer, one single measure of spirits, a $4\frac{1}{2}$ oz glass of wine or a $2\frac{1}{2}$ oz glass of fortified wine (for example sherry). Each unit contains nine grams of alcohol, and whether the alcoholic drink is mixed with other drinks, or is taken with meals, makes no difference at all to its potential for causing damage.

The fact that some people seem to be able to drink prodigious amounts of alcohol without overt signs of being ill should not be taken as proof that it is safe to drink to this level. Many of these heavy drinkers have damage that can only be recognized by careful testing.

People who drink more than the recommended safe amounts, but without evidence of alcohol related problems, are usually described as heavy drinkers; they are advised to reduce intake as a preventive measure. People with actual problems related to drinking should seek help before they develop symptoms of addiction and dependence.

The common symptoms of addiction are: the morning shakes; *delirium tremens* (confusion and hallucinations); confusion when the individual stops drinking. Many other symptoms are, in addition, caused by the alcohol damaging the body (see margin).

CAUSES Most experts believe that alcoholism is a social habit out of control. By contrast, many drinkers think of alcoholism as a disease – which conveniently releases them from responsibility.

There is some evidence to suggest that alcoholism may run in families, but this may be more environmental than genetic. Apart from the added danger of damage in women, it is impossible to determine who, on the individual level, is most at risk from what level of drinking. Certain occupations (including seamen, people running premises where alcoholic drinks are consumed and people in high stress occupations) are, however, associated with increased alcoholism.

TREATMENT

As there is no specific cause, there is no magic pharmacological treatment for alcoholism – other than avoiding alcohol. The immense value of Alcoholics Anonymous in the rehabilitation process cannot be overstated. Various drugs are used to help the patient get off alcohol and prevent withdrawal symptoms.

Tranquillizers *(see **anxiety,** page 84)* are given for a week or two to prevent the symptoms of withdrawal when alcohol is stopped.

How they work: by calming the patient down and suppressing the central nervous system, giving relief from sweating, anxiety, shaking and hallucinations which are common features of withdrawal from any addictive drug such as alcohol.

Disulfiram can be used to try and prevent the alcoholic starting to drink again.

How it works: by interfering with the normal breakdown of alcohol in the body and allowing the accumulation of a toxic chemical in the body. This makes the patient feel nauseous and vomit if alcohol is taken with the pills, which thus discourages alcohol consumption.

QUESTIONS TO ASK THE DOCTOR

- Have I any signs of physical damage?
- Do I need specialized help?

SIDE EFFECTS

Tranquillizers: These are only prescribed during drying out. They may make you drowsy, unsteady and excessively tired, but risk of other long-term problems is insignificant given the short duration.

Disulfiram: Very few side effects unless you drink alcohol – see HOW IT WORKS.

SELF-MANAGEMENT

- If you think you have been drinking too much, but are unsure if you have damaged yourself, talk it over with your doctor. If it seems there are no signs of damage but you want help to limit your drinking, try a self-help group such as Alcoholics Anonymous.
- If you have symptoms of addiction and dependence on alcohol, do not stop drinking suddenly. See your doctor, but in any case, gradually reduce your intake.

criticizing your drinking?

- Have you ever felt bad or guilty about your drinking?
- Have you ever had a drink first thing in the morning to steady your nerves or to get rid of a hangover?

Two or more positive answers strongly suggests a drink problem.

AFTER DRYING OUT

Once you are dried out, you may need help either to keep your drinking under control, or to abstain altogether. In addition to the self-help groups mentioned above, there are many professional counseling agencies, some based in hospitals, others in the community.

PATIENT'S EXPERIENCE

"I started drinking in college and it has gradually increased over the years. I have lost a few days from work and my wife says I drink too much. Recently, after a heavy bout of drinking, I vomited some blood. This gave me a shock, so I stopped drinking, and felt very nervous and shaky. My doctor said I have an enlarged liver, and had me admitted to a hospital. A short treatment with tranquillizers was prescribed: they made me sleepy, but I stopped shaking. I am now seeing a counselor and have stopped drinking entirely. I feel much better, but still miss alcohol."

NAMES YOU WILL HEAR
Generic name: prochlorperazine; **trade names:** Compazine, Stemetil, Anti-Naus, Mitil, Vertigon. **Generic name:** cinnarizine; **trade name:** Stugeron. **Generic name:** diazepam; **trade names:** Valium, Alupram, Atensine, Evacalm, Solis, Tensium, Valrelease. **Generic name:** betahistine dihydrochloride; **trade name:** Serc. **Generic name:** promethazine; **trade names:** Mepergan, Phenergan, Avomine, Progan, Prothazine, Histantil, Lenazine, Prohist, Profan.

WHAT IS DIZZINESS?

''Dizziness'' and ''vertigo'' are both terms used to denote a feeling of reeling: the patient senses a rotatory movement either of themselves going round and round, or of the environment rotating (''the room is spinning around''). The sense of balance is lost to some extent; in true vertigo, the patient may fall to one side in particular as a result of the false impression of movement.

CAUSES True vertigo is caused by problems in the sensory apparatus (the vestibular system and labyrinths of the inner ear) concerned with balance and co-ordination of movement. These problems include Menière's disease, labyrinthitis, arterial and nervous conditions, certain drugs and some infections. It may be accompanied by nausea, and sometimes by changes in hearing – deafness and ringing in the ears (tinnitus). These may be mild in degree, or severe and disabling. It is diagnosed by positional and caloric tests of middle ear function.

Dizziness of a more general kind, not localized to one side or direction, may be caused by anxiety and hyperventilation (accompanied by nausea and faintness), as when blood pressure is low and standing up produces temporary faintness and dizziness (postural hypotension); or when blood glucose is low (hypoglycemia).

PRESCRIPTION DRUGS

Vestibular sedatives such as phenothiazines can suppress or at any rate diminish the symptoms of vertigo as can **antihistamines** (eg cinnarizine). The latter may be given by mouth or by injection or suppository if vomiting prevents oral intake. They lessen nausea, vomiting and vertigo.

How they work: by acting on the brain.

Tranquillizers such as diazepam may sometimes be used to treat dizziness associated with anxiety.

How they work: *see **anxiety**, page 84.*

In Menière's disease, **betahistine dihydrochloride** may help in the early stages, along with the vestibular sedatives mentioned above; later, an operation may be needed if attacks become frequent and disabling.

OVER-THE-COUNTER TREATMENTS

Some of the antihistamines, for example chlorpheniramine (Chlor-trimeton) are available and used in motion sickness/travel sickness (chlorpheniramine, promethazine). In pregnancy, and for all other uses, a doctor should be consulted first. Self-treatment of travel sickness is perfectly appropriate, but not of dizziness; dizzy spells and falls related to dizziness should be investigated by a doctor.

QUESTIONS TO ASK THE DOCTOR

- Is there a known cause for my dizziness?
- How long is the dizziness likely to last?
- How long should I take the pills?
- Will they make me sleepy?
- Is it safe to take them if I get pregnant?
- What about driving?

SIDE EFFECTS

Phenothiazines, although very effective, do have side effects especially if taken over long periods continuously; watch for involuntary movements. *See* ***schizophrenia,*** *page 120.* **Antihistamines** also commonly produce side effects: a dry mouth, difficulty in urinating, sometimes blurred vision, or temporary impotence in men. None of the drugs should be taken in pregnancy. They have an additive effect with alcohol.

SELF-MANAGEMENT

- Notice carefully whether any particular position of head or neck makes attacks come on or get worse.
- Fatigue may worsen or precipitate symptoms: try to relax; lie down and stay down if necessary until symptoms have abated.
- If you have postural hypotension (a doctor can diagnose this by taking your blood pressure while you are sitting or lying down and again when you stand up), take great care when getting out of bed; make a gradual transition from lying down to standing up.

If you are having repeated falls for no known reason, see your doctor.

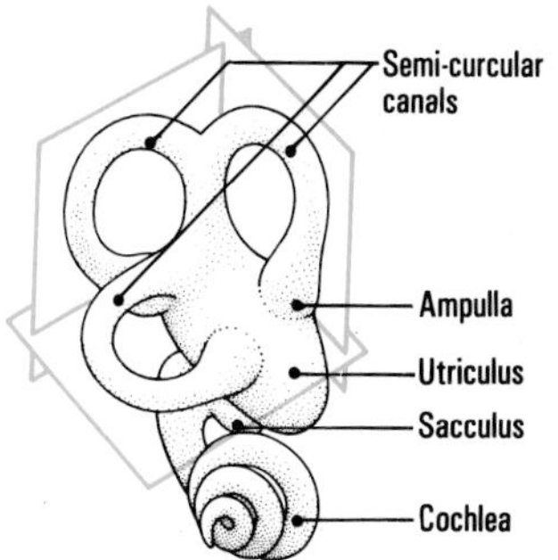

The balance system of the inner ear: *the three semi-circular canals are filled with fluid. Its movements – in response to bodily movements – are detected by extremely sensitive hairs projecting into the canals from the cells which line them.*

PATIENT'S EXPERIENCE

"I woke up one morning and found that I could not get out of bed. Each time I tried, I had the most terrible sensation – everything whirled round and round and I felt awfully sick. I thought I was going to pass out every time I lifted my head off the pillow. I had to be taken to the emergency room by paramedics. The doctor came and said I had an infection, labyrinthitis, due to a virus, and that it would get better in two weeks or so. She gave me some pills, prochlorperazine, to calm down the vertigo sensation and they did make it a bit better right away. But it was three weeks before I really felt I could go outdoors by myself."

DOCTOR'S EXPERIENCE

"I hadn't realized how disabling vertigo can be till I saw this patient in the emergency room when I was a trainee. And then I saw two more patients with labyrinthitis in the same week – it was a "mini-epidemic", presumably due to a virus going round. Sometimes, though, it is difficult to determine the cause of giddiness and "dizzy spells" and we have to send patients to be investigated by a specialist. Fortunately prochlorperazine works as a vestibular sedative for vertigo due to many different causes, so we can use it as a first-aid measure."

NAMES YOU WILL HEAR
Generic name: aspirin; **trade names:** Ascriptin, Ecotrin, Measurin, Aspirin, Astrin, Bi-Prin. **Generic name:** acetaminophen; **trade names:** Phenaphon, Panadol, Tempra, Tylenol, Pamol, Calpol, Tylenon, Paracin, Parmol, Panado, Ceetamol, Atosol, Exctol, Ennagesic, Ilvamol. **Generic name:** codeine phosphate; **trade names:** Codeine Linctus, Codeine Syrup, Uniflu, Codlin, Paveral. **Generic name:** mefenamic acid; **trade names:** Ponstel, Ponstan, Ponstan Forte. *See also* ***pain, page 106.***

WHAT IS HEADACHE?

– Site, severity, frequency and character vary enormously. Even so, most people can distinguish between an ordinary headache and the rare, atypical one which should be reported to a doctor.

CAUSES Ordinary headaches are probably caused by small blood vessels dilating or contracting under the control of nerves. These blood vessels are probably on the surface of the membranes surrounding the brain. Alterations in these areas probably account also for tension headache, pre-menstrual headaches and migraines *(see pages 99 and 100).*

Tension headaches are aching, rather than sharp pains, and are localized to muscles in the scalp, cheeks, jaw, temples, and the back of the neck, sometimes with a feeling of a tight band around the head. There is often difficulty getting off to sleep, and sometimes nervous indigestion as well. Often, tension headaches occur in known ''worriers''; but sometimes they are the first sign of stress at work or within the family.

Other causes of headache are problems in the teeth, ears, sinuses *(see* ***sinusitis,*** *page 262);* the nerves, joints and muscles of the head, neck and face. For example: neuralgic pain is usually a shooting pain in a localized area – this might follow an attack of shingles. Temporal arteritis is a rare cause of headache and only occurs after the age of 50; it is associated with tenderness over the scalp, severe headache and painful throbbing over blood vessels at the temples. A blood test is necessary to confirm the diagnosis. If untreated, it may cause blindness. Infections such as meningitis, typhoid and encephalitis are uncommon causes of headache, but should be considered if there is severe headache in someone who is also ill with fever, vomiting, diarrhea or drowsiness.

A very severe headache (''worst ever'') with vomiting or drowsiness may possibly, but not definitely, signal a grave problem: see a doctor immediately.

High blood pressure, contrary to popular belief, is not a common cause of headache.

PRESCRIPTION DRUGS

Analgesics are available both on prescription and over-the- counter. **Aspirin** and **acetaminophen** are both effective in headache, and can be combined with **codeine** for extra effectiveness. *See* ***migraine,*** *page 100* and ***pain,*** *page 106.*

Tranquillizers are sometimes used for tension headache *(see* ***anxiety,*** *page 84).*
Mefenamic acid can be used for headache as well as for period pain – *see page 190.*

Because headache is usually a recurrent problem, drugs which are potentially addictive, such as tranquillizers and opiate-related drugs, should be avoided in favor of simple painkillers.

Occasionally, antibiotics, anti-epileptic drugs such as carbamazepine, antidepressants, or steroids may be used to treat the underlying cause of the rarer forms of headache.

OVER-THE-COUNTER TREATMENTS

Aspirin maybe a stronger remedy than acetaminophen, which has fewer side effects. *See* ***common cold,*** *page 134* and ***pain,*** *page 106.*

QUESTIONS TO ASK THE DOCTOR

- What sort of headache have I got?
- How long should I take the pills?
- Should I come back for a further check-up if it doesn't improve?

SIDE EFFECTS

Acetaminophen is very safe up to eight pills a day: side effects are extremely rare, except in people with kidney or liver disease. **Aspirin:** Reduce dose, or take it with milk or antacids, if you get indigestion or heartburn, as it irritates the stomach. Ringing in the ears is a sign that the dose should be reduced. Buffered aspirin preparations such as ascriptin cause less gastric irritation, and allow rapid absorption, but still share aspirin's potential for adverse effects on blood platelets and in aspirin-sensitive asthmatics, Enteric-coated aspirin also causes less stomach irritation, but absorption is delayed. **Codeine:** Constipation can be kept to a minimum by drinking plenty of water and increasing the fiber content of the diet.

The more powerful painkillers sometimes cause drowsiness.

SELF-MANAGEMENT/SELF-HELP

See section on ***stress,*** *page 88* and on ***anxiety,*** *page 84.* Any method of relaxing/distracting yourself from everyday problems will help a tension headache – you will have noticed how these go away when you are busy doing something you enjoy. Exercise, rest and diet can all help.

PATIENT'S EXPERIENCE

"I know some people hate to take pills at all, but I find that taking a couple of acetaminophen as soon as I notice a headache coming on seems to stop it right away – and then I can cope better."

DOCTOR'S EXPERIENCE

"People worry that headaches mean they have high blood pressure, or even a brain tumor. This isn't so. The rare, serious kinds of headache are completely different from run-of-the-mill headaches – they're much more severe and disabling."

Simple analgesics, ergotamine, propranolol, methysergide

NAMES YOU WILL HEAR
Generic name: aspirin; **trade names:** Ascriptin, Ecotrin, Measurin, Asprin, Astrin, Bi-Prin. **Generic name:** acetaminophen; **trade names:** Anacin 3, Phenaphon, Panadol, Tempra, Tylenol, Pamol, Calpol, Tylenon, Paracin, Parmol, Panado, Ceetamol, Atosol, Exctol, Ennagesic, Ilvamol. For further trade names of these drugs, *see also **pain,** page 106.*
Generic name: aspirin and metoclopramide combination: **trade name:** Migravess. **Generic name:** ergotamine; **trade names:** (sublingual form) Ergomar, Ergostat; (with caffeine) Cafergot; (aerosol form) Medihaler Ergotamine; Migril, Dihydroergot, Lingraine. **Generic name:** methysergide; **trade names:** Sansert, Deseril. **Generic name:** pizitofen; **trade name:** Sanomigran. **Generic name:** propranolol; **trade names:** Inderal, Angitol, Apsolol, Bedranol, Berkolol, Sloprolol, Cardinol.
Of the drugs mentioned only acetaminophen and aspirin are available without prescription

WHAT IS MIGRAINE?

– An intermittently recurring headache usually affecting only one side of the head at a time. It is often preceded by visual disturbances (flashing lights, jagged, bright or colored lines, partial loss of vision) and accompanied by nausea and vomiting. However, many migraine sufferers do not experience the warning symptoms, and the pain can affect both sides of the head.

The problem may affect anyone, but it is rare before the age of 15 or 16. It troubles people mainly in their 20s and 30s, and tends to become less severe with age. Attacks rarely occur for the first time in people over the age of 50. It does not only afflict ''intelligent'' individuals; it does tend to run in families.

Don't assume that all severe headaches are migraine *(see **headache,** page 98).*

CAUSES The basic biochemical trigger is not known, but many precipitating factors are well recognized: for example, a period of hard work followed by relaxation (weekend migraine); stress; body changes prior to menstruation; certain foods (e.g. fish, chocolate, cheese); alcohol; oral contraceptives; hunger. However, none of these factors will necessarily cause an attack of migraine, even in combination.

It is possible that the symptoms preceding the headache result from a transient decrease in blood supply to areas of the brain. The headache may be due to a subsequent widening of blood vessels in the scalp.

TREATMENT

In an acute attack: As soon as possible after noticing the warning features of an attack, take either **soluble aspirin** (three tablets of 325 mg each) or **acetaminophen** (three tablets of 500 mg each) in a glass of milk or water. Taking pain-killing pills in this way, before the headache develops, prevents a full-blown migraine attack in many people. It is important to take the pills as soon as possible because during an attack the stomach empties more slowly than usual, only a small dose of the drug being absorbed.
How they work: *see **pain,** page 106; **headache,** page 98.*

The pain-relieving effect of aspirin or acetaminophen may be increased by taking **metoclopramide** in addition.
How it works: by making the stomach empty quicker than usual.

If this combination therapy is ineffective, try **ergotamine** eg as Cafergot – take 2 pills at start of attack,

and, if needed, one per hour after that to a maximum of 6, and no more than 10 total in a week.
How it works: Ergotamine is a powerful constrictor of blood vessels. See SIDE EFFECTS.
Preventive measures: If the migraine attacks are frequent – say more than one a week – regular long-term treatment with **propranolol** may be effective.
How it works: not fully understood, but the drug does affect blood vessels.

Another effective prophylactic drug is **methysergide** (initially 0.5 mg as a test dose increasing to a maximum of 2 mg three times a day).
How it works: by antagonizing some of the chemicals produced in excess during a migraine attack. Methysergide should be used only as a last resort.

OVER-THE-COUNTER TREATMENTS

Aspirin and **acetaminophen:** The choice is a matter of personal preference: *see **pain,** page 106* and ***common cold,** page 134.*

Apart from these simple analgesics, there are of course dozens of proprietary combinations available for migraine: most of them include combinations of some of the drugs mentioned above. The large number of products available indicates that there is no 100 per cent effective treatment. Migraine sufferers should be able to reduce attacks to one a month with a doctor's help and the drugs mentioned under TREATMENT.

A drawback of the combination products is that they often do not contain full-strength doses of the most important agents.

SIDE EFFECTS

Aspirin and **acetaminophen:** *see **pain,** page 106.*
Metoclopramide should not be taken during the first three months of pregnancy, and preferably not at all during pregnancy, to avoid any possibility of risk to the fetus. It should not be taken with certain tranquillizers as it has an additive effect: consult your doctor.
Ergotamine and **methysergide** should not be taken during pregnancy or while breast-feeding; or by patients with coronary artery disease, high blood pressure or poor blood supply to the brain or legs. Exceeding the stated dose can cause permanent damage to the circulation or the kidneys.
Propranolol should not be taken by asthmatics or those with wheezy bronchitis or heart failure: it aggravates these conditions.

PATIENT'S EXPERIENCE

"I used to get terrible migraine, just like my mother. They often came on with my periods, starting as flashing zig-zag lines. Then came the headache, so bad that I had to lie still in a darkened room. Sometimes the headache lasted two or even three days. I found ergotamine helped the headache if I took it soon enough. Sometimes it works better if my doctor gives me metoclopramide as well. I still get attacks from time to time – but at least I can cope with them."

SELF-HELP

■ It is worthwhile to try to identify a specific trigger of migraine and then to minimize your exposure to it. Dietary changes help in a few people in the long term, so systematic omission of certain foods is worthwhile in trying to find a cause. Keep a diary of attacks and try to trace the cause. ■ See if stopping the oral contraceptive pill lessens the frequency or severity of attacks.
■ Don't get overtired, hungry or drunk – all may cause migraine.
■ During an attack, rest in a quiet darkened room. After sleep the pain is nearly always less severe.

NAMES YOU WILL HEAR

Opiates

Generic name: morphine; **trade names:** Roxanol, Nepenthe, MST Continus, Duromorph, Cyclimorph. **Generic name:** diamorphine; **common name:** heroin; usually prescribed by generic name. **Generic name:** pethidine, meperedine; **trade names:** Demerol, Pethilorfan, Pamergan, Pethoid, Demer-Idine; usually prescribed by generic names. **Generic name:** methadone; **trade names:** Dolophene, Physeptone. **Generic name:** codeine; **trade name:** prescribed by generic name in USA. **Generic name:** propoxyphene; **trade names:** Darvon, Dolene. **Generic name:** oxymorphone; **trade name:** Numorphan. **Generic name:** hydromorphone; **trade name:** Dilandid. **Generic name:** dipipanone; **trade names:** Diconal, Wellconal. **Generic name:** dihydrocodeine; **trade names:** DF 118, Aust Fortruss, Paracodin, Rikodeine, Tuscodin. *See also* ***pain,*** *page 106.*

Stimulants

Generic name: dexamphetamine; **trade names:** Dexidrine, Durophet. **Generic name:** diethylproprion; **trade names:** Tepanil, Apisate, Dospan, Dietec, D.I.P., Nobensine- 75, Regibon. *See also* ***fatigue,*** *page 90.*

Anti-psychotic drugs

*Drugs marked * are available as longer lasting depot injections.*

Generic name: chlorpromazine: **trade names:** Thorazine, Largactil, Dozine, Chloractil, Procalm, Promacid, Protran, Chlorprom, Chlor-Promanyl, Klorazin. **Generic name:** trifluoperazine; **trade name:** Stelazine. **Generic name:** thioridazine; **trade names:** Mellaril, Novoridazine, Thioril. **Generic name:** haloperidol*; **trade names:** Haldol, Serenace. **Generic name:** fluphenazine*; **trade names:** Permitil, Prolixin, Modecate, Moditen, Anatensol. **Generic name:** flupenthixol*; **trade names:** Depixol, Fluanxol.

WHAT IS DRUG ABUSE?

– Strictly speaking, taking drugs for non-medical reasons, for example curiosity, because friends take them, or to induce an altered state of mind. The drugs are usually obtained illicitly, but some prescribed drugs are also misused. The principal drug types involved are: opiates, cocaine and other stimulants, hallucinogenic drugs and cannabis.

CAUSES Either ''accidental'' (a young person is introduced to drugs by a 'pusher' or an underlying psychological problem. For many, the sense of belonging to a group which takes drugs is more important props than the drug itself.

OPIATE ABUSE

Morphine, meperidine, methadone and **hydromorphone** are used medically, in controlled doses, as strong painkillers. When taken non-medically, they induce a euphoric sense of well-being and of unconcern about practical necessities. They are smoked, sniffed, taken by mouth or injected. At first they often cause nausea, sickness, and drowsiness. The dangers are: taking too much – overdose can cause unconsciousness or death, especially if mixed with alochol or tranquillizers; addiction – see below; health hazards associated with injecting – see below.

Opiate addiction is not invariably the result of opiate misuse, but it is impossible to predict who will become addicted. Anyone dabbling is at risk. Taking opiates can be an intense experience, and it is easy to try them again . . . and again . . . then find you need more to gain the same effect; within a few months, often much sooner, the user is addicted. Smoking opiates can lead to addiction, just as injecting them. An addict takes opiates to ward off withdrawal symptoms as much as for pleasure.

TREATMENT

– Almost always involves counselling to help the addict understand his or her underlying problems. The hardest part is often making the decision it really is time to stop. Different clinics have different approaches, but there are three basic lines of treatment:

Detoxification: The addict stops taking illicit drugs and medicines are prescribed as necessary to help with the withdrawal symptoms on a one-to-two-week basis. A typical regime for the heroin addict could be hypnotics for insomnia plus codeine phosphate for diarrhea. In case of opiate addiction, the illicit drug may be prescribed in reducing doses.

Short-term prescription over several months. The addict is switched from illicit to prescribed opiates; then the prescribed dose is slowly reduced to minimize withdrawal symptoms. The idea is to provide a legal supply of drugs to free the addict from the hassle of the black market; and to provide time in which to sort out problems before withdrawing.

Maintenance prescription: the opiate is prescribed indefinitely until the addict wants to stop. This line is out of favor with most doctors now.

Prescribed opiates are 100 per cent pure and in known quantities. By contrast, illicit opiates are contaminated with additives, and the amount of drug in any weight sold may vary. Some opiates, for example, methadone, are long-lasting and only need to be taken once a day, while others, such as heroin, last only six to eight hours. The trend is to give addicts longer-acting drugs, such as methadone, in syrup which cannot be injected and has no street value.

SIDE EFFECTS

All **opiates,** prescribed or illicit, can cause constipation, nausea, difficulty in passing urine, depression and loss of interest in sex. They are sedative: an overdose can cause coma or death, especially if mixed with alcohol or tranquillizers. There can be withdrawal symptoms if they are stopped suddenly.

SELF-MANAGEMENT

Remember: there is more to coming off – and staying off – opiates than going through withdrawal symptoms. Think why you take opiates: To relieve anxiety? To be part of a group? Because you are bored? To forget about problems at home or work? How will you manage without them?

To stop taking opiates:

■ Steadily reduce the amount taken to as little as possible. ■ Get rid of any surplus drugs. ■ Plan when you will stop – you will need to be somewhere you feel comfortable and safe, away from other drug users. ■ Stay away from areas and people associated with drugs. Self-help groups may help. Withdrawing is like having a dose of flu – you may feel feverish, have aches and pains, a runny nose, diarrhea and find it difficult to concentrate or sleep well. Expect three to five bad

TERMS YOU WILL HEAR

Tolerance

The body will get used to certain drugs, making physical adaptations to compensate for their presence. Thus if the dose has to be increased to maintain the effect, the body is said to have developed tolerance to a drug.

Withdrawal symptoms

Stop taking a drug to which the body has built up a tolerance, and there will be a period (usually several days to several weeks) while the body readapts to life without the drug. The pattern of withdrawal symptoms is different for different drugs. Heroin, for instance, normally makes the new user drowsy and constipated; if taken regularly, these effects are less pronounced because the body adapts. If the drug is stopped, the user will probably have difficulty in sleeping, and suffer from diarrhea until the body re-adapts.

Addict

Essentially a lay term for someone who has repeatedly taken a drug over a period of time, and as a result, craves it. The addict will go to great lengths to ensure continued supplies; thinking about the drug takes precedence over most other things in life. Depending on the drug misused, either psychological or physical dependence, or both, may be involved.

Physical dependence

Compared with addiction this is a technical term, but what it describes is not much different: having taken a drug regularly, the user's body adapts to it; if the drug is stopped, there are withdrawal symptoms.

Psychological dependence

The drug user depends on a drug for a sense of well-being; physical dependence and/or addiction is not necessarily implied.

days, starting 24-48 hours after you stop; after that things will improve. Look after yourself – even spoil yourself. Buy easily prepared food and drinks, and plan interesting activities to take your mind off yourself. Once you are over the first two weeks, you should be physically well again; rest-lessness and difficulty sleeping may last longer, but they will stop. Be careful with alcohol and tranquillizers – don't switch one addiction for another.

CANNABIS ABUSE

Cannabis marijuana is usually smoked, though recently an injectable form has appeared which is often contaminated with hepatitis viruses. The typical effect is feeling relaxed or ''high''. It can induce altered sensations so that music appears to sound differently or time to pass more slowly. Feelings of being unreal or anxious are not uncommon. Spatial judgement is impaired; driving or operating machinery is hazardous. Regular or heavy use is risky. Some use cannabis to escape problems, which may intensify them in the long run. It can cause or aggravate psychotic illness, manifested, typically, by excitement, confusion, aggression and delusional ideas.

HALLUCINOGENIC DRUG MISUSE

Commonly used drugs are **LSD, "magic mushrooms"** and **phencyclidine (PCP – Angel Dust)** Many ''mushrooms'' are extremely poisonous and eating the wrong ones will cause death. Once taken, usually by mouth, the effects – ''the trip'' start in 20 mins to 2 hours; they may last for several hours. It is a common experience that after the effects have subsided people may experience unpleasant ''flash backs'', often provoked by other drugs. During a trip, the subject may see, hear, smell and feel the world in a more intense way that may seem mystical at the time. However, perception becomes dangerously distorted, and many have died while, for example, attempting to fly from a high building. Phencyclidine in low doses produces agitation; excitement and disorganized thinking. The painkilling effects of this drug often enable the victim to exert far greater force than the body can normally tolerate. This leads to violent encounters with the police. The resultant injuries and the convulsant effects of the PCP often result in the death of the drug abuser.

SELF-MANAGEMENT

Realize that taking hallucinogenic drugs can amount to

putting your life at risk: see HALLUCINOGENIC DRUG MISUSE.

The effects usually wear off in 12 hours. If someone has a bad trip, stay with them, take them somewhere peaceful, reassure them it will soon be over, that it is a drug effect, no more, no less, and that they are not going mad. Seek medical help if the drug user is acting dangerously. Avoid violent restraint.

STIMULANT ABUSE

Cocaine is usually sniffed as a powder; **amphetamines** are sniffed, injected or taken as pills. Diet pills may also be misused. The main effects are to induce a sense of well-being, to reduce fatigue and to reduce appetite. Small doses can cause insomnia, irritability, over-talkativeness and paranoid suspicions. Stomach pains, palpitations and repetitive thinking occur. Individuals vary widely in the amounts they can take without complications. Cocaine use definitely leads to addiction.

SIDE EFFECTS

If **stimulants** are taken regularly, tolerance develops, and the edginess and insomnia get worse. As the drug wears off, it is common to feel depressed and this may be severe enough to lead to suicide.

Amphetemine or cocaine can also cause psychotic illness similar to schizophrenia *(see page 120)*, though short-lived by comparison. This tends to be the result of heavy or regular use, but some people are ultra-sensitive to these drugs. Taking **cannabis** or **LSD** at the same time can increase the risk. Cocaine, by damaging the heart, may cause sudden death, even in professional athletes.

QUESTIONS TO ASK THE DOCTOR

- Can I talk to you in confidence about illicit drugs?
- Is my drug-taking making me ill?
- Can I withdraw from drugs at home?
- If I get pregnant will the drugs affect the baby?
- Will you help me explain to my family?

SELF-MANAGEMENT

■ If you feel tired and in low spirits when you stop amphetamine or cocaine, this will pass in a few days. Think of it as repaying the debt for the extra energy and high spirits conferred by the stimulant. ■ Seek the support of someone not involved with drugs. ■ Analyze why you started taking the stimulant, and have taken it so often.

DOCTORS' EXPERIENCE

"I can't trust drug-takers at all. They're very difficult to help. I believe that if they want to stop they have to do it themselves."

AFTER WITHDRAWAL

■ You will feel good about yourself, but beware: as time goes on, you may start to feel low, and wonder whether it was worth it. This is the time you will need support and encouragement to put into practice alternative ways of coping with problems. ■ If you relapse after coming off, don't get disheartened; at least you have made a start. Think over what went wrong, and try to plan your next attempt more carefully. With time, being off drugs will just seem normal.

Analgesics
Narcotics, narcotic derivatives, antagonists

NAMES YOU WILL HEAR
Simple analgesics
Some preparations in this list are combinations, for example Veganin, but aspirin is still the main ingredient, and they are thus classified here as simple analgesics. Given here is a fuller list of trade names for many common painkillers than elsewhere in the book.

Generic name: aspirin containing aspirin or acetylsalicylic acid; **trade names:** Acriptin, Ecotrin, Measurin, Excedrin, Bufferin, Aspirin APC Mixture, Analgesic Dellipsoids D6, Anodyne Dellipsoids D4, Asagran, Bayer Aspirin, Breoprin, Caprin, Hypon, Laboprin, Levius, Nu-seals, Paynocil, Safapryn, Trancoprin, Veganin, Bi-prin, Codral Junior, Elsprin, Novosprin, Prodol, Provoprin, Rhusal, Sedalgin, Solusal, SRA, Winsprin, Acetophen, Asadrine C-200, Astrin, Coryphen, Entrophen, Neopirine-25, Nova-Phase, Novasen, Rhonal, Sal-Adult, Sal-Infant, Supasa, Triaphen-10, Aquaprin, Aspasol, Aspegic. **Generic name:** soluble aspirin; **trade names:** Alka Seltzer, Disprin, Antoin, Aspar, Claradin, Codis, Migravess, Myolgin, Solprin. Buffered or with antacid: Aloxiprin, Palaprin (Paloxin S.A.), Trisilate. **Generic name:** acetaminophen; **trade names:** Anacin-3, Liquiprin, Phenaphen, Panadol, Tempra, Tylenol, Valadol, Acetaminophen, Cafadol, Calpol, Disprol, Dolvan, Lobak, Medised Suspension, Medocodene, Myolgin, Neurodyne, Norgesic, Paldesic, Pamol, Panadeine, Panasorb, Paracodol, Paradeine, Parahypon, Parake, Paralgin, Paramax, Paramol, Para-seltzer, Pardale, Paxidal, Pharmidone, Propain, Salzone, Solpadeine, Syndol, Ticelgesic, Tinol, Unigesic, Bramcetamol, Calpon, Ceetamol, Dolamin, Dymadon, Pacemol, Panamax, Paracet, Parasin, Paraspen, Parmol, Placemol, Atasol, Campain, Exdol, Robigesic, Rounox, Tivrin, Ennagesic, Fevamol, Napamol, Paraprom, Pyralen, Repamol, Sedapyren. **Generic name:** acetaminophen in combination with

WHAT IS PAIN?

– An unpleasant sensory and emotional experience associated with actual or potential tissue damage, or described in terms of such damage. This definition recognizes the psychological factors which can affect pain tolerance and threshold, differentiating pain from the five senses of taste, smell, vision, hearing and taste.

A large proportion of consultations with a doctor are made because of pain. Obviously the doctor will try and identify the cause of the pain, and treat this, whereupon the pain will go. He may give something for the pain itself, or the underlying condition; sometimes both can be treated with the same drug, for example, an anti-inflammatory agent – indeed most simple painkillers have this property.

These two pages deal with minor pain and its relief, the next two with stronger painkillers.

Pain relating to specific areas of the body is dealt with under separate headings. *See* for example ***headache,*** *page 98,* ***period problems,*** *page 190,* ***strains and sprains,*** *page 234,* ***migraine,*** *page 100,* ***ear infections,*** *page 256,* ***cancer,*** *pages 202-13* and ***sunburn,*** *page 278.*

PRESCRIPTION DRUGS

Simple analgesics are usually given by mouth as pills, but can be given as suppositories, or rarely by direct application as lotions or creams to the skin. They are often combined with other medications. Many types are available, but none has consistently been proved best. **How they work:** by blocking the inflammation caused by injury. Damaged tissues release prostaglandins, substances which irritate nerve endings thereby causing pain. Analgesics inhibit the formation of prostaglandins, reducing inflammation and pain.

OVER-THE-COUNTER TREATMENTS

These will contain aspirin, ibuprofen or acetaminophen, often in combination with other substances, which do not normally offer any advantage. Aspirin is so widely available because people are used to it: many of the alternatives are in fact safer. Aspirin is a potent drug, with significant side effects; acetaminophen is milder, with fewer side effects. Choice is often a matter of habit, and is learned from parents or others during childhood. Auto-suggestion does have a role in relieving pain too. These drugs have an excellent effect in relieving minor pains which do not require a doctor's attention. But if pain persists, or side effects occur, see a doctor soon.

QUESTIONS TO ASK THE DOCTOR

- Are there any special risks for me in taking simple painkillers?
- Is there medication available that I can take less often?
- Should I carry on with my daily routine despite the pain, or do I need to rest?

SIDE EFFECTS

Aspirin: nausea, indigestion, dizziness, ringing in the ears. If there is bleeding, asthma, skin rashes, confusion, stop taking it and see a doctor. Aspirin may also cause liver or kidney damage with prolonged use. Unless the circumstances are exceptional, it must not be used in people with a history of stomach ulcers,bleeding problems, severe indigestion, asthma, liver or kidney disease, severe allergies, pregnancy, lactating mothers or children under 12. In the latter, evidence suggests that it may be a factor in Reye's Syndrome, a rare but serious form of liver failure and neurological damage.

Special problems: indomethacin causes headache; phenylbutazone and oxphenbutazone may rarely cause life threatening blood disorders.

Acetaminophen's side effects are rare and mild. **Minor:** skin rashes, allergies. **Major and very rare:** liver damage, only in acute or chronic overdose.

SELF-MANAGEMENT

- Local measures: bruises, sports injuries – cold compresses; torn muscles or stiffness – local heat (lamp, rubs, heating pads); massage to stimulate blood flow and relax tense muscles.
- Exercise: gentle to start with, then building up can help minor injuries and nagging ailments: surrounding muscles are strengthened, ligaments stretched, blood flow and healing stimulated.
- Keep a supply of simple analgesics handy; they should be a type which you know from experience don't upset you. If the condition is long-term, take them in time to prevent the pain breaking through.
- Rest helps after an acute injury; *see **strains and sprains**, page 234.*
- If the pain is prolonged, consider safe "alternative" techniques like acupressure or transcutaneous nerve stimulation. Consult your doctor for sources of help.

aspirin; **trade names:** Benorylate: Benoral, Winolate.

NSAIDs

Generic name: diflunisal; **trade name:** Dolobid. **Generic name:** fenoprofen; **trade names:** Nalfon, Fenopron, Progesic. **Generic name:** meclofenamate; **trade name:** Meclomen. **Generic name:** ibuprofen; **trade names:** Motrin, Advil, Nuprin, Medipren, Rufen, Apsifen, Brufen, Ebufac, Fenbid, Ibuslo, Ibumetin, Lidifen, Nurophen, Paxofen. **Generic name:** indomethacin; **trade names:** Indocin, Artracin, Imbrilon, Indocid, Indoflex, Indolar, Indomod, Mobilan, Rheumacin, Arthrexin. **Generic name:** ketoprofen; **trade names:** Orudis, Alrheumat, Oruvail. **Generic name:** mefenamic acid; **trade names:** Ponstel, Ponstan, Ponstan Forte. **Generic name:** methyl salicylate ointments, creams; **trade names:** Oil of Wintergreen, Balmosa, Bengué's Balsam, Dubam. **Generic name:** naproxen sodium; **trade names:** Naprosyn, Synflex, Laraflex. **Generic name:** nefopam; **trade name:** Acupan. **Generic name:** oxphenbutazone; **trade names:** Oxalid, Tandacote, Tandalgesic, Tanderil, Oxbutazone, Tandearil, Artzone, Buteril, Fibutrox, Otone. **Generic name:** phenylbutazone; **trade names:** Azolid, Butazolidin, Butacote, Butazone, Parazolidin, Tibutazone, Butacal, Butalan, Butarex, Butoroid, Butoz, Buzon, Algoverine, Butagesic, Intrabutazone, Malgesic, Nadozone, Neo-Zoline, Phenbutazone, Butrex, Panazone. **Generic name:** piroxicam; **trade name:** Feldene. **Generic name:** salsalate; **trade name:** Disalcid. **Generic name:** sodium salicylate; **trade names:** Entrosalyl, Ancosal, Ensalate, Rhumax. **Generic name:** sulindac; **trade name:** Clinoril. **Generic name:** tolmetin; **trade names:** Tolectin, Tolectin DS. **Generic name:** suprofen; **trade name:** Suprol.

Continued on page 108

Narcotics, narcotic derivatives, antagonists

NAMES YOU WILL HEAR
Class 1
Generic name: morphine; **trade names:** Roxanol, Nepenthe, MST Continus, Duromorph, Cyclimorph, Haustus Linct., Brompton Cocktail. **Generic name:** diamorphine; **common name:** heroin; usually prescribed by generic name. **Generic name:** opium; **trade names:** prescribed by generic name. **Generic name:** papaveretum; **trade name:** Omnopon. **Generic name:** oxymorphone; **trade names:** Numorphan, Hydroxymorphone, Dilaudid. **Generic name:** pethidine, meperedine; **trade names:** Demerol, Pethilorfan, Pamergan, Pethoid, Demer-Idine; usually prescribed by generic name. **Generic name:** anileridine; **trade name:** Leritine. **Generic name:** dextromoramide; **trade name:** Palfium. **Generic name:** dipipanone; **trade name:** Diconal. **Generic name:** oxycodone; **trade names:** Roxicodone, Endone, Proladone, Supeudol. **Generic name:** phenazocine; **trade name:** Narphen. **Generic name:** levorphanol; **trade names:** Levo Dromoran, Dromoran. **Generic name:** methadone; **trade names:** Dolophine, Physeptone. **Generic name:** propoxyphene; **trade names:** Propoxyphene, Cosalgesic, Co-Proxamol, Dextrogesic, Distalgesic, Dolasan, Doloxene, Napsalgesic, Paxalgesic, Algaphan, Algodex, Darvon-N, Depronal SA, Novopropoxyn, Pro-65, 642 Tablets.

SEVERE PAIN

Pain can be classified as follows:
Acute – minor: headache, period pains, sunburn and minor injuries/strains and sprains. *See pages 98, 190, 274 and 234.*
– major: heart attack, post-operative, labor, kidney or gall stones; may need medical treatment with potent drugs.
Chronic – trauma: low back, fractures, crash injuries.
infection: after shingles.
degenerative: arthritis, gout.
vascular: arteriosclerosis, migraine.
neurological: trigeminal neuralgia.
cancer: tumors, secondary deposits.
psychological: anxiety, tension, stress, depression.

As pain may be acute or chronic, minor or severe, intermittent or continuous, many different treatments are available. These two pages deal with drugs commonly used for moderate to severe pain, including that caused by cancer.

PRESCRIPTION DRUGS

Class 1: morphine or **morphine-like narcotics.** These are the most potent, and are either naturally occurring for example opium, or synthetic, for example methadone.
Class 2: narcotic derivatives. Not as potent as Class 1, and less likely to produce addiction and major side effects.
Class 3: antagonist drugs. Also less addictive, but may be quite strong. They produce minor side effects in quite a large number of people.

Unless the pain is expected to be very severe (for example after major surgery or a heart attack), the doctor will usually start with Class 2 drugs (for example codeine, propoxyphene). If the pain persists, stronger drugs may be used, often tailored to the expected duration of pain. Of these, morphine, meperidine and methadone last about four hours. M.S. Contin (a slow-release morphine preparation) oxycodone and buprenorphine last longer. They can be given orally, or, if swallowing is a problem, under the tongue, rectally, intramuscularly, intravenously, subcutaneously or by epidural infusion. Some anesthetic agents can be inhaled – *see* ***anesthetics,*** *page 130.* The drugs *must* be given at regular intervals, according to their length of action, if the pain is expected to persist. Dose is gauged individually for the particular pain. The correct dose is that which stops the pain.

OVER-THE-COUNTER TREATMENTS

Not available.

QUESTIONS TO ASK THE DOCTOR

- What are the side effects?
- How long can I take them without risk of addiction, and how often?
- Will I be able to stop them easily?
- Can I take more if the dose is ineffective (particularly with cancer)?
- What can I do/What should I avoid?

SIDE EFFECTS

Narcotics: constipation (laxatives are essential if narcotics are given for more than two days); nausea and vomiting; drowsiness. These last two usually settle after one week. Confusion, nightmares, sweating, flushing, dizziness due to low blood pressure, and itching. These effects are rarer, and may settle. Depression of breathing can be dangerous especially in the elderly. Addiction. This last is not regarded as a problem in terminal illness. Narcotic derivatives: very similar to narcotics, but addiction and breathing problems are much rarer.

Buprenorphine: much less addictive than other narcotics. Less constipation, and fewer problems with breathing. Conveniently dissolves under the tongue. Incidence of vomiting, sweating and dizziness higher than with Classes 1 and 2.

MANAGEMENT OF SEVERE PAIN

Very dependent on cause. Self-management strategies may play a part with some types: ask your doctor. Medical treatment is often directed at the cause, and unfortunately this can mean that actual pain is poorly treated. Insist on adequate painkilling drugs in labor, after surgery or a heart attack, and for cancer pain. In chronic non-cancer pain, a high chance of addiction, major side effects, or increase in pain on stopping medicine means that most doctors are rightly reluctant to give all but codeine-type preparations. Even these are better stopped after three months if not fully effective.

TIMING

It is important, especially in cancer pain (see margin), that painkillers are given in time to stop the pain "breaking through". If painkillers are regularly used to *prevent* pain, then a lower dose may well suffice.

Class 2

Generic name: codeine; **trade names:** generally prescribed by generic name in the USA; elsewhere Codlin, Paveral. **Generic name:** codeine combined with aspirin; **trade names:** Anodyne Dellipsoids D4, Hypon, Safapryn-Co, Veganin. **Generic name:** codeine combined with soluble aspirin; **trade names:** Antoin, Codis, Myolgin. **Generic name:** codeine combined with acetaminophen; **trade names:** Medocodene, Neurodyne, Panadeine Co, Paracodol, Paradeine, Parahypon, Parake, Paralgin, Pardale, Pharmidone, Propain, Solpadeine, Syndol. **Generic name:** dihydrocodeine; **trade names:** DF 118, Onadex 118, Paramol 118, Rikodeine, Tuscodin, Co-Dydramol, Paracodin, Fortuss. **Generic name:** ethoheptazine; **trade names:** Equagesic, Zactipar, Zactirin.

Class 3

Agonist/antagonists

Generic name: pentazocine; **trade names:** Talwin, Fortagesic, Fortral, Sosegon. **Generic name:** meptazinol; **trade name:** Meptid. **Generic name:** buprenorphine; **trade names:** Buprenex, Temgesic, Buprex. **Generic name:** butorphanol; **trade name:** Stadol. **Generic name:** nalbuphine; **trade name:** Nubain.

MANAGEMENT OF CANCER PAIN

The causes of the pain must be identified, and treated accordingly:
- Bone/soft tissue pain: aspirin-like drugs, radiotherapy, calcitonin, rest.
- Pain from organs: Start with codeine, going on to morphine if no effect. Give sufficient doses, by the clock. Nerve blocks or steroids (cortisone) may be needed.
- Nerve pain: stabbing – anticonvulsants; burning – amitriptyline. May also respond to nerve blocks or radiotherapy. Other options may include antacids, laxatives, antibiotics, muscle relaxants.

NAMES YOU WILL HEAR
Generic name: phenytoin; **trade names:** Dilantin, Epanutin, Dantoin, Toin Unicelles. **Generic name:** carbamazepine; **trade name:** Tegretol. **Generic name:** sodium valproate; **trade name:** Depakene, Epilim. **Generic name:** ethosuximide; **trade names:** Zarontin, Emeside. **Generic name:** phenobarbital; **trade names:** Luminal, Gardenal, Maliasin, Nova-Pheno. **Generic name:** primidone; **trade names:** Mysoline, Midone, Sertan. **Generic name:** clonazepam; **trade name:** Klonopin, Rivotril. **Generic name:** clobazam; **trade name:** Frisium. **Generic name:** diazepam; **trade names:** Valium, Alupram, Atensine, Evacalm, Solis, Tensium, Valrelease.

WHAT IS EPILEPSY?

– A tendency to have fits, seizures or convulsions: the three terms mean the same.

The condition results from disturbance of normal electrical activity in the brain – something like a short circuit. Normal communication between brain cells is disrupted and a variety of aberrant discharges are produced. There are three main types of seizure:

Generalized tonic clonic or ''grand mal'' seizures: Here the electrical disturbance passes over the whole brain. There is a loss of consciousness; the patient becomes rigid and may cry out. He or she falls to the ground; the limbs jerk as muscles alternately contract and relax. Sometimes the patient loses bladder control or bites the tongue. Recovery follows spontaneously over a few minutes, although a dazed or confused state may persist for an hour or two.

"Partial" or "temporal lobe" seizures: These occur when the electrical discharge is confined to one part of the brain only – commonly one of the temporal lobes. The patient can be quite unaware of what happens: involuntary movements, loss of speech, confusion or complicated automatic actions all occur. Sometimes the event may be confined to a momentary loss of concentration; occasionally it develops into a generalized tonic-clonic convulsion. ''Partial'' fits vary greatly from person to person.

Absence or ''petit mal'' **seizures:** Found primarily in children, these are short periods of interrupted or clouded consciousness, easily mistaken for day dreaming. The child stops what he/she is doing, remains motionless and stares into space. The episodes last only seconds but they may be frequent throughout the day and disrupt his/her educational performance.

Epilepsy is not inherited in any direct sense apart from a few rare instances. Even if both parents are epileptics, the chance of offspring having fits is only increased very slightly.

Driving regulations for epileptics vary from state to state. In general a patient with a history of one or more seizures in the last three years may be denied a driver's license.

Children with epilepsy are usually educated in normal schools. They can take part in most activities except climbing and underwater diving. Epilepsy carries a real stigma which at times can seem almost medieval: people need educating about this condition. If required to fill in a form with a question about fits when applying for a job, be truthful, but if possible return the form to the firm's medical department or officer rather than the personnel department: you may find a more understanding attitude.

Between episodes, the brain usually works normally. Epilepsy can affect every age from infancy to the elderly.

CAUSES There are a large number. It is thought that the most common is previous brain damage. This may be a consequence of a difficult birth, a brain infection, a head injury or even a stroke. Very rarely, it is the first sign of a brain tumor. Many years can elapse from the time of the injury to the onset of epilepsy, which usually takes the form of partial seizures. However, in most cases, no specific cause can be identified.

INVESTIGATIONS

The electroencephalogram (EEG), an amplified measure of the brain's electrical activity, will identify abnormal discharges coming from a scar and can sometimes pick up evidence of low seizure threshhold. Unfortunately, an EEG may be normal in people with epilepsy and abnormal in some others who have never had a fit. Brain scans can detect an area of brain damage which may be responsible for the fits. Occasionally this enables the malfunctioning part to be removed surgically and the epilepsy cured.

PRESCRIPTION DRUGS

Anticonvulsant drugs There is a considerable overlap in the action of the various drugs listed; initial choice depends on the type of epilepsy and the clinical response, but it is usually between a well-tried drug such as **phenytoin, carbamazepine** or **sodium valproate.** Sometimes the first drug chosen will not suit an individual while an alternative will. There is still, unfortunately, an element of trial and error in these decisions.

Current medical thinking suggests that for most people a single drug in the right dose causes fewer long term problems than a combination, and offers equal or improved benefit. Nevertheless, a few patients seem to require more than one drug. Although many individuals require life-long treatment, the condition can remit and therapy may be slowly withdrawn over a number of months without recurrence of the fits. The decision to withdraw treatment is a difficult one but the longer the person is seizure-free, the more he/she is likely to re-

PATIENT'S EXPERIENCE
"Prior to an attack, I get a sudden sensation of fear and panic. I am paralysed during the seizure. I've no idea what I'm doing except fighting feelings of torture with pictures of bad memories and nightmares: it's like flickering, broken-up film sequences. As I come round, I can hear voices around me but cannot move or speak or see. I want to shout out to everyone to "leave me alone". During recovery, I feel lost. I don't know what I'm doing, where I am, or what time of day it is. After the struggle, I just want to sleep."

FIRST AID IN AN ATTACK
Generalized tonic-clonic or "grand mal" seizures
What to do:
1 Note the time. **2** Clear a space round the person having the attack and remove sharp objects which might cause injury. **3** Cushion the head, loosen collar and remove spectacles. **4** Remove false teeth if this is easily done (see 3 below). **5** As soon as the attack appears to be settling, turn the patient on their side to aid breathing. **6** At the end of the attack, reassure the patient and talk to them quietly until full recovery takes place.

What not to do:
1 Don't move the patient while the fit is in progress unless they are in acute danger. **2** Don't restrict movements. **3** Don't force anything between the teeth. **4** Don't give anything to drink. **5** Don't try to rouse the patient.

Partial or "temporal lobe"
The patient may wander around aimlessly with a glazed expression, so accompany them, and gently lead them away from any source of danger. Don't interfere unnecessarily. Afterwards, calm reassurance will be greatly appreciated. Don't try to stop the attack.

main in permanent remission. This is particularly so for children who develop the disorder in adolescence but have no evidence of brain damage or a family history of epilepsy.

How they work: All the anticonvulsants act on the brain to increase the seizure threshhold and prevent the spread of the abnormal electrical discharge. They are wholly successful in about 80 per cent of patients. A minority, however, will continue to have fits no matter what drug or combination is used – although their frequency may be reduced. This is particularly true of people with brain damage and in those who do not take their medication regularly. There is no doubt that frequent seizures can themselves cause brain damage and so perpetuate the disorder. Effective daily treatment is important in preventing this outcome.

OVER-THE COUNTER TREATMENTS
None.

QUESTIONS TO ASK THE DOCTOR
- What type of epilepsy do I have?
- Is there any evidence of brain damage?
- What possible side effects can I expect from my treatment?
- Will I have to take medication all my life?
- What should I tell my friends, family and employer?
- Can I drive?
- Will I pass on epilepsy to my child?
- Will my child have to go to a special school?

SIDE EFFECTS
At the start of treatment, the dose is gradually increased until the fits come under control, or, if they are infrequent, until a satisfactory blood level is obtained. This is to avoid the dampening effect of the drug on the other electrical activities of the brain which are concerned with alertness, concentration and memory. At high dosage, all the **anticonvulsants** can cause some degree of drowsiness. Some patients become sedated before the beneficial effects are obtained and so must try an alternative preparation.

There are few other predictable side effects of these drugs. **Phenytoin** can cause gum overgrowth, which can be prevented by scrupulous dental hygiene. **Sodium valproate** can produce a tremor. All may rarely cause damage to the liver or to the bone marrow in susceptible individuals. This is an allergic response, usually occurs within three months of starting treatment, is rever-

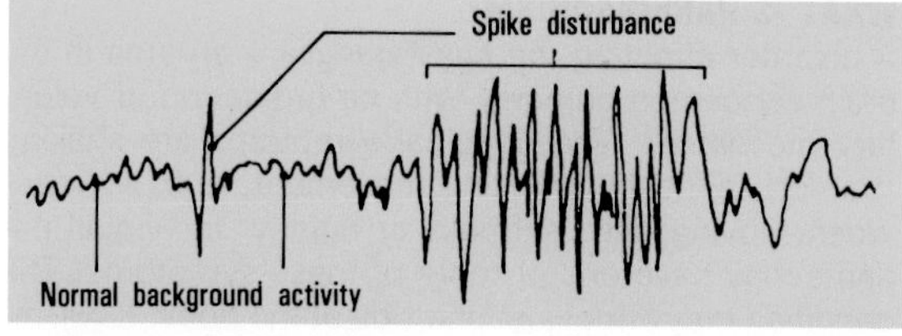

Examples of abnormalities *on the EEG that can help in the diagnosis of epilepsy.*

sible, and can be anticipated by carefully monitoring the patient's general health.

Anticonvulsants taken during pregnancy: there is a small risk (less than six per cent) that these drugs will affect the fetus. Discuss the problem fully with your doctor. Usually there is no reason why an epileptic should not plan her family normally.

Some of the anticonvulsant drugs, particularly carbamazepine, phenobarbitone and phenytoin, increase the turnover of hormones, and so bigger doses of the oral contraceptive pill may be required than that normally prescribed.

HOW TO PREVENT SEIZURES

- Take the medication regularly: control of fits is greatly helped by maintaining a consistent level of the drug in the blood and brain. If you have a complicated life or are just forgetful, you should probably be prescribed a drug which can be taken once or, at most, twice a day. If you forget to take your pills on time, have the dose as soon as you remember and follow-up with the next dose at the usual time.
- Some children only have fits when they develop a high fever. Simple measures such as tepid sponging and giving acetaminophen elixir can keep the temperature down. If this is not effective, parents can be taught to administer diazepam into the child's rectum at signs of twitching.
- Have as little alcohol as possible: it can cause seizures. It can also act in concert with medication to make the patient feel drunk very quickly. It may also make you forget to take your tablets.
- Fits can be triggered off by stimuli such as flashing lights, loud noises or hunger. Tiredness can also make an individual more susceptible. A healthy, sensible lifestyle is important. Some people find boredom, anxiety, depression or stress make them worse. Keep busy, realistic and positive.

WHEN SOMEONE HAS A SEIZURE

- See the advice in the margin of this page.

PARKINSONISM

Levodopa, anticholinergics, bromocriptine, amantadine, selegiline

NAMES YOU WILL HEAR

Preparations containing levodopa
Generic name: levodopa; **trade names:** Larodopa, Berkdopa, Brocadopa. **Generic name:** levodopa and benserazide; **trade names:** Madopar 62.5, Madopar 125, Madopar 250, Prolopa. **Generic name:** levodopa and carbidopa; **trade name:** Sinemet.

Anticholinergics
Generic name: trihexyphenydyl HCl; **trade names:** Artane, Bertex, Broflex, Anti-Spas, Aparkane, Novohexidyl, Trixyl. **Generic name:** biperiden; **trade name:** Akineton. **Generic name:** orphenadrine; **trade names:** Disipal, Norflex. **Generic name:** methixene; **trade name:** Tremonil. **Generic name:** procyclidine; **trade names:** Kemadrin, Arpicolin, Procyclid.

Dopamine agonists
Generic name: bromocriptine; **trade name:** Parlodel.

Other agents
Generic name: amantadine; **trade name:** Symmetrel. **Generic name:** selegeline; **trade name:**.Eldepryl.

WHAT IS PARKINSONISM?

A disorder affecting the basal ganglia – an area in the brain concerned primarily with co-ordination of voluntary movement. The principal symptoms are shaking (tremor), difficulty imitating movement, and slowness when moving; also stiffness or rigidity. Individual patients may have one or more of these symptoms. The condition may affect just one side of the body. It will require treatment for life. Although more than half the sufferers are disabled by the disease in time, this is not universal: with medical treatment patients may live full lives for five or ten years, possibly more.

CAUSES Nerve cells containing the neurotransmitter dopamine die at an unusually rapid rate in Parkinsonian patients. This results in an imbalance of nerve signals, and hence the symptoms. In some patients, symptoms of Parkinsonism may be due to the administration of drugs (for example metoclopramide) used to treat other medical problems such as dizziness or vomiting, and which act by blocking dopamine receptors. Stopping these drugs will usually give improvement. Previous brain damage by carbon monoxide or other chemicals may underlie some cases. In most cases of true Parkinsonism the cause is unknown.

PRESCRIPTION DRUGS

Levodopa (L-dopa): often given in combination with another drug (in the same pill) to prevent breakdown of the L-dopa outside the brain and increase its effect.
How it works: by increasing the amount of dopamine in the brain.
Anticholinergic drugs counteract the relative excess of the transmitter acetyl choline present as a result of lack of the dopamine-containing neurones. They seem to help the tremor more than the rigidity.
Dopamine agonists: drugs such as **bromocriptine** act directly on dopamine receptors. They have not been an outstanding success, primarily because of adverse side effects and lack of specificity – they affect all parts of the brain.
Amantadine is a milder-acting alternative to L-dopa. Sometimes used as an initial treatment, so as to leave the other drugs in reserve. **Selegiline** is used in combination with L-dopa to treat late complications.

The response to treatment is variable. Over 75 per cent of patients respond to drugs. About a third can hope to return virtually to normal for some period of time; the remainder must expect varying success. A small proportion do not respond to treatment at all, or find the side effects worse than the disease. For these, physiotherapy may sometimes be beneficial.

OVER-THE-COUNTER TREATMENTS

None.

QUESTIONS TO ASK THE DOCTOR

■ Am I taking drugs which might be adding to my symptoms?
■ Should I take a full dose to start with, or increase to the dose you prescribe over a few days?
■ How long should I take what you are prescribing?
■ Should I look for any particular side effect?
■ Should I increase the dose if the drugs don't work?
■ Would physiotherapy exercises help?

SIDE EFFECTS

Nausea may occur when starting **L-dopa.** This can be reduced by taking tablets with meals and by gradually increasing the dose to an optimum level. Odd uncontrolled movements, particularly of the face or limbs, indicate overdosage. Episodes of relative immobility may occur (the 'on-off' phenomenon). **Anticholinergics** may cause dry mouth, difficulty in focusing, difficulty passing urine and constipation. *See also* ***asthma,*** *page 74.* **Bromocriptine** may cause nausea, dizziness and confusion.

L-dopa also carries some more serious, though rare side effects including dizziness on standing, a tendency to fall, constipation, difficulty with memory and occasionally hallucinations. Adjustment of dose (in consultation with a doctor) may be helpful in either case.

SELF-MANAGEMENT, SELF-HELP

■ Symptoms are helped by taking the medication regularly. If symptoms are bad first thing in the morning, consider taking pills in bed before getting up to get a "booster effect" for dressing and washing.
■ Many sufferers tire by the end of the day, so consider planning your day around times of peak drug effect.
■ Try simple aids such as Velcro fasteners instead of buttons, a higher chair and a stick for walking.
■ Don't stop anti-cholinergic drugs suddenly as this may cause "freezing up" or severely restricted movement.
■ Accept that other illness experienced while on these drugs may upset response to treatment and stabilization may take some days.

PATIENT'S EXPERIENCE

"I first noticed difficulty doing delicate tasks with my right hand two years ago. The shake gradually became worse and affected my foot. My doctor started treatment with pills and my shake became much less obvious. I felt sick after taking them at first, but this stopped when I took them with food. I still find my hand shakes at times, particularly when I am anxious. My walking is also slower than it used to be. I notice my symptoms are worse if I forget my pills, but currently manage my shopping and light housework without too much trouble."

NAMES YOU WILL HEAR

Tricyclic antidepressants
Generic name: imipramine; **trade names:** Tofranil, Janimine, Imiprim, Tramil, Melipramine, Prodepress, Simipra, Impril, Novopramine, Panpramine. **Generic name:** amitriptyline; **trade names:** Elavil, Limbitrol, Tryptizol, Lentizol, Domical, Laroxyl, Tryptanol, Saroten, Amiline, Deprex, Levate, Meravil, Novotriptyn, Amilent, Trepiline, Tryptanol. **Generic name:** desipramine; **trade names:** Norpramin, Pertofrane, Pertofran. **Generic name:** dothiepin; **trade name:** Prothiaden. **Generic name:** nortriptyline; **trade names:** Parmelor, Allegron, Aventyl, Nortab, Nortrilin.

Atypical (novel) antidepressants
Generic name: mianserin; **trade names:** Solvidon, Norval, Tolvon, Lantanon. **Generic name:** maprotilene; **trade name:** Ludiomil. **Generic name:** trazodone; **trade names:** Desyrel, Molipaxin.

Monoamine oxidase inhibitors (MAOIs)
Generic name: phenelzine; **trade name:** Nardil. **Generic name:** tranylcypromine; **trade name:** Parnate.

Lithium salts
Generic name: lithium carbonate; **trade names:** Eskalith, Lithane, Lithobid, Camcolit, Priadel, Liskonum, Phasal, Lithicarb, Manialith, Carbolith, Lithizine, Lentolith, Quilonum Retard. **Generic name:** lithium citrate; **trade name:** Litarex.

WHAT IS DEPRESSION

The term is used in two different ways: **1** to signify a *symptom* – a patient's report of the subjective experience of low mood; **2** to describe an *illness* in which, apart from low mood, a group of symptoms occur together. While the symptom of depression is a common experience to everybody and in itself does not require treatment, depressive illness is distressing and dangerous, and usually requires medical attention.

The characteristic symptoms of depressive illness are depressed mood (feeling ''blue'', ''under the weather'', being ''fed up'', sad or gloomy), weepiness, difficulty in concentration, loss of interest in one's work, hobbies and family, a feeling of hopelessness, low self-esteem, loss of appetite for food and sex, disturbed sleep. If the symptoms persist, the patient loses weight as a result of poor appetite and reduced eating. In severe forms, the patient may blame him- or herself for mistakes, wrong-doings or even crimes not committed; suicide may be contemplated.

Depression is typically an episodic illness; an episode usually lasts for a few weeks or months. Although most patients would recover eventually without treatment, treatment is often necessary to shorten the depressive episode or to prevent a recurrence.

CAUSES An episode of depression may be the result of some adverse event (usually a significant loss, such as death) in the patient's life (reactive depression). Depression may also be secondary to some hormonal change (for example post-natal depression) or to some disease of the brain or body (for example depression in dementia or in a patient suffering from a brain tumor). In some patients, however, the symptoms may appear for no apparent reason (endogenous depression). Endogenous depression often occurs several times in a lifetime (recurrent depression). In some patients suffering from recurrent depression, episodes of depression alternate with episodes of complete well-being (unipolar depression). In some patients, however, episodes of depression may alternate with episodes of elation and over-activity (mania) and with episodes of normal mood: manic depressive illness, manic depression or bipolar depression. Endogenous depression might be due to some malfunction of brain chemistry, and it may be inherited.

PRESCRIPTION DRUGS

Antidepressants: these are frequently prescribed either by the family doctor or the psychiatrist. There are three major groups in current use: **1** tricyclic antidepressants; **2** novel (or atypical) antidepressants; **3** monoamine oxidase inhibitors (MAOIs). All are taken in tablet or capsule form. Most can be taken in one daily dose.

How they work: It is believed that antidepressant drugs act by modifying the effects of certain natural chemicals (''monoamines'') in the brain. Since monoamines also occur outside the brain, for example in the gut, blood vessels and glands, antidepressants can have undesired side effects.

These drugs do not have an immediate effect: it may take two or three weeks before the patient experiences significant improvement. The **tricyclic antidepressants** are the most commonly used, and their effectiveness in depressive illness is well established. The novel or **atypical antidepressants** are chemically different from the tricyclics. Their initial advantage was that they had fewer effects outside the brain, and thus fewer side effects; however recent experience has shown that severe side effects can occur. The **monoamine oxidase inhibitors** are usually prescribed when the other two classes of drugs do not work.

Lithium: Patients suffering from recurrent episodes of depression, either of the unipolar or bipolar kind, can benefit from long-term maintenance treatment with a lithium. If a patient is responsive to lithium, further episodes of depression and/or mania will not occur, or will occur less frequently or in a much milder form. Lithium is usually supplied in tablet form, and can be taken once daily at bedtime.

How it works: Lithium salts normally do not occur in the body. However, lithium, a simple element, is similar to sodium, an important constituent of body fluids. Lithium can to some extent be a substitute for sodium in the body, and this may result in the stabilization of mood. It is not known how this effect is brought about. Lithium is usually prescribed by a psychiatrist, and the patient taking it needs follow-up, with regular checks of the amount of lithium in the blood.

OVER-THE-COUNTER TREATMENTS

No established antidepressants are sold without a prescription.

QUESTIONS TO ASK THE DOCTOR

- How long should I take the antidepressant/lithium?
- How long will it take before the drug works?
- Can I drink alcohol or take other pills as well?

PATIENTS' EXPERIENCES

"When my wife died, I just could not take it in. We were very close and I never thought that she might die before me. I was numb and emotionally paralyzed for several days. Then I had these attacks of anguish and crying, and couldn't sleep: I paced up and down all night. I couldn't concentrate, and couldn't cope with the most trivial tasks. I thought that was the end: better if I join her. Then my daughter asked me to move in with them for a month or so. This really helped: we talked a lot about my wife and I had a lot of comfort from being with my loved ones. This was two years ago. I still keep thinking of her, but at least I can remember the good times we spent together."

"I have had depression for the past 20 years. It always comes in the spring, and lasts for two months. I do not know why I get depressed: everything is fine, and then it suddenly descends on me like a black cloud. I just wake up one morning and cannot face the day. It is an effort to get up, and it takes a long time to get dressed. I really feel useless and think everybody would be better off if I died. Then my sleep goes: I wake up in the small hours and think how useless I am. During the day I cannot do anything, I cannot concentrate to read the papers. I don't enjoy my food and cannot be bothered about sex. My doctor usually prescribes amitriptyline: it definitely helps me sleep. I usually feel much better after two weeks, but I am not really well for about two months. I do not like the drug: it makes my mouth dry and I occasionally feel dizzy, but I always ask for it because it helps."

■ Is there anything I should avoid eating while taking the pills?
■ Can I drive a car? ■ Will the pills affect my work?
■ What happens if I cannot tolerate the antidepressant/lithium? Is there an alternative?
■ May I become pregnant while on the drug?

SIDE EFFECTS

Antidepressants are usually prescribed for several months. The beneficial effects usually develop gradually during the first few weeks of treatment: very often the patient does not experience much improvement during the first week. Some of the side effects, on the other hand, appear at the beginning of treatment, and many of them may subside after a few weeks. It is therefore important that the patient does not give up the antidepressant on the grounds that it does not work and causes unpleasant side effects. If the patient perseveres, the depression should gradually lift, and the side effects will become less and less troublesome. After the depression has lifted, most doctors prefer their patients to continue with the medication for six to eight months: it has been shown that continued medication reduces the risk of relapse.

The most common side effects of the **tricyclic antidepressants** are dry mouth, blurred vision, constipation, occasionally difficulties in passing urine, dizziness and drowsiness. Some patients may complain of increased sweating or slight shakiness of the hands. Patients with a history of heart disease need careful monitoring. At the start of treatment with all these drug types your doctor will advise you on the safety of driving a car or operating machinery. The novel or **atypical antidepressants** are less likely to produce some of these side effects; with some of the drugs (eg trazodone) drowsiness and dizziness may occur.

The **monoamine oxidase inhibitors** usually cause a drop in blood pressure resulting in dizziness: this symptom normally dissipates with time. Patients taking these drugs should avoid certain foods, in particular aged meats or cheeses, pickled herrings, sour cream, Chianti wine, sherry or beer, liver, canned figs, raisins, bananas, avocados, chocolate, soy sauce, fava bean pods, yeast extracts or tenderized meat. They can result in a dangerous increase in blood pressure. Patients are given a card listing all foods to avoid. They must avoid *all* other drugs or medicines, unless these have been cleared with the doctor, especially other antidepressants, opiates and decongestants.

Lithium salts have to be taken over many years for the prevention of the recurrence of depression. Side effects include nausea, diarrhea, shakiness of the hands, increased thirst and passing more than the usual quantity of urine. These side effects are usually mild if the level of lithium in the blood is not too high. Patients on lithium salts have to drink adequate amounts of water (usually three pints per day), especially if there is an excessive loss of fluid (for example as a result of diarrhea or hot weather). Consequences of a wrongly adjusted dose are serious, including convulsions.

SELF-MANAGEMENT

As adverse events in one's life can lead to depression it is important to learn how to cope with stress.

■ Try to share your distress with someone close to you: sharing *can* relieve anxiety and distress; 'bottling things up' *can* increase the anguish.

■ Do not medicate yourself: do not use alcohol or other people's sedatives. These drugs do not solve problems and they can lead to serious complications.

■ If your sleep is disturbed, try taking a walk for a couple of hours before bedtime. *See page 93*

■ If symptoms of depression persist, or you cannot cope with your daily life, go and see your doctor. Your doctor will take your complaints seriously: he or she *can* help you decide whether you are suffering from a 'normal' reaction to an adverse event or whether you are suffering from depressive illness.

HELPING A DEPRESSED RELATIVE

Don't underestimate the distress of true depressive illness. While some patients are able to describe their feelings and experiences, others may find it difficult to put their anguish into words.

■ Appreciate that depression is an illness and the patient cannot help some of his feelings, thoughts and behavior. Do not reproach the patient for being unaffectionate or selfish: the patient is already plagued by feelings of self-blame and guilt. It is no use saying "Pull yourself together", or "It is up to you".

■ Treat the patient as a normal person with understanding and compassion. Try to involve the patient in family activities, but do not apply too much pressure.

■ The patient has a low self-image. Try to emphasize achievements, and give praise as appropriate.

■ The patient may not appreciate what is wrong, and may even refuse to see a doctor. In such a case contact the family doctor yourself; suicide is a risk.

PATIENTS' EXPERIENCE

"The doctor says that I have manic depression. My mother had it too. Every year, three or four times, I feel very low, just cannot be bothered about anything and feel suicidal; these depressions may last for two to three weeks. Every year, once or twice, I go 'high'; feel very well, have lots of energy, could do anything, don't need any sleep or food and spend a lot of money. These 'highs' last for a couple of weeks each time. Two years ago the psychiatrist persuaded me to try lithium. I was reluctant to do so because you have to take it for years, but I am glad that I agreed. For the past two years I have been depressed only twice. The only thing is, I have to go to the clinic once every two months. I also have to remember to take the pills at bedtime. At first I had some nausea and diarrhea, but now I hardly notice I am on lithium."

SAFETY

If a patient is on pills, help him to remember to take them. Keep an eye on the pills: some patients may take an overdose of antidepressants in a desperate moment. It may be necessary for you to dispense the pills on a daily basis.

Anti-psychotic drugs, anti-Parkinsonian drugs

NAMES YOU WILL HEAR
Anti-psychotic drugs
*Drugs marked * are available as longer lasting depot injections.*
Generic name: chlorpromazine; **trade names:** Thorazine, Largactil, Dozine, Chloractil, Procalm, Promacid, Protran, Chlorprom, Chlor-Promanyl, Klorazin. **Generic name:** trifluoperazine; **trade name:** Stelazine. **Generic name:** thioridazine; **trade names:** Mellaril, Melleril, Novoridazine, Thioril. **Generic name:** haloperidol*; **trade names:** Haldol, Dozic, Fortunan, Serenace. **Generic name:** Droperidol; **trade name:** Droleptan. **Generic name:** fluphenazine*; **trade names:** Prolixin, Permetil, Modecate, Moditen, Anatensol. **Generic name:** flupenthixol*; **trade names:** Depixol, Fluanxol. **Generic name:** Zuclopenthixol*; **trade name:** Clopixol.

Anti-Parkinsonian drugs
Generic name: trihexyphenidyl; **trade names:** Artane, Bentex, Broflex, Anti-Spas, Aparkane, Novo Hexidyl, Trixyl. **Generic name:** benztropine; **trade names:** Cogentin, Bensylate. **Generic name:** orphenadrine; **trade names:** Disipal, Biorphen, Norflex, Norgesic. **Generic name:** procyclidine; **trade names:** Kemadrin, Arpicolin, Procyclid.

WHAT IS SCHIZOPHRENIA?

– A common, and serious mental illness. The symptons vary widely, but fall into two main groups: 1 bizarre perceptions and 2 loss of drive and interest in life.

Typical bizarre perceptions are: hallucinations (hearing voices, seeing or feeling things when no one is present); difficulties in thinking clearly; delusions – firmly believing in something which is untrue and out of the ordinary. Paranoid delusions are common, typically the belief that people are against one. These perceptions may feel so real to sufferers that they actually respond to them. Patients may talk back to imaginary voices, or try to protect themselves from people they believe wish to harm them. The schizophrenic loses the ability to distinguish reality from what is imagined.

The second group of symptoms include: apathy; self-imposed isolation; loss of emotion; difficulties in relating to people.

Symptoms can develop slowly over a period of years, or rapidly, as a reaction to stress. Relatives and friends will probably notice changed, sometimes bizarre behavior. The outcome of the illness is variable: some have only one episode; others recover from a first episode and have further symptoms when stressed, while a proportion never fully recover from the symptoms and are permanently disabled. Not all cases need hospital admission; but some inevitably require institutional care, even against their will, because of self-neglect, or potentially dangerous behavior.

CAUSES Not known, but a biochemical abnormality affecting part of the brain is suspected. The illness can run in families, but the pattern of inheritance is not clear-cut. Theories of family interaction causing schizophrenia promoted in the past are now discounted. Once a person has had schizophrenic symptoms, however, the tendency to relapse can be affected by family attitudes and relationships.

OTHER PSYCHOTIC ILLNESSES

Schizophrenia-like symptoms can develop as a consequence of drug or alcohol misuse, or as a long-term complication of certain types of epilepsy. The drugs most commonly implicated are amphetamines and cannabis.

Also in this category are miscellaneous individual psychoses in which an unfounded idea develops out of proportion to reality: for example delusional jealousy; delusions about body size or shape; paranoid beliefs.

PRESCRIPTION DRUGS

Schizophrenia and other psychotic illnesses share similar drug treatments; however, management of associated problems such as excessive drinking, marriage problems, drug abuse, isolation and deafness is of course just as important.

Anti-psychotic drugs are used both to treat psychotic episodes and to prevent relapses. There are many types. They can be taken by mouth as tablets or syrup, or by injection. Depot preparations are given as injections to release the drug slowly into the body, one injection lasting several weeks. Anti-psychotic drugs are not addictive, but it is always better to reduce them slowly rather than stopping them suddenly.

How they work: by acting on certain nervous pathways in the brain. They have a calming action, and they damp down the bizarre perceptions. Doses needed to treat an acutely disturbed person are usually greater than those needed to prevent a relapse.

Anti-Parkinsonian drugs are used to treat the side effects of anti-psychotic drugs (see below), not the psychiatric symptoms. As they can have side effects themselves, their use is kept to a minimum. Despite these drawbacks they can be particularly helpful while high doses of anti-psychotic drugs are being given, or for the first few days after a depot injection. They are not addictive.

How they work: by acting on certain nervous pathways in the brain to balance the effect of anti-psychotic drugs on muscle tone and movement.

Anti-depressant drugs: Depression and mood changes are not uncommon in association with schizophrenia, and treatment with anti-depressants may well be combined with anti-psychotic drugs. *See **depression,** page 116.*

OVER-THE-COUNTER TREATMENTS

None.

QUESTIONS TO ASK THE DOCTOR

- For how long should I take the drug(s)?
- Should I stop them when I feel better?
- May I just take them when I need them?
- Should I drive?
- What else can I do to help myself?

SIDE EFFECTS

Anti-psychotic drugs have a number of side effects but there is considerable variation between the different drugs and it is often possible to find one that suits the

PATIENTS'EXPERIENCES

"When I first came to the hospital it was like a nightmare. I was convinced the government was plotting against me and everyone at work knew. Can't remember it properly now. The pills must have helped, but I couldn't pee even when I wanted to, and it was difficult to walk easily. That's all sorted out now with changes in the drugs; but it was frightening."

"I don't know why I still need injections – I'm okay – the psychiatric nurse comes every three weeks – but I don't really mind."

RELATIVES' EXPERIENCES

"I know my wife better than any psychiatrist does. I've looked after her over 12 years of these breakdowns. She kept well with just one tablet at night but the doctor insisted on weaning her off it. Now here we are, I'm just recovering from major heart surgery and she's ill again and in the hospital.

When she first went into the hospital the drugs made her like a zombie. They were dreadful those first few months. She's much better now, she's only on a small dose."

"We'd been doing it all wrong with Terry, but we learned a lot from the relatives' group, from the others. We spoiled him because he'd been ill and because he was so odd, but the other children got fed up with us and they all left home very young. He could be awful to the girls. Now he's in his own apartment we still worry about him and what will happen. But I'm getting on much better with my husband and the family come round again now."

Anti-psychotic drugs, anti-Parkinsonian drugs

HOSPITAL STAFF'S EXPERIENCE
"Bill used to just stay in his room, lying in bed and he wouldn't do anything. We all thought he was on far too much medication and asked for it to be reduced. When it was cut down he went mad and was up all night talking to himself, shouting obscenities or pacing around the streets. We've got to find a balance for him when he settles down."

IF THE DRUGS DON'T SEEM TO HELP
■ Don't despair. Recovery is often slow and can take months or years, rather than days or weeks. Find sanctuary: somewhere you feel safe and unafraid, where you can cope with any demands made, somewhere that understand what you are going through. Hospitals have traditionally provided such a haven, but so can friends, some lodgings or hostels, cafés, sheltered workshops, and so on. Adapting to the effects of the illness, and regaining confidence, take time.

individual even if several produce side effects which are unacceptable.

In the first few days of treatment they tend to cause a dry mouth, blurred vision, constipation and difficulty in passing urine. Fainting is a risk, especially in the elderly. These side effects normally wear off as the body gets used to the drugs.

More seriously, they can increase the tendency to have epileptic fits in those who have had them before, and occasionally in those who have not. They can also cause weight gain, and chlorpromazine, in high doses, makes the skin sensitive to sunlight: a sun-screen *(see page 278)* should be used to prevent burning. Jaundice and damage to blood cells are further serious, but rare, complications.

The most troublesome side effect of the anti-psychotics is on muscle tone and movement. In the first few days of treatment, muscle spasms can occur, typically at the back of the neck, or in the tongue or eye muscle. Restlessness of the limbs may be experienced, too. Most common of all is a slowing of movements and a stiffness in the limbs and face muscles. This drug-induced Parkinson's syndrome starts after some days or weeks of treatment, and fortunately responds to anti-Parkinsonian drugs.

Long-term treatment with anti-psychotics can cause abnormal muscle movements, particularly of the face (tardive dyskinesia). Sucking or chewing movements are typical. They are most likely if high doses of drugs are used over long periods, and may not cease, even if the drugs are stopped

Is treatment worth all this trouble? Families and friends of schizophrenics, with first-hand experience of the miseries of mental illness, usually have few doubts. The side effects are not invariable, and in the short-term, the potential benefits of treatment usually outweigh them. Long-term complications, including tardive dyskinesia, are another matter: careful supervision is essential.

Anti-Parkinsonian drugs cause drowsiness, dry mouth, blurred vision, constipation and difficulty in passing urine, but these tend to pass in a few days. The elderly may become confused. If taken regularly over a long period, the drugs can increase the risk of tardive dyskinesia developing (see above).

Anti-depressive drugs: *see **depression**, page 116.*

SELF-MANAGEMENT

Resist the inclination to carry on without professional

advice. Precisely because the perception can seem so real, it is difficult for the sufferer to gauge the extent of the problem, or the need for help.

To prevent further attacks:

■ Don't fight against the drugs. They do prevent further episodes and they will keep symptoms at bay. Balance the disadvantages in taking them against the risk of a further breakdown. Consider the possible consequences of this at home or work; bear in mind that next time it might be admission to the hospital. Discuss the options with your doctor or psychiatrist.

■ Try to steer a middle course between becoming isolated or lonely and seeing people who worry or annoy you.

■ Aim for a middle way also between being stretched by work or responsibilities and giving up routines and responsibilities. Try to keep active and get out of the house at least once a day.

Ideas for friends and relatives:

It is difficult to give general advice which will be helpful in specific circumstances, but:

■ Living with someone suffering from schizophrenia can be draining: friends and relatives may need help and support themselves. Remember this is available from self-help groups, and from professionals such as family doctors, psychiatrists, psychiatric nurses or social workers.

■ Remember that negative symptoms such as loss of drive and ability to respond to other people are just as much a part of the illness as the bizarre perceptions. Don't view apathy as laziness. Encourage the schizophrenic to participate in things, but accept the handicaps and don't behave like a school marm.

■ Don't argue with delusional ideas: it is probably best to accept them and change the subject: "Well, it may seem as if the TV's affecting you, but anyway it's supper time now."

■ Getting on with other people, particularly those close to them, can be difficult for schizophrenics. Don't press them; if in doubt, let them be. If you are getting irritated or worried, the schizophrenic will often sense it, and this can make things worse. Can you spend less time together, develop other interests for yourself, or talk about it with an objective outsider?

■ Remember, the drugs are *not* addictive, and they are often used to prevent relapse. Don't press for them to be stopped just because a schizophrenic seems well.

DOCTORS' EXPERIENCES

"If John had stayed in the boarding house with the landlady looking after him, and carried on pottering down to the workshop in the week, he would have been fine without any drugs at all. But when his landlady fell ill he went back home to his parents; they expected too much of him."

"I feel guilty and embarrassed when I talk to patients who have tardive dyskinesia as a result of their drug treatment. It almost makes it worse that they don't seem to either notice or care."

"It's always difficult to decide when to advise coming off anti-psychotic drugs. The statistics about relapse rates and risk factors don't help much with individual patients, and if someone does break down again, they often lose insight into what's happened and don't come for help."

Antidepressants, tranquillizers, hypnotics, vasodilators

NAMES YOU WILL HEAR

Anti-depressants
Generic name: amitriptyline; **trade names:** Elavil, Limbitrol, Tryptizol, Lentizol, Domical, Laroxyl, Tryptanol, Saroten, Amiline, Deprex, Levate, Meravil, Novotriptyn, Amilent, Trepiline. *See also **depression,** page 116.*

Tranquillizers
Generic name: chlorpromazine hydrochloride; **trade names:** Largactil, Dozine, Chloractil, Procalm, Promacid, Protran, Chlorprom, Chlorpromanyl, Klorazin. *See also **anxiety,** page 84.*

Hypnotics
Generic name: chloral hydrate; **trade names:** Chloralex, Chloradorm, Chloralix, Dormil, Elix-Nocte.

Vasodilators
Generic name: cyclandelate; **trade names:** Cyclospasmol, Cyclobral. **Generic name:** isoxsuprine hydrochloride; **trade names:** Defencin, Duvadilan, Vasodilan. **Generic name:** naftidrofuryl oxylate; **trade name:** Praxilene. **Generic name:** co-dergocrine mesylate; **trade name:** Hydergine.

WHAT IS SENILE DEMENTIA?

– Loss of mental function to the extent that it causes problems in daily living. It does not involve loss of consciousness, but intellect and memory, especially recent memory, gradually deteriorate. There may also be impaired judgement or impaired abstract thinking (for example difficulty in defining words), personality changes and speech difficulties.

The doctor must be at pains to exclude any other medical cause for these symptoms: drugs, infections, emotional disorders, pain, nutritional deficiencies, eye and ear problems and heart failure can aggravate the symptoms and once these factors have been identified and treated there can be a vast improvement.

CAUSES Usually, degeneration of brain cells. Premature degeneration of brain cells is known as Alzheimer's Disease, but sometimes this label is extended to include brain degeneration in all age groups. What ultimately causes this degeneration in the brain is unknown. Thyroid disease and lack of vitamin B12 may cause dementia.

One cause of brain damage in the elderly is relatively identifiable: poor blood supply to the brain due to chronically narrowed blood vessels. This is often associated with a history of high blood pressure and/or stroke. In some cases there is a mixture of brain degeneration and reduced blood supply.

Senile dementia progresses gradually, although in patients where the disease is caused by narrowed blood vessels, deterioration may be in identifiable steps as new areas of the brain suffer reduced blood flow.

PRESCRIPTION DRUGS

In old people, drugs often have more marked side effects, some of which may result in aggravation of the dementia. Therefore it is important never to use a drug without a definite reason; to use as small a dose as possible; and to avoid using more than one drug.

Antidepressants: Depression is common in old people, especially when mobility is restricted or when eyesight or hearing fail. It may be difficult to distinguish at first between dementia and depression, so expert assessment is worthwhile. Alternative interests should be encouraged, and old people should be made to feel useful even if they can only perform simple tasks. If they live alone, they should be encouraged to go out. These general measures can lessen the need for antidepressants. Drugs used in the treatment of depression

are discussed in detail under ***depression,*** *page 116.* Amitriptyline is the one most commonly used in the old because it has relatively few side effects.
Tranquillizers may be necessary: *see* ***anxiety,*** *page 84;* but equally, they may not. A few kind and reassuring words can be better than any medicine. The knack is to probe for the cause of the anxiety and treat that. Is the anxiety over an animal left alone at home? Or a minor physical symptom such as constipation? Pinning down the cause can be difficult when the patient is confused and cannot communicate effectively, but it is worth trying.
Hypnotics: Difficulty sleeping is all too common in the elderly. It is normal for older people to need less sleep, and they need reassurance that just a few hours at night may be enough for them, especially if they catnap during the day. *See* ***insomnia,*** *page 92* for the drugs used.
Vasodilators are controversial drugs in this context. The drugs listed are thought to have a selective effect on blood vessels in the brain – but many doctors mistrust them. Certainly they should only be used when there is good reason to believe that dementia is due to narrowing of blood vessels in the brain. Psychological test results have suggested the drugs give some improvement, but the results in practice so far are inconclusive.
How they work: by dilating the blood vessels in the brain; however, the drug may succeed only in dilating healthy blood vessels, diverting blood away from vessels already narrowed. Symptoms can thus be made worse.

OVER-THE-COUNTER TREATMENTS

No generally available remedies have any significant effect on senile dementia, despite the claims of advertising. Don't be persuaded to spend money on such drugs; if you are tempted, ask your doctor first for advice.

QUESTIONS TO ASK THE DOCTOR

- What plans can I make for the patient's care?
- If the patient remains with the family, what outside support can the family get?
- What about alternative accommodation?

SIDE EFFECTS

Drug reactions and interactions between drugs are much more common in the elderly because:
– Most drugs are broken down in the liver or excreted by the kidneys. Decreased liver and kidney function is common in older people and this means that drugs are

PATIENT'S EXPERIENCE

"My husband was fit and active until he was 66. Then he gradually became more forgetful and seemed to lose touch with what was going on around him. At first I paid little attention: most people have some difficulty remembering things as they get older. But soon it became embarrassing. He had retired from a highly responsible job only a year before; but now I could see that he was not capable of working on the committees he was still involved with. I had a private talk with our doctor, who asked to see my husband. The doctor confirmed my suspicions: George was suffering from an early onset of senile dementia. He gave me all the advice he could. For example, we have some good friends, and although I had been embarrassed about George's behavior, once I had explained the problem to them, they were understanding. Some of the men carried on taking him golfing as they had done before, although it can't have been easy as he had to be looked after like a child. He was unable to drive on his own; he kept getting lost.

It was difficult for me. He didn't look like an old man. I couldn't leave him alone: he would wander away from the house and as he had no road sense, I was always terrified he would be knocked over by a car.

The doctor was a help, even though there was nothing he could do to treat the condition. He suggested having George admitted to a hospital so that I could get away for a while; but it did not work out because George had become totally dependent on me. Even if my daughter came to look after him for an afternoon, he kept on asking when I would be home and got very agitated.

Over the next year and a half the strain became too much. It was intolerable being alone with him, yet I was reluctant to go out with him or invite friends around. Eventually, I decided to take up my other daughter's offer of a small separate house on their farm. It means that I

Continued on page 127

Antidepressants, tranquillizers, hypnotics, vasodilators

not eliminated efficiently. Side effects are therefore more frequent.
– If the patient is confused, he or she may forget having taken a pill, and take the dose twice.
– The patient may not take the pills, and the doctor may increase the dose on the grounds that the drug is not working. If the patient then takes the increased dose, there may be side effects.

Antidepressants: *See* ***depression,*** *page 116.* The monoamine oxidase group are not usually used in the elderly because of the high risk of side effects.

Tranquillizers: *See* ***anxiety,*** *page 84.* Tranquillizer drawbacks specific to the elderly include falls – potentially serious because of brittle bones; confusion; depression; memory failure and incontinence. An additional problem is that these side effects may not be recognized as a result of the drugs, but attributed to deteriorating mental function.

Hypnotics can have a reverse effect in the elderly (ie keep them awake) particularly if they are in pain. So, give something for the pain first; when it has eased, use the sleeping pill. An old person who has had a sleeping pill is especially likely to have a fall if they try to get up during the night. *See* ***insomnia,*** *page 92.* Note that chloral hydrate, though still commonly prescribed for the elderly in some countries, is not generally used in the USA.

Vasodilators bring a risk of excessive fall in blood pressure. This leads to dizzy spells or fainting, and in the extreme, a reduced blood supply to the brain can be followed by a stroke. Vasodilators can also cause skin rashes, nausea, palpitations and insomnia. They are not usually used in patients who have recently had strokes nor in those with heart disease or severe anemia.

SELF-MANAGEMENT

■ Patients with memory loss do better if pressure to remember is removed. So, set them up with memory aids: note pads, a notice board, a clock with large digits, an easily read calendar. An established routine also gives a sense of security.

■ Symptoms can suddenly become worse if the old person is moved to unfamiliar surroundings such as a hospital.

■ Symptoms can also suddenly worsen if the patient becomes physically ill, depressed, or has side effects from drugs. Thus any sudden deterioration in mental condition should be investigated by the doctor.

■ Symptoms are often exacerbated by alcohol.

■ Many old people, especially (but not only) those living alone, have a restricted diet. Vitamin deficiencies, anemia and malnutrition can all aggravate dementia. These factors must be carefully evaluated, and the diet supplemented with vitamins and iron if necessary.

■ Loss of vision or hearing can aggravate symptoms.

■ Remove all unnecessary medicines: confused old people, like children, can accidentally take dangerous overdoses, even of aspirin, iron or acetaminophen.

■ The patient should see the doctor regularly for reviews of drugs. Don't allow an old person to have indefinite refills of prescriptions, even though it is convenient. Symptoms may be due to accumulation of drugs in the body, not progression of the disease.

■ If using tranquillizers and sleeping pills, guard against falls by making the route to the bathroom as unobstructed as possible, or put a pot or bedpan in an easily accessible position in the bedroom. A night light can help.

■ Living arrangements may have to be adapted so that stairs need not be used.

■ Social support is important. Visits by the doctor and visiting nurse will help to define problems in the home and their possible solution.

■ Temporary admission to hospital or nursing home can give family carers a rest or holiday. This change in environment may upset an old person, but their memory for recent events is short. It is essential for care-givers to have a break, otherwise the quality of the care that they can give deteriorates.

■ Recent onset of urinary incontinence should be investigated for the possibility of a bladder infection. Urinary incontinence can be distressing, but gentle persuasion to use absorbent pads inside underwear pays dividends. *See* ***urinary incontinence,*** *page 188.*

■ Old people often prefer life in their own homes to the safe but unhappy existence in an institution. Their point of view should at least be considered in milder cases of dementia.

■ Markedly confused patients can be like young children and the same precautions apply: safety in the kitchen; protection of open fires; locking away medicines; help with crossing the street.

■ Some confused elderly patients may wander away from home. Make sure the patient has their name and address in a pocket or on a bracelet that cannot be removed. Regular exercise may be a solution: the elderly person is less likely to wander if tired.

am close to the family, and my husband is able to walk more safely and there are things on the farm which interest him. It appears to be working well, but life is still a strain.

Not everyone is so lucky. This move however, does underline the fact that care of the old ought to be shared: if one person tries to do it alone, the quality of care becomes deplorable."

MULTIPLE SCLEROSIS

Steroids, immune suppressants, baclofen, dantrolene, carbamazepine, diazepam

NAMES YOU WILL HEAR

Steroids

Generic name: methyl prednisolone; **trade names:** Solumedrol, Codelsol, Delta Phorical, Deltacortril, Deltalone, Deltastab, Precortisyl, Prednesol, Sintisone, Nisolone, Delta-Cortef, Deltasolone, Prelone, Lenisolone, Meticortilone, Predeltilone. **Generic name:** dexamethasone; **trade names:** Decadron, Oradexon.

Immune suppressants

Generic name: azathioprine; **trade names:** Azathioprine Tablets, Imuran. **Generic name:** cyclophosphamide; **trade names:** Endoxana, Endoxan-Asta, Cytoxan, Procytox, Endoxan.

Others

Generic name: baclofen; **trade name:** Lioresal. **Generic names:** dantrolene; **trade name:** Dantrium. **Generic name:** carbamazepine; **trade name:** Tegretol. **Generic name:** diazepam; **trade names:** Valium, Alupram, Atensine, Evacalm, Solis, Tensium, Valrelease.

WHAT IS MULTIPLE SCLEROSIS (MS)?

– Patchy damage to the insulating sheath of myelin around nerves – see diagram. As a result, nerve signals are no longer conducted. In young people, MS tends to come in attacks lasting between weeks and months; each attack indicates damage to a group of nerves in one part of the central nervous system. As each attack settles, the symptoms usually improve and apparently full recovery may occur especially after early attacks.

In older people, or young people who have had the disease for some time, MS tends no longer to occur in attacks, but to follow a slowly progressive course.

To make a diagnosis of MS, the clinician needs to have sound evidence for multiple attacks occurring in different parts of the nervous system or occurring at different times. If a single attack of inflammation or damage has occurred in only one part of the nervous system, there is no basis for a diagnosis – although the patient may go on to develop MS.

CAUSE Ultimately unknown. There is a weak genetic component; people with a certain gene pattern are prone to develop MS, although it rarely occurs in more than one member of a family. There is also an environmental factor, possibly a virus encountered during the first 20 years of life. MS is more common in whites than in black people. However, if a black person is born in or moves to a temperate climate zone before the age of 15, the risk of developing MS rises; the reverse is true for whites moving from temperate to hotter climates.

PRESCRIPTION DRUGS

Short courses of **steroids:** these drugs, including prednisolone, dexamethasone or ACTH probably shorten the duration of minor attacks; however, they have no effect on the long-term outcome. Thus most physicians reserve steroids for severe attacks.

Immune suppressants such as azathioprine can benefit patients who experience frequent attacks. Their use is a comparatively recent development, and the object is to reduce the frequency of attacks.

How they work: by acting on the immune system, preventing the body from breaking down myelin.

Others alleviate specific symptoms: Impotence, depression, urinary incontinence, constipation, pain and dizziness/vertigo, blurring of vision and weakness are common at various stages of MS, treatment of which is dealt with on *pages 172, 116, 188, 28, 106 and 98.*

Spasticity or increased stiffness in the legs is common and may be helped by baclofen, dentrolene, carbamazepine or diazepam.

OVER-THE-COUNTER TREATMENTS

None.

QUESTIONS TO ASK THE DOCTOR

- What about my work?
- Can I continue being active?

SIDE EFFECTS

Steroids given in short courses for this condition have no serious side effects.

Immune suppressants have substantial serious side effects, especially bone marrow suppression. Sore throat, mouth ulcers or serious infections may reveal this. Azathioprine can also cause mild gastro-intestinal upset. Report these and any other side effects to your doctor immediately. No patient should start this type of treatment without full discussion of the risks.

Baclofen can cause gastro-intestinal upset, drowsiness and faintness. **Dantrolene** can give transient drowsiness, fatigue and diarrhea; a possibly serious side effect may be liver malfunction and tests should be conducted six weeks after starting treatment. **Carbamazepine** may cause dizziness, marrow damage, major toxic reactions, drowsiness, gastro-intestinal upset and a rash. For ***diazepam**, see page 84.*

SELF-MANAGEMENT

Most doctors advise MS patients to avoid saturated fats (mainly animal fats and dairy produce) and to switch to a diet rich in polyunsaturated fats; there is some evidence that this improves myelin repair and thus the long-term outlook. Regular gentle exercise is important, and physiotherapy can be of considerable benefit. See also HOME ADAPTATIONS in margin.

SELF-HELP IN AN ATTACK

It is usually best to rest. The trigger for most attacks is unknown. They are slightly more likely to occur following childbirth, and some follow viral infection such as flu. In general, however, most attacks occur without warning.

It is important to remember that 60 per cent of patients are working ten years after onset. Only 20 per cent end up in a wheelchair. The outlook is not as bleak as commonly conceived.

PATIENT'S EXPERIENCE

"Ten years ago I had an attack of blurred vision in my left eye. It cleared over three months. Then three months ago I noticed increasing difficulty with walking due to stiffness in my legs. It was at this stage that my doctor diagnosed MS and put me on baclofen. Since then my walking has been a little easier."

Basic nerve structure

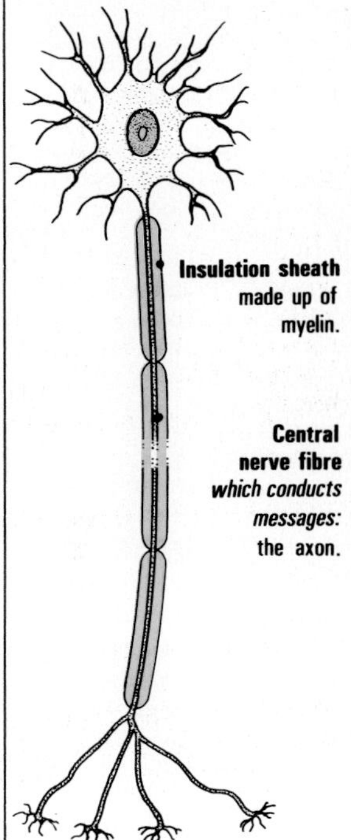

HOME ADAPTATIONS

Home assessment by an occupational therapist can provide a considerable range of aids to improve mobility and increase independence, as well as advice on how to prevent the complications associated with immobility. These are frequently the most important issues in caring for MS patients.

NAMES YOU WILL HEAR

Premedication

Generic name: diazepam; **trade names:** Valium, Alupram, Atensine, Evacalm, Solis, Tensium, Valrelease. **Generic name:** lorazepam; **trade names:** Ativan, Lorazepam. **Generic name:** papaveretum; **trade name:** Omnopon. **Generic name:** papaveretum and hyoscine; **trade name:** Omnopon and Scopolamine. **Generic name:** morphine; **trade names:** Roxanol, Nepenthe, MST Continus, Duromorph, Cyclimorph. **Generic name:** pethidine, meperedine; **trade names:** Demerol, Pethilorfan, Pamergan, Pethoid, Demer-Idine; usually prescribed by generic name. **Generic name:** atropine sulfate; **trade names:** Atropine Sulfate. **Generic name:** hyoscine hydrobromide; **trade name:** Scopolamine.

Intravenous induction agents

Generic name: thiopental sodium or thiopental sodium; **trade names:** Pentothal, Intravel Sodium. **Generic name:** methohexital sodium; **trade names:** Brevital, Brietal. **Generic name:** midazolam; **trade names:** Versed, Hypnovel. **Generic name:** diazepam; **trade names:** Valium, Alupram, Atensine, Evacalm, Solis, Tensium, Valrelease.

Inhalation agents

Generic name: halothane; **trade name:** Fluothane. **Generic name:** enflurane; **trade name:** Euthrane. **Generic name:** isoflurane; **trade name:** Forane. **Generic name:** nitrous oxide; **trade name:** Nitrous Oxide.

Muscle relaxants

Generic name: succinylcholine chloride; **trade names:** Quelecin, Sucostrin, Scoline, Anectine. **Generic name:** alcuronium chloride; **trade name:** Alloferin. **Generic name:** pancuronium bromide; **trade name:** Pavulon. **Generic name:** vecuronium; **trade name:** Norcuron. **Generic name:** atracurium besylate; **trade name:** Tracrium.

WHAT ARE ANESTHETICS?

– The drugs used to produce ''anesthesia'', a state of freedom from pain during surgical operations. Some examinations are also carried out under anesthesia, for example of the bladder (cystoscopy) and some X-ray procedures. Anesthesia may be ''general'', in which case the patient is unconscious during the procedure, or ''local'', when the nerves to the part to be operated on are ''frozen'' and the area feels numb and sometimes cannot be moved. The patient may be conscious during a local anesthetic, or sedated.

PRESCRIPTION DRUGS

Premedication is given by mouth or injection before the patient leaves the ward. Its purpose is to provide relief from anxiety, a measure of sedation, and sometimes loss of memory; it may also cause a dry mouth.

How they work: by acting on various parts of the brain. Drugs which dry the mouth act on the autonomic nervous system – which controls involuntary functions such as digestion and salivation.

The **intravenous induction** agents are most commonly given by injection into a vein, usually by the anesthesiologist, to induce unconsciousness. If a patient really dislikes injections, or if a suitable vein is difficult to find, an inhalation agent is the alternative.

Modern anesthesia is not just a single state produced by a single drug, but is comprised of different aspects, provided by different drugs administered during the course of an operation. In addition to unconsciousness, the aim is to provide pain relief, by means of analgesics; and also physical relaxation, by means of muscle relaxants. Using these procedures, an anesthesiologist can maintain an unconscious, pain-free patient at a relatively light level of anesthesia. This means that the patient recovers consciousness more quickly after surgery, and suffers fewer of the adverse effects of deep anesthesia.

How they work: General anesthetics depress the brain, producing unconsciousness, but they can also depress other body functions, such as those of heart, lungs and blood vessels and this is why the state of anesthesia needs to be continually monitored. **Local anesthetics** block nerves and stop pain impulses from the surgical operation site from passing along these nerves to reach the brain. The drugs are injected near the nerves, and during the injection, the patient may feel tingling or ''pins and needles'', and occasionally, transient pain. These drugs can also be applied to the skin, eyes and linings of body orifices such as the mouth, nose, anus and urethra. Such preparations are used before minor procedures such insertion of a catheter; removal of a foreign body from the eye; insertion of a drip.

How they work: a complex chemical process involving ion changes across nerve membranes.

OVER-THE-COUNTER-TREATMENTS

The pain of a sore throat or painful hemorrhoids can be relieved by the use of proprietary preparations which contain local anesthetic as one of the constituents.

QUESTIONS TO ASK THE DOCTOR

These questions are better put to an anesthesiologist rather than to a general practitioner. They are especially important before having an anesthetic as an outpatient.

- Will I have a local or a general anesthetic?
- How long must I not eat or drink before the anesthetic?
- When will I be able to resume normal activity?
- When will I be able to drive my car?
- Should I stop smoking before the anesthetic?
- Should I continue to take my usual pills?

SIDE EFFECTS

Even after a long **general anesthetic** for major surgery, recovery of consciousness will be quite rapid, although there may be disorientation and drowsiness afterwards. Some, probably a minority, suffer nausea and vomiting – but this is not a major problem of modern anesthetics. Likewise, some patients feel "hung-over"; others not at all. After **minor outpatient surgery,** recovery is usually fast and complete, but there will nevertheless be some who suffer headache, sickness, sore throat and soreness at the site of injection. These are usually mild and short-term. There is also the remote, but real chance that a patient may react adversely to an anesthetic, and here the consequences can be grave. In practice, this risk is tiny, provided the anesthesiologist has the appropriate background information about the patient – see BEFORE GOING INTO THE HOSPITAL. The range of modern anesthetics available means that there is a safe one for almost everybody.

SELF-MANAGEMENT

- You may not be allowed a drink immediately after a general anesthetic; if you are, take just a few sips. If you feel no nausea, then drink larger amounts.

Analgesics
Generic name: morphine; **trade names:** Roxanol, Nepenthe, MST Continus, Duromorph, Cyclimorph. **Generic names:** pethidine, meperedine; **trade names:** Demerol, Pethilorfan, Pamergan, Pethoid, Demer-Idine. **Generic name:** fentanyl citrate; **trade names:** Sublimaze, Thalamonal.

Local anesthetics
Generic names: lignocaine hydrochloride, lidocaine hydrochloride; **trade names:** Xylocaine, Xylotox, Lidothesin, Lignostab. **Generic name:** bupivacaine hydrochloride; **trade name:** Marcain.

PATIENTS' EXPERIENCES

"I had the premedication at breakfast-time and to my astonishment, after a two-hour operation, I was feeling back to normal at lunch-time: clear-headed, wide-awake and not even queasy. It was nothing like my last operation ten years ago."

PRE-SURGERY NERVES

If you are especially anxious about an operation, you could have a sleeping pill the night before: your family doctor will advise. Don't drive yourself to the hospital; allow plenty of time for the journey so that you can arrive calmly. Don't take any alcohol the evening before going into hospital.

ILLNESS BEFORE ANESTHESIA

Telephone the hospital if you have an illness within four weeks of admission for a procedure under anesthesia. This applies to any illness, even a common cold. You will be advised on whether the operation should be postponed.

BEFORE GOING INTO THE HOSPITAL

Make a note of everything you can remember about illnesses; previous anesthetics; all drugs you are taking, especially steroids; any allergies to anything, even bandaids; any problems which you or any member of your family has had with anesthesia.

Infections

The body is prone to infections by many different organisms. Sometimes these are viruses which establish themselves inside cells (for example influenza); sometimes they are caused by bacteria and occasionally by parasites. In tropical countries, parasitic diseases are common, but the only one of real concern in developed countries is malaria. This disease is on the increase in the West, due largely to the growth of air travel.

Some infections are dealt with in this book under the part of the body affected rather than here. For example pneumonia, page 78 and cystitis, page 142.

See also: *Pneumonia and pleurisy, page 78; tuberculosis, page 80; middle and external ear infections, page 256; sinusitis, page 262; laryngitis, page 266; red eye and dry eye, page 268; acne, page 274; fungal infections, page 284; scabies and nits, page 286.*

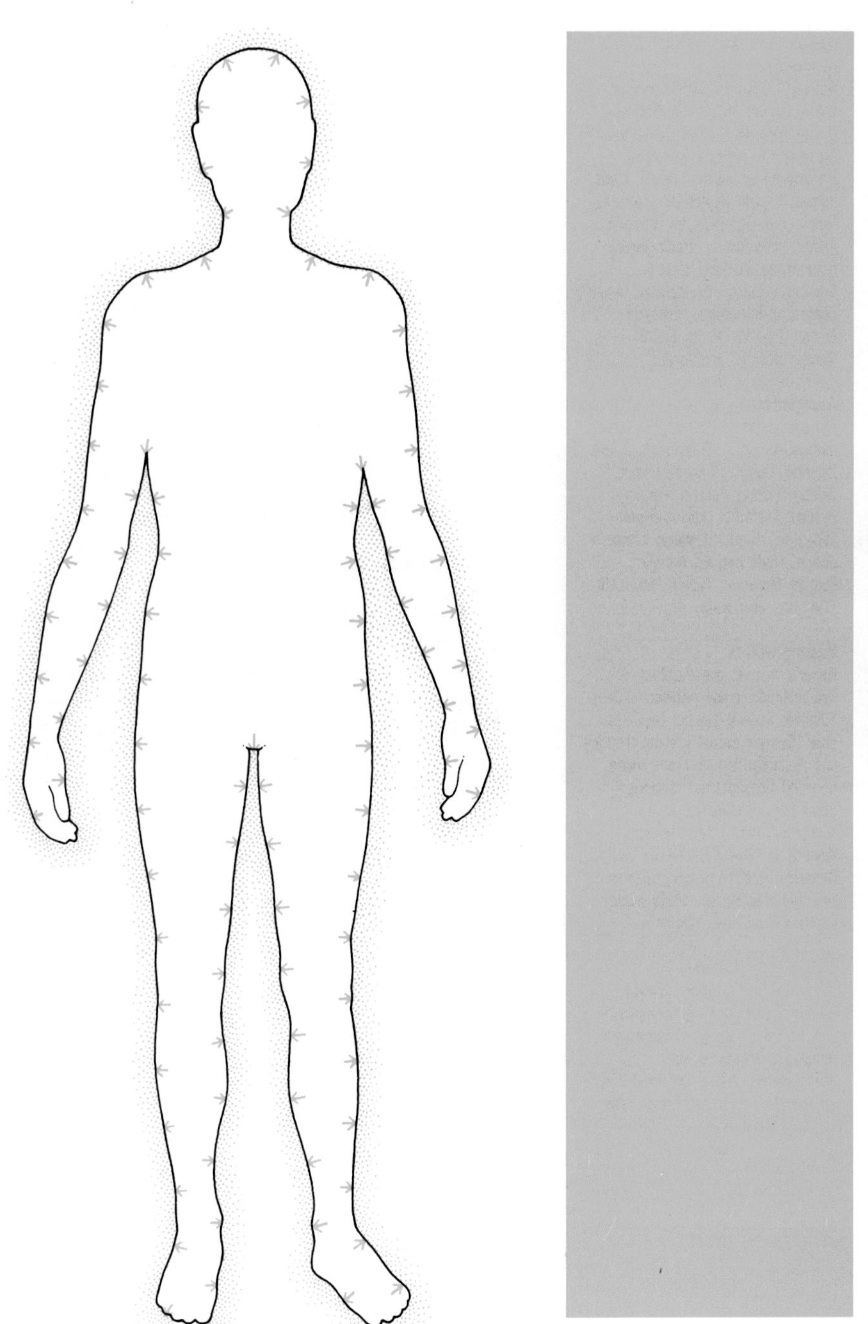

Antibiotics, analgesics/antipyretics, decongestants, nasal decongestants

NAMES YOU WILL HEAR

Antibiotics

Generic name: amoxycillin sodium; **trade names:** Augmentin, Polymox, Triniox, Wymox, Amoxil, Moxacin, Moxilean, Novamoxin, Penamox. **Generic name:** co-trimoxazole; **trade names:** Septra, Septra DS, Bactrim, Fectrim, Nodilon, Septrim. **Generic name:** erythromycin; **trade names:** Benzamycin, Erymax, Ilotycin, Arpimycin, Erycen, Erythroped, Retcin, Erythrocin, Erythromid, EpMycin, Erostin, Emu-V, Ethryn, Eromel, Illocap, Illosone, Rythrocaps.

Analgesics

Generic name: acetaminophen; **trade names:** Anacin 3, Phenaphon, Datril, Panadol, Tempra, Tylenol, Pamol, Calpol, Tylenon, Paracin, Parmol, Panado, Ceetamol, Atosol, Exctol, Ennagesic, Ilvamol. **Generic name:** aspirin; **trade names:** Ascriptin, Ecotrin, Measurin, Aspirin, Astrin, Bi-Prin. *See also* ***pain,*** *page 106.*

Decongestants

Generic names: pseudoephedrine hydrochloride; **trade names:** Actifed, Sudafed, Sudelix, Drixora Repetabs, Eltor. **Generic name:** pseudoephedrine and diphenhydramine; **trade name:** Benadryl Decongestant. **Generic name:** pseudoephedrine and chlorpheniramine; **trade names:** Sinutab, Sudafed Plus, Isoclor. **Generic name:** phenylpropanolamine and chlorpheniramine; **trade names:** Comtrex, Triaminic, Contac.

Locally-acting nasal decongestants (nose drops)

Generic name: phenylpropanolamine and brompheniramine; **trade name:** Dimetapp. **Generic name:** phenylephrine; **trade names:** 4-Way Dristan Mist, Neo-synephrine, Vicks Syrup. **Generic name:** ephidrine hydrochloride; **trade name:** Ephidrine Nose Drops. **Generic name:** normal saline 0.9% nose drops; **trade name:** Normal Saline Nose Drops.

WHAT IS A COMMON COLD?

– A viral infection of the nose and throat. The illness begins suddenly with sneezing, a sore throat and a profuse watery discharge from the nose. There may be associated fever and general malaise. These symptoms usually last two or three days. Secondary infection by bacteria may occur, causing sinusitis *(page 262),* ear infection *(page 256),* laryngitis *(page 266),* tonsillitis *(see below),* or pneumonia *(page 78).*

CAUSES A number of different viruses are usually responsible. Infection occurs from contact with other people who have the virus, which is spread via moisture droplets, either breathed or sneezed out. Cold weather does not cause colds, but rapid changes in body temperature may make the body more susceptible to viral infection. Overcrowding also favors spread of the virus. Infection by one of the common cold viruses does not give immunity to others.

PRESCRIPTION DRUGS

Antibiotics should not be used at the onset of a cold. In the elderly and the very young, in patients with chronic diseases like asthma, chronic bronchitis or heart disease, there may be a temptation to use antibiotics to prevent the development of bacterial infections which could rapidly result in serious illness. Antibiotics do not, however, shorten the duration of a common cold, as they have no effect on the viruses causing it. Antibiotics are used for the treatment of bacterial sinusitis, ear infection, laryngitis, tonsillitis and pneumonia if they develop during a cold.

How they work: by killing bacteria responsible for infection. *See* ***pneumonia*** *and* ***pleurisy,*** *page 78* and ***drugs in children,*** *page 196.*

OVER-THE-COUNTER TREATMENTS

Analgesics/antipyretics such as apirin and acetaminophen help to lower the temperature (antipyretic effect) and ease muscle pains and headache. Their action only lasts four to six hours and they should be repeated regularly if the temperature is high.

How they work: *see* ***pain,*** *page 106.* Children under 12 should be given acetaminophen, *not aspirin:* see **SIDE EFFECTS.** For adults, the choice between the two can be entirely personal. Aspirin may be more effective, both as a painkiller and as an antipyretic but it can have serious side effects (see below).

Decongestants are meant to dry up the nasal secretions,

reduce swelling of the nasal passages, and so unblock the nose.
How they work: by constricting the blood vessels in the nose, thus limiting the secretions and reducing swelling of the membranes in the nose. They are not always effective.
Decongestant nose drops also help to reduce nasal secretions and unblock the nose.
How they work: in the same way as decongestants taken by mouth. Normal saline (salt water) nose drops work by loosening the mucus in the nose, thus helping to unblock the nasal passages.

It is best to choose single-ingredient medicines rather than those with analgesic and decongestant combined. Some ingredients need to be given more frequently than others and the doses in a combination treatment are not always in the right concentration. An active ingredient gives more flexibility of timing and dose.

All of these medicines may be used together, and antibiotics can be combined with any of them, too.

QUESTIONS TO ASK THE DOCTOR

■ What will happen if my temperature goes up? How can I get it down?
■ How long will the cold last?
■ How long should I take the medicine(s)?

SIDE EFFECTS

All medicines have side effects so it is important to take only those medicines which are absolutely necessary to relieve significant symptoms and promote recovery. Taking excess drugs for minor illnesses such as the common cold may result in side effects which are worse than the illness.

Antibiotics: *see* ***pneumonia*** *and* ***pleurisy,*** *page 78.*
Acetaminophen has no common side effects when taken in the correct dose, except in patients with severe liver or kidney disease. Because it has an effect on the liver, it is not advisable to take it with alcohol. Skin rashes occur occasionally.
Aspirin can cause nausea, ringing in the ears and even deafness. These effects are not usually seen except in very high doses and will disappear as soon as the drug is stopped. It also causes indigestion due to gastric irritation, which can be minimized by taking the drug after food. Occasionally it causes such severe irritation to the stomach that vomiting or bleeding results. This complication usually occurs on high doses, but some

PATIENT'S EXPERIENCE
"I came home from work with a slight tickle in my throat. Soon after, I started sneezing a lot and my nose was running. I took some of the common cold treatment we had in the medicine chest and went to bed. I couldn't sleep because my nose was blocked and during the night I became feverish. I was afraid to take any more medicine, as it said that it should be taken every eight hours. The next day I was feeling a bit better but my four-year-old daughter had the same symptoms. My wife called the doctor. He said give her a dose of acetaminophen and by the time we got her to his office she was a bit less feverish. He told us to run a bath and let her play in it, slowly letting in more cold water until it was quite cool. She was happy to play in the bath for nearly half an hour and by then her temperature had returned to normal. He mentioned that the temperature often goes up in the late afternoon and that she should have more acetaminophen and another cool bath then, and again during the night if necessary."

people are more sensitive than others. Aspirin should not be taken with alcohol, as both have this effect on the stomach and the risk of vomiting blood is increased.

Occasionally, a patient has an allergic reaction to aspirin. This manifests itself as a skin rash, and wheezing with difficulty breathing. If this occurs, aspirin should not be taken again. Aspirin should not be given to children under age 12 years, except on instruction by the doctor. Reye's syndrome, a serious disease of brain and liver, has occurred in some children given aspirin for fever. Aspirin should not be taken during pregnancy and should be used with caution in patients with asthma, liver or kidney disease.

Decongestants usually contain two active compounds. One of these acts on the blood vessels in the nose and in other parts of the body; they should not be used in patients with high blood pressure, heart disease, diabetes, thyroid disease nor in patients on some drugs for the treatment of depression. They should not be given to babies under one year since they may cause hyperactivity. Many decongestants also contain antihistamines which cause drowsiness, and should not be taken when driving or working in a potentially dangerous environment. This effect is made worse by drinking alcohol. Do not take decongestants during pregancy: their antihistamine content has been associated with fetal abnormality and they may constrict blood supply to the placenta.

Nose drops can cause irritation to the membranes inside the nose, which in turn may cause more congestion. If used for long periods (two weeks or more), they can cause permanent damage to the sensitive membrane inside the nose. These drugs should not be given to babies (see above). It is safe to give babies normal saline nose drops, but even these are only indicated if there is extreme difficulty in feeding.

SELF-MANAGEMENT

In older children, and in adults, the common cold is usually mild: it is often not necessary to see a doctor.

■ Bed-rest is not essential. A day or two spent quietly at home, however, will tend to shorten recovery time and lessen the spread of the infection.

■ The temperature may be high, and this should be brought down with aspirin or acetaminophen (see above), particularly in children under six, in whom there is always a risk of "febrile convulsions". Bring the fever down immediately, even if the doctor has already been called. A cool (not cold) bath is often useful, indeed necessary, if the fever is running high. It lowers the temperature for four to six hours, and may need to be repeated. Patients often feel dramatically better once the temperature has returned to normal, so it is doubly worthwhile treating fever early and effectively. The patient will probably feel more inclined to eat and drink when the temperature is lowered, and vomiting is less likely.

■ The temperature is more likely to go up in the late afternoon and early evening and this should be anticipated. It is better to put a child into a cool bath *before* he or she starts feeling uncomfortable. Repeat the cool bath during the night if necessary: the child will often sleep for a few hours if the temperature is down to normal.

■ Don't hesitate to treat the symptoms of headache and muscle pains with acetaminophen or aspirin.

■ Decongestants are useful if the blocked nose is so severe that it interferes with rest.

■ Drink plenty of fluids, particularly water or fruit drinks: a high temperature can lead to dehydration.

■ Food intake is less important than fluid intake, as the illness does not usually last for long. Children, in particular, should be allowed to eat whatever they like.

■ Colds in babies up to about six months are particularly distressing. The blocked nose may interfere with feeding. Ephedrine nose drops are too strong; but normal saline nose drops will liquify the mucus in the nose and usually help to unblock it. If this does not work, a baby can be given milk with a spoon for a while. Breast feeding should be continued whenever possible. If the mother has some resistance to the infecting virus, antibodies from the mother's milk will pass on some resistance to the baby and help speed recovery. Clear fluid should also be offered as well as milk, especially if the temperature is high: again, the object is to prevent dehydration.

Controlling the temperature is very important. A baby with a cold should be dressed in cool, loose clothing – a top and a diaper are usually all that is necessary. Acetaminophen should be given in the correct dose for age and frequent cool baths may be necessary. Cooling a baby in this way is not dangerous; but a high temperature left untreated can be serious because of the risk of convulsions.

■ The patient should start feeling better after two or three days. If recovery is delayed, it it worth consulting a doctor.

TONSILLITIS

– Can be confused with the common cold. It is an infection of the tonsil glands, which guard the entrance to the gullet at the back of the mouth. There is usually a sore throat and it may be painful to swallow. A gargle with salty water (one teaspoonful per pint) or with dilute aspirin solution is often the best treatment, although in severe cases a doctor may have to prescribe an antibiotic.

NAMES YOU WILL HEAR

Influenza vaccine
Generic name: influenza vaccine; **trade names:** Fluvirin, Influvac.

Antibiotics
Generic name: amoxycillin sodium; **trade names:** Augmentin, Polymox, Triniox, Wymox, Amoxil, Moxacin, Moxilean, Novamoxin, Penamox. **Generic name:** co-trimoxazole; **trade names:** Septra, Septra DS, Bactrim, Fectrim, Nodilon, Septrim.

Analgesics
Generic name: acetaminophen; **trade names:** Anacin 3, Phenaphon, Datril, Panadol, Tempra, Pamol, Calpol, Tylenon, Paracin, Parmol, Panado, Ceetamol, Atosol, Exctol, Tylenol, Ennagesic, Ilvamol. **Generic name:** aspirin; **trade names:** Ascriptin, Ecotrin, Measurin, Aspirin, Astrin, Bi-Prin. *See also* ***pain,*** *page 106.*

WHAT IS INFLUENZA?

– An acute, highly infectious disease which tends to occur in epidemics. The symptoms are those of a general illness, and include fever, headache and muscle pains, with or without nausea and vomiting. Sneezing, sore throat and a profuse watery discharge from the nose can also occur, as in the common cold. The patient usually feels distinctly unwell.

Severe consequences of influenza can include complications such as inflammation of the heart muscle or brain. Secondary infection by bacteria can occur too, causing sinusitis, ear infection or pneumonia *(see pages 262, 256 and 78).*

Most patients are ill for a few days, then recover rapidly. Some have a more prolonged convalescence with mental and physical lethargy, even depression, lasting weeks or even months (post-viral syndrome).

CAUSE The influenza virus, of which there are many different strains. Infection by one strain does not result in immunity to others. The virus is spread in the same way as for the ***common cold,*** *page 134.*

PRESCRIPTION DRUGS

Influenza immunization may be a good idea for the elderly, and for patients with chronic diseases such as asthma, chronic bronchitis, heart disease or a generally lowered resistance to infection. Such individuals are more likely to develop the severe complications and secondary bacterial infection. People who cannot take time off work might also benefit. The vaccine is given by injection in autumn – the start of the flu season.
How it works: For a flu vaccine to be effective, it is necessary to predict which strains of virus are likely to be in circulation. Each year the World Health Organization recommends which should be included in the vaccine; it ought then to protect against about 70 per cent of infections by these strains. The effect lasts for about 12 months.
Antiemetics, in liquid form, are useful against the vomiting, when and if it occurs. Because the side effects of these drugs are significant they should only be used in cases of persistent vomiting, and not if a patient just feels a little nauseous. This applies especially to children, in whom the side effects are commoner than in adults.
How they work: by acting on the brain, suppressing the stimulus to vomit.
Antibiotics are not usually used at the beginning of the il-

lness; their use is discussed in ***common cold,*** *page 134*.

OVER-THE-COUNTER TREATMENTS

*See **common cold,** page 134.*

QUESTIONS TO ASK THE DOCTOR

*See **common cold,** page 134.*

SIDE EFFECTS

Influenza vaccine can cause a painful local reaction at the injection site. It can also cause fever and malaise, within a few hours or days of the injection, but these are usually mild. Severe, but rare, reactions can occur in patients allergic to egg protein, or to antibiotics contained in the vaccine.

Antiemetics cause a dry mouth, skin rash and drowsiness. They should not be taken while driving or working in a potentially dangerous environment. The drowsiness is made worse by alcohol. Muscle stiffness and spasms can also occur. These are usually associated with high doses, but children, and some adults, are especially sensitive; however, an antidote is available. **Antiemetics** should not ever be used on children under 22 lbs (10 kg) or on patients who are dehydrated – the side effects would be more likely to occur than usual.

For side effects of **antibiotics,** *see **penumonia and pleurisy,** page 78,* and for analgesics, *see **common cold,** page 134.*

SELF-MANAGEMENT

Generally the illness is more severe than the common cold: the temperature is usually higher, headache and muscle pains more severe. Nausea and vomiting are frequent in influenza, but rare in the common cold. This in mind, self-treatment as in ***common cold,*** *page 134*, applies equally well to influenza.

■ Remember that all medicines have side effects: if treating yourself, only take those medicines which are absolutely necessary to relieve significant symptoms and promote recovery. ■ It is impossible to isolate patients with influenza and thus there is no way to prevent them passing on the virus. The patient is most likely to pass on the virus the day before the symptoms begin. ■ The patient should start feeling better after three or four days, but an early return to full activities can delay recovery and should be avoided. If there is a delay in recovery beyond two weeks, consult a doctor.

PATIENT'S EXPERIENCE

"When I hear that influenza occurs in epidemics, I can believe it. Half the people in my office were down with it when I started feeling ill. My muscles were so painful that I could hardly walk and by the time I got home, I had a high temperature and a headache. My wife was so worried that she called the doctor. He listened carefully to my heart and chest and said that things were not too bad, as I was generally quite fit. He prescribed aspirin every four hours and a cool bath, and after that I felt better – but weak. It was four or five days before I felt well enough to get up. The doctor suggested that I did no physical exercise for a month, and I must say I didn't feel like it. Even once I was back at work, I found that I got tired easily. I was moody and depressed for months afterwards, which I believe is common.

I have my own small business and can't afford to take much time off. Next year all of us at the office will have flu vaccinations."

POST-VIRAL SYNDROME

Depression, continuing weeks or even months, is in most cases mild, but occasionally requires drug therapy. If it is significantly interfering with work and social life, discuss it with your doctor. Even the most severe cases resolve over a few months, and the condition does not predispose to recurrent bouts of depression.

WHEN TO CALL THE DOCTOR

A doctor should see elderly, young and chronically ill patients. For the few cases where lethargy continues for weeks or even months afterwards, there is no specific treatment, though rest is important.

NAMES YOU WILL HEAR

Antiviral agents
Generic name: idoxuridine; **trade name:** Herpid, Herplex. **Generic name:** acyclovir; **trade name:** Zovirax.

Simple analgesics
Generic name: acetaminophen; **trade names:** Phenaphon, Panadol, Tempra, Tylenol, Pamol, Calpol, Tylenon, Paracin, Parmol, Panado, Ceetamol, Atosol, Exctol, Ennagesic, Ilvamol. **Generic name:** aspirin; **trade names:** Ascriptin, Ecotrin, Measurin, Aspirin, Astrin, Bi-Prin. **Generic name:** ibuprofen; **trade names:** Motrin, Apsifen, Advil, Ebufac, Brufen, Fenbid, Medipren, Nuprin, Ibumetin, Lidifen, Paxofen. **Generic name:** naproxen sodium; **trade names:** Naprosyn, Anaprox, Synflex, Laraflex. *See also* ***pain,*** *page 106.*

Compound analgesics
Generic name: acetaminophen and propoxyphene hydrochloride; **trade names:** Darvocet N-50, N-100, Wygesic. **Generic name:** acetaminophen plus codeine; **trade name:** Tylenol Codeine #1, #2, #3, #4. **Generic name:** calamine lotion; **trade name:** Calamine Lotion.

WHAT IS SHINGLES?

– An infection caused by the chicken pox virus, *herpes zoster*. The virus lies dormant in the nerves of the body for many years after the chicken pox infection, but can suddenly become activated, spreading down a nerve, causing a painful, itchy rash in the area of the skin supplied by that nerve. Often the pain, which can be severe, will precede the skin rash by a day or two. Small blisters appear, which last for some weeks. Usually several adjacent nerves on one side of the body are affected. The rash stops exactly in the mid line, which is where the nerve itself ends. Occasionally, a nerve of the face and eye is affected. Blisters developing on the cornea of the eye may lead to scarring and impaired vision if not treated promptly. General symptoms include nausea, lethargy and loss of appetite.

The rash may increase over about a week, but once improvement begins, it is unlikely to reappear in other areas, or spread further. The pain usually subsides as the rash improves, but occasionally (and especially in older people), the pain may last for many months.

The *herpes zoster* virus is not the same as *herpes simplex,* which causes cold sores and genital herpes.

CAUSE Why the virus is suddenly activated is not always known, but shingles is more common in patients with impaired immunity.

PRESCRIPTION DRUGS

Antiviral agents are of limited use: viruses live within the body cells and as a result are relatively inaccessible. Thus topical acyclovir is of limited usefulness. Taken by mouth it is more likely to reduce the duration of pain during the severe phase and decrease the incidence of prolonged pain afterwards; they may also alleviate the eye pain.

How they work: by preventing the virus from multiplying.

Analgesics: Pain is the most serious problem with shingles, and its treatment, particularly in older patients, is important. As the pain can last for months, depression, loss of appetite and general debility may occur if the pain is not adequately treated. Aspirin and acetaminophen may not be sufficient, in which case a doctor will suggest something stronger.

How they work: *see* ***pain,*** *page 106,* and ***rheumatoid arthritis,*** *page 242.*

Compound analgesics are an option if, as is possible, the pain is really severe. Doctors do not, however, like using them because the disadvantages usually outweigh the advantages. The advantages are that each ingredient may be used in a lower dose, thus decreasing side effects. Sometimes the drugs in the preparation enhance each others' effect, giving better pain relief than that normally expected from the sum of the component parts. The disadvantages are that some ingredients need to be given more frequently than others, and the doses of the various ingredients are not always in the correct concentration.

How they work: *see **pain**, page 106,* and ***rheumatoid arthritis**, page 242.*

OVER-THE-COUNTER TREATMENTS

If the drugs your doctor has given are failing to control the pain, be sure to go back to discuss it. Some of the drugs already prescribed may contain aspirin or acetaminophen, and if you treat yourself with these drugs in addition, overdose may result. Calamine lotion will help dry the blisters and stop the itch.

QUESTIONS TO ASK THE DOCTOR

- How long will it last? How long is it contagious?
- Would antiviral drugs be useful?

SIDE EFFECTS

Antiviral agents: idoxuridine solution can cause stinging on application and overuse can damage the skin. Acyclovir used locally can cause stinging on application or occasionally redness or drying of the skin. If given as a tablet it can cause nausea, headache, fatigue, impaired liver and kidney function, and also blood and nerve abnormalities.

Analgesics: acetaminophen and aspirin: *see **common cold**, page 134.* Ibuprofen and naproxen: *see **pain**, page 106* and ***rheumatoid arthritis**, page 242.*

The side effects of the **compound analgesics** are those of their component parts. Codeine phosphate causes constipation. Propoxyphene is a narcotic analgesic and carries a slight risk of abuse and addiction. It should be used with caution in patients with asthma, lung, kidney or liver disease. Side effects include nausea, constipation, retention of urine, and suppression of breathing.

SELF-MANAGEMENT

- Relief of pain is essential: remember to take analgesics on time. Delaying until pain is severe makes you feel much worse.
- If you are depressed, discuss this with your doctor: it is not unusual, or a sign of weakness.

PATIENT'S EXPERIENCE

"I was a fit 66-year-old when I developed shingles. I noticed an itchy sensation on my left side and a day later the skin was red and very painful. I felt generally ill, as if I had 'flu. Then blisters appeared on the skin and the pain became very severe. My doctor confirmed that it was shingles. The pain dominated my whole day and I lived for the moment that I could take the next dose of painkiller. Neither acetaminophen or ibuprofen gave much relief. The one that really worked was Tylenol no. 3, but the effect wore off just before the next dose was due. The pharmacist also recommended calamine lotion to dry the blisters.

What worried me most of all was that the inflammation and blistering might extend inside my abdomen: the pain certainly seemed to penetrate right into me. My doctor reassured me that this was not the case.

The pain made me feel sick. I was tired all the time and did not feel like eating. My neighbor came in every day and brought me a light meal of salad and cheese or fish. I was grateful for this: left on my own, I would not have bothered to eat. Over a few weeks, the pain eased a little. My doctor was sympathetic: however, he said that he did not feel that I needed an antidepressant unless things really got too much for me. In the end, it did improve – but even now, a year later, I can still feel the pain sometimes."

PASSING ON SHINGLES

Shingles can only be passed on as chicken pox, and only to those people who have not had chicken pox.

Shingles typically occurs in people who have once had chicken pox, usually becoming apparent when they are debilitated or immunocompromised

Antibiotics, sodium bicarbonate

NAMES YOU WILL HEAR
Antibiotics
Generic name: sulphamethizole; **trade names:** Microsul, Urolucosil, Urolex, Uroz, Thiosulfil, S-Methizole, Thiosulfil. **Generic name:** ampicillin; **trade names:** Omnipen, Polycillin, Principen, Ampifen, Penbritin, Pentrexyl, Vidopen, Austrapen, Bristin, Amcill, Ampicin, Ampilean, Biosan, Ampil, Famicilin, Pentrex, Petercillin, Synthecillin. **Generic name:** co-trimoxazole; **trade names:** Septra, Bactrim, Fectrim, Nodilon, Septrin. **Generic name:** nalidixic acid; **trade names:** NegGram, Mictral, Uriben. **Generic name:** nitrofuroantoin; **trade names:** Furadantin, Macrodantin.

WHAT IS CYSTITIS?

– An inflammation of the bladder. It may be accompanied by, or mimicked by urethritis, an inflammation of the tube by which urine passes from the bladder out of the body. Typical symptoms are painful and frequent urination, lower abdominal pain, blood in the urine and a high temperature.

CAUSES The root cause is either infection or bruising. The infection may be present in the kidneys or bloodstream and descend to the bladder, but more commonly it ascends from the urethra.

PRESCRIPTION DRUGS

Antibiotics: the common remedy. Many types are available; those listed here are particularly suited to treating cystitis; typically taken in pill form.
How they work: By killing bacteria responsible for infection. However, some bacteria can become resistant to some antibiotics; the antibiotic becomes ineffective, and a different one has to be prescribed. Antibiotics also have a tendency to kill not only the 'target' bacteria, but others as well; as some bacteria are naturally helpful in fighting harmful bacteria, a course of antibiotics can leave you without natural defenses.
Sodium bicarbonate helps relieve discomfort of cystitis.
How it works: by neutralizing acid in the urine.

OVER-THE-COUNTER TREATMENTS

Potassium citrate used to be a commonly recommended treatment but is no longer advised because if the kidneys are damaged a dangerous build-up of potassium could occur.

QUESTIONS TO ASK THE DOCTOR

- How long should I take the antibiotics?
- How soon will the symptoms go?
- How will I know whether they are working?
- What happens if I am allergic to the antibiotics?

SIDE EFFECTS

Antibiotics are usually prescribed for less than one week, but for recurrent cystitis you may take them for several weeks. Antibiotics can make you feel under-the-weather and lethargic; some people are allergic to them, and may develop a rash. Report this to a doctor immediately.
Potassium citrate: A helpful treatment, but it tastes awful, and could make you vomit.

SELF-MANAGEMENT

If you have had cystitis once, work against future infection – and the need to take antibiotics:

■ After using lavatory paper in the usual way, soap hands and gently clean anus; rinse hands, then pour a bottle of warm water over anus away from vagina.

■ Wear cotton underpants and change them daily. Avoid wearing panty hose. Rinse underwear well and do not use strong detergents or bleach.

■ Always pass urine within 15 minutes of sexual intercourse and then wash the uro-genital area with cool water. Rest – if possible.

■ Drink as little alcohol as possible, and if you do, try to have long drinks, and some bland liquid afterwards.

■ Drink 1-2 quarts of bland liquid or water daily.

SELF-HELP IN AN ATTACK

As soon as the attack begins:

1 Get a couple of heating pads. **2** Drink one pint of cold water and let your stomach settle. **3** Take one teaspoon of bicarbonate of soda mixed in water or jelly. **4** Take two strong painkillers. **5** Fill a pitcher and glass with bland liquid; keep them by you and drink often. **6** Once each hour drink strong coffee. **7** Try to put your feet up, or go to bed. Take your jug and glass, but before resting, drink another half pint of fluid. **8** Put one heating pad on your back and the other high up between your legs, resting against the uretheral opening. **9** Every time you pass water, wash the surrounding area and gently pat it dry. **10** Continue to drink half a pint of liquid every 20 minutes.

The key to self-help is to drink large amounts of fluid, and to take sodium bicarbonate to make the urine less acid. However, if your kidneys do not function normally, this could be dangerous. Before attempting to manage subsequent attacks, get your doctor to measure your kidney function.

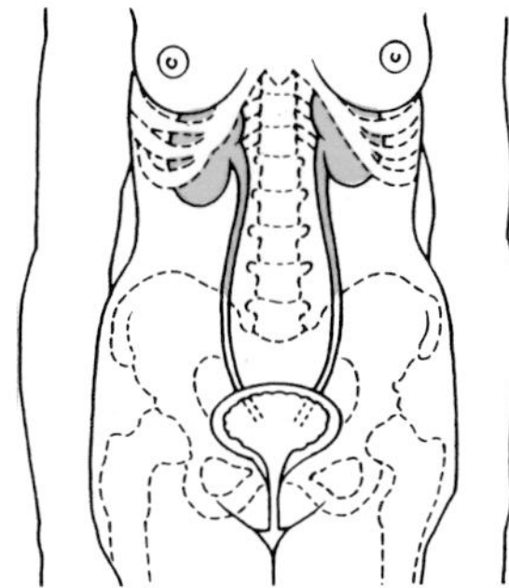

The kidneys *produce and excrete urine. Waste materials in the blood are extracted in the kidneys and transformed into urine. This passes via the ureter tubes to the bladder where it is stored until the bladder fills up. It then passes through a valve to the urethra, down which it passes to be expelled from the body.*

PATIENT'S EXPERIENCE

"My first treatment for cystitis was a month's course of antibiotics which made me really sick. A few weeks later, back came the cystitis, and more antibiotics were prescribed. Over the next few months I had to take 14 different types of pills. After a variety of investigations, including cauterizing of my urethra, I was prescribed yet more antibiotics. In the end, it was my doctor who said 'try passing water after intercourse'. After all that fruitless medication, it was this simple advice which worked."

NAMES YOU WILL HEAR
Generic name: ampicillin; **trade names:** Omnipen, Polycillin, Principen, Ampifen, Penbritin, Pentrexyl, Vidopen, Austrapen, Bristin, Amcill, Ampicin, Ampilean, Biosan, Ampil, Famicilin, Pentrex, Petercillin, Synthecillin. **Generic name:** oxytetracycline; **trade names:** Abbocin, Terramycin, Oxycycine, Beta-cycline, Oxytet, Berkmycen, Imperacin. **Generic name:** doxycycline; **trade names:** Vibramycin, Dioxin, Doxylor, Doxatet.

SYPHILIS, GONORRHEA, NSU

Syphilis is an infection spread by sexual intercourse. Several weeks after the disease has been contracted, a painless ulcer appears on the sex organs, and the lymph glands in the groin may become enlarged. A skin rash may follow later. Eventually the disease attacks the heart and nervous system.

Gonorrhea causes a discharge or leakage of pus from the urethra (water passage) in men, together with a burning sensation in the penis during the passage of urine. Symptoms usually appear a few days after infection has occurred. Women with gonorrhea usually have no symptoms, but may infect their partner, or a child born at the time of an active infection.

NSU (non-specific urethritis) also causes discharge and burning in men, but the symptoms are often quite mild and occur several weeks after the infection has been acquired. Women with NSU usually have no symptoms. However, if a woman has had sexual contact with a man with NSU, both partners should be treated in order to prevent them from re-infecting each other and also to prevent spread of the infection into her Fallopian tubes which can lead to infertility. *Chlamydia* is one of the organisms which can cause NSU.

Crabs (pubic lice) may be regarded as sexually transmitted disease: *see **scabies and nits,** page 286.*

PRESCRIPTION DRUGS

There is no alternative to treatment with **antibiotics** for these conditions.

Penicillin injections (typically given in the form of ampicillin) are used to treat syphilis. Approximately 14 injections may be required, depending on the stage of the infection.

Penicillin injections or tablets are used to treat gonorrhea, usually in a single high dose. Probenecid may be given to improve the effect of the penicillin.

Nowadays, a substantial number of gonorrhea cases fail to respond to penicillin because the organisms develop resistance to the drug. A specialist may be needed to advise on alternative therapy.

Tetracyclines are used to treat NSU, in treatments at least one week's duration. There are several different types of tetracycline.

Erythromycin is an alternative to tetracycline for the treatment of NSU.

QUESTIONS TO ASK THE DOCTOR

- How did I get this infection?

■ Have you checked me for any other sexually transmitted diseases?
■ How long must I avoid sexual intercourse?
■ How will I know I have been cured?
■ Does my partner need to be treated?

SIDE EFFECTS

Some patients are allergic to **penicillin** – it may cause a rash. Patients receiving penicillin for syphilis frequently develop a reaction early in the course of treatment: this is known as the Herxheimer reaction, which is not caused by allergy, and treatment can normally continue.

Tetracyclines and **erythromycin** may cause nausea. Most tetracyclines should be taken well before meals, and they should not be used in pregnant women because they can damage the developing bones and the teeth of the fetus.

SELF-MANAGEMENT

■ Take the full course of treatment as prescribed.
■ Don't have sex until you have been cleared.
■ Ensure that your partner(s) have been treated.
■ Restrict alcohol to minimize nausea, which could impair the treatment.
■ Take this opportunity to consider the health implications of your sexual lifestyle. Remember that condoms reduce the risk of transmission of infection, but do not guarantee protection.
■ Remember that symptoms from these conditions will rapidly improve once the infection has been treated.
■ Men with NSU may find that alcohol makes the symptoms worse.

PATIENT'S EXPERIENCE

"I had casual sex – just once – away one weekend. Two weeks later I noticed a burning sensation when I urinated. My doctor said I had cystitis and prescribed antibiotics which didn't work. When I went back, the doctor then said that it might be gonorrhea, and gave me some different pills. By now I was really worried, so I went to a sexually transmitted disease clinic, and had some tests. They told me I had NSU. This got rapidly better on treatment. But that, unfortunately, wasn't the end of it. The clinic also asked to see my regular girlfriend. She was angry at first, but agreed to be treated once it was explained that she might be carrying the infection without knowing it."

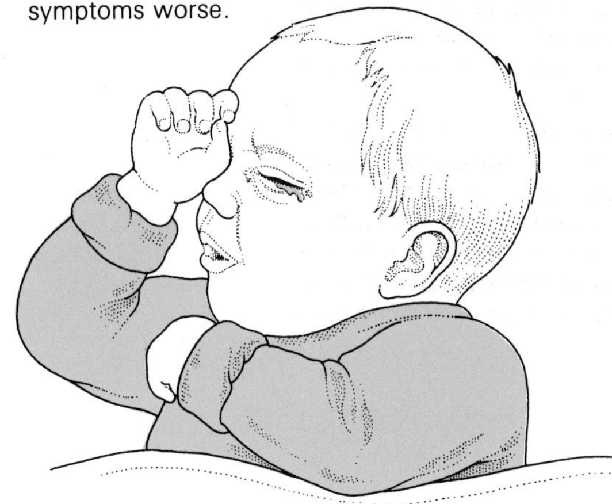

The unacceptable face of STD: *a baby can become infected with gonorrhea during birth; the resulting conjunctivitis may lead to blindness. Im some states, including California, it is a legal requirement to put drops of silver nitrate into the newborn's eyes to prevent the infection – regardless of the mother's standing and health.*

Fungicides, antibiotics, antiviral agents, podophyllin

Generic name: metronidazole; **trade names:** Flagyl, Vaginyl, Tichozole, Neo-Tric. **Generic name:** nystatin; **trade names:** Mycostatin, Nystan, Canstat. **Generic name:** clotrimazole; **trade name:** Nilstat, Canesten. **Generic name:** econazole; **trade names:** Ecostatin, Gyno-Pevaryl. **Generic name:** ketoconazole; **trade name:** Nizoral.

VAGINAL DISCHARGE, HERPES, GENITAL WARTS

Vaginal discharge: A certain amount of discharge may be quite normal, but an abnormal discharge is likely to be excessive, to smell unpleasant, and to cause irritation or itching. A retained tampon is sometimes the cause.

A yeast infection also known as thrush can bring about a thick white discharge and irritation, common after a course of antibiotics, and in diabetics. Some men carry the yeast organism which causes thrush and can re-infect their partner unless they are treated.

Trichomonas, or TV, causes a watery and highly irritating discharge. It is almost always sexually transmitted (men carry it without symptoms) and male sexual partners should therefore be treated too.

Anerobic vaginosis is a mixed infection causing a vaginal discharge, more noticeable after intercourse. It is not usually acquired sexually.

Herpes is caused by a virus which most of us carry in our bodies and is responsible for cold sores around the lips. Similar sores can also occur on the sex organs, and these can be acquired sexually. A first attack of herpes can be painful with multiple sores on the genitals and swelling of the lymph glands in the groin. The condition often recurs, although recurrent attacks tend to be far less severe than the original one. There is no cure, and sufferers may get recurrent attacks; but attacks can decrease in frequency over the years.

Genital warts are caused by certain strains of wart virus (papillomavirus or HPV), and are spread sexually. It may take weeks or months before they appear. Wart infection can result in abnormality in the cancer smear and this can progress in time to cancer of the cervix. Patients with genital warts may therefore need specialist advice and treatment. *See also* ***viral warts,*** *page 282.*

PRESCRIPTION DRUGS

Fungicides: Nystatin or imidazoles (eg clotrimazole) are used to treat thrush, given in the form of vaginal tablets and cream. Nystatin taken by mouth only clears the bowel. Ketoconazole by mouth can be given for severe resistant thrush, but see below.

Metronidazole is used to treat trichomonas and anerobic vaginosis – given either as a single large dose by mouth or as a short treatment.

Acyclovir, the antiviral agent, can be taken by mouth as a five-day treatment for a severe first attack of herpes. It is far less effective as a cream. For severe recurrent herpes it can be taken regularly to suppress attacks.

Genital warts are painted carefully with **podophyllin solution,** which inhibits the wart virus inside skin cells. The treatment may need to be repeated two or three times a week for several weeks. Other treatments for warts include cryotherapy (freezing), cautery, laser treatment and surgery. *See also* ***viral warts,*** *page 282.*
How they work: all these preparations kill the organism responsible, or prevent it from multiplying.

QUESTIONS TO ASK THE DOCTOR

- Will I infect my sexual partner?
- How long will the treatment last?
- What happens if the treatment doesn't work?

SIDE EFFECTS

Some vaginal tablets for thrush may suit some patients better than others, but treatment is usually safe.
Ketoconazole pills can cause liver damage and should therefore only be used for severe resistant thrush.
Metronidazole can cause nausea, and severe vomiting if taken with alcohol. It should be avoided in the first three months of pregnancy.
Acyclovir has few side effects, but should not be taken in pregnancy.
Podophyllin may cause skin irritation, especially if spilled on healthy skin. It should be washed off four to six hours after application.

SELF-MANAGEMENT

- Thrush: avoid unnecessary antibiotics, wear loose cotton underwear, avoid irritants (including detergents). If recurrent, has your partner been checked?
- TV: Ensure your partner has been treated before resuming sex.
- Herpes: Obtain definite diagnosis and advice from a specialist. Identify and avoid anything that could cause recurrences – and this includes stress. Look after your general health, rather than waste time on unproven remedies. Make sure you understand when you should avoid sex – it often helps if your partner also understands your condition. Ignore myths and old wives' tales about the condition: they are rarely correct.
- Warts: Persist with the treatment until you are cured. Use condoms to prevent spread to your partner. Have regular Pap smears.
- Thrush and TV: Bathe in plain or slightly salty water; avoid irritants. Use non-pasteurized yogurt on the vagina if no other treatment is available: it can be a fairly effective temporary measure.

PATIENT'S EXPERIENCE

"I was having recurrent herpes; it made me depressed and anxious. The doctor told me I had wasted time on quack remedies and sent me to a herpes counsellor. To my surprise she spoke as much about organizing my life and looking after my health generally as about the condition itself. I tried to get a firmer grasp on my life, and after a while I realized that no drug treatment was necessary. I started taking better care of myself generally. I found I could discuss the problem with my boyfriend; we have a good relationship. Soon the herpes started to improve, and now I only get an attack once or twice a year, usually when I have a heavy cold."

MALARIA

Chloroquine, proguanil, quinine, mefloquine Maloprim, Fansidar

NAMES YOU WILL HEAR
Generic name: chloroquine; **trade names:** Aralen, Nivaquine, Avloclor. **Generic name:** proguanil; **trade name:** Paludrine. **Generic name:** pyrimethramine plus dapsone; **trade name:** Maloprim. **Generic name:** pyrimethramine plus sulfadoxine; **trade name:** Fansidar. **Generic name:** mefloquine hydrochloride; **trade name:** usually prescribed by generic name. **Generic name:** amodiaquine; **trade name:** Camoquin.

At the root of malaria *is a parasite called* Plasmodium. *Swallowed by a mosquito, it multiplies in the insect's stomach, producing hundreds of cells which migrate to the saliva glands. When the mosquito bites a human, the parasite enters the bloodstream and quickly makes its way to the liver, where it again multiplies, and can live for years. From the liver, the parasites enter the bloodstream periodically, invading the red blood cells, again developing and multiplying. When mature, they rupture the red blood cells – which causes fever.*

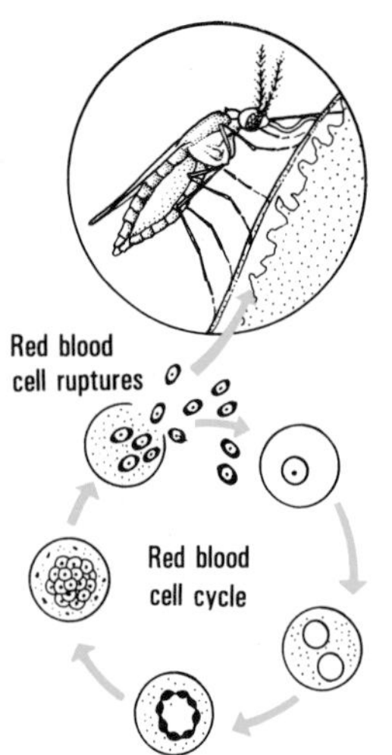

Plasmodium divides and multiplies

WHAT IS MALARIA?

– A common tropical infection, responsible for the deaths of well over a million people in Africa alone every year. Fever and illness follow infection after one week or more, but sometimes illness may be delayed many months or even years. Apart from fever, symptoms may include any of the following: shivering, headaches, vomiting, cough, diarrhoea, drowsiness or confusion. The disease is impossible to diagnose conclusively without laboratory tests. Anyone with the above symptoms either during or after a trip to a malarial area should suspect they have the infection. There are four major varieties of malaria: all cause chills and fever, but one, *Plasmodium falciparum*, causes severe illness, and is commonly fatal if not treated quickly.

Two of the four species of malaria have a stage of the parasite that may remain dormant in the liver for months or years. Malaria due to these species – *P. vivax* and *P. ovale* – may recur several times over a period of years, even after treatment of the acute infection with standard drugs. This calls for further medication – see under **PRESCRIPTION DRUGS.**

CAUSES A single-celled parasite called *Plasmodium* that invades red blood cells, carried from person to person by mosquitoes.

PRESCRIPTION DRUGS

Resistance to antimalarial drugs is becoming an increasing problem, especially in the case of *P. falciparum*. Consequently drug use has to be revised frequently and only broad generalizations can be presented here.

Preventive: tablets, typically **chloroquine** or, especially where *P. falciparum* is likely, the pyrimethamine/sulfadoxine combination known as Fansidar is taken regularly by any visitor to a malarial area, starting a week before the visit and continuing until a month after leaving the area. The actual drugs recommended depend on the place(s) to be visited, and the current patterns of drug resistance; up-to-date advice is essential.

How they work: malarial drugs interfere with the metabolism of the parasite, but exactly how is not fully understood.

To treat an attack: An acute attack must be treated quickly with a drug to which the parasite is sensitive. Chloroquine and quinine have a major role, but there are alternatives and the choice depends on the area in which

the malaria was contracted. The method of giving the drug depends on the severity of the attack: tablets are usually effective for mild or moderate illness, but intravenous therapy is needed for severe cases.
How they work: see **Preventive,** above.

OVER-THE-COUNTER TREATMENTS

Aspirin or acetaminophen will help the symptoms, but have no effect on the parasite.

QUESTIONS TO ASK THE DOCTOR

■ What is the latest recommendation for preventive pills for the countries I will be visiting?
■ What variety of malaria parasite has been found in my blood test? Do I need extra treatment to eliminate parasites from the liver?
■ Are there other diseases like yellow fever or hepatitis where I am going that I should be immunized against?

SIDE EFFECTS

Chloroquine and **paludrine** taken for prevention cause very few unwanted effects. Weekly chloroquine should not be taken for more than six years, as it may then begin to damage vision. Occasionally, **Maloprim, Fansidar** and **amodiaquine** have dangerous effects on the bone marrow and skin and are therefore not recommended for prevention except in unusual circumstances. **Quinine** (taken to treat an attack) commonly causes a high-pitched ringing sound in the ears, but this is not dangerous and does not affect hearing.

SELF-MANAGEMENT

The malarial parasite develops resistance to antimalarial drugs. Treatment is therefore varied on a local basis. So before you set out on a trip, find out the currently recommended treatment for that area. Your doctor will advise. Be sure to take preventive pills *regularly*; continue for a month after leaving the malarial area. Avoid mosquito bites by sleeping under a mosquito net and wearing protective clothing out of doors, especially around dusk. Insect repellant gives no guarantee against bites and possibly a false sense of security.

SELF-HELP IN AN ATTACK

It is essential to seek medical attention urgently as soon as you think you may have malaria: do not wait to see how things go. If, however, you are far from medical facilities, take the appropriate pills as soon as fever develops. Drink plenty of fluids.

PATIENT'S EXPERIENCE

"I had travelled extensively in Africa for 20 years and decided I was probably immune to malaria by now, so I didn't take a preventive course during a visit to central Africa. When I got home, I developed a fever, but decided not to bother the doctor. After three days, I was delirious and my skin was becoming yellow. My wife rang our doctor; he ordered me to hospital where I lay unconscious for nearly a month. When I came around, I had lost all my memory of the past two years; it is only slowly returning. The doctors say I am lucky to have survived such a severe bout of malaria. If I had reported the fever immediately, the illness would have probably amounted to a few days of feeling under the weather, and if I had taken preventive measures, it need never have happened at all."

CAUTION

Attacks of malaria are often particularly severe in infants and pregnant women. Treatment in the latter is complicated because certain drugs such as primaquin tetracycline and pyrimethamine cannot be used. Even though quinine, chloroquine and Fansidar have been used safely by pregnant women, they should be discouraged from travelling to malarial areas if possible.

NAMES YOU WILL HEAR

Antibiotics

Generic name: benzylpenicillin (penicillin G); **trade name:** Crystapen. **Generic name:** gentamicin; **trade names:** Garamycin, Cidomycin, Genticin, Lugacin, Alcomicin, Refobacin. **Generic name:** chloramphenicol; **trade name:** Chloromycetin. **Generic name:** co-trimoxazole; **trade names:** Septra, Septra DS, Bactrim, Fectrim, Nodilon, Septrin. **Generic name:** ampicillin; **trade names:** Omnipen, Polycillin, Principen, Ampifen, Penbritin, Pentrexyl, Vidopen, Austrapen, Bristin, Amcill, Ampicin, Ampilean, Biosan, Ampil, Famicilin, Pentrex, Petercillin, Synthecillin.

Anticonvulsants

Generic name: phenobarbitol; **trade names:** Luminal, Gardenal, Maliasin, Nova-Pheno. **Generic name:** diazepam; **trade names:** Valium, Alupram, Atensine, Evacalm, Solis, Tensium, Valrelease. **Generic name:** phenytoin; **trade name:** Epanutin.

Analgesics

Generic name: acetaminophen; **trade names:** Anacin 3, Phenaphon, Panadol, Tempra, Tylenol, Pamol, Calpol, Parasin, Parmol, Panado, Ceetamol, Atosol, Exctol, Ennagesic, Ilvamol. **Generic name:** aspirin; **trade names:** Ascriptin, Ecotrin, Measurin, Aspirin, Astrin, Bi-Prin. *See also **pain,** page 106.*

WHAT IS MENINGITIS?

– An inflammation of the membrane covering the brain. It causes fever, irritability, drowsiness, headache, vomiting, and a painful, stiff neck. Occasionally convulsions occur. It is much more common in children than in adults. It can be fatal.

CAUSES Principally viruses and bacteria. Some types of meningitis are contagious. Viral meningitis is caused by a number of different viruses, including the one which causes mumps. This is the less severe form of the disease and recovery is usually complete. Bacterial meningitis is caused by a number of different bacteria. Brain damage or death may result, particularly in the young, and in severe cases.

Which type of meningitis the patient has developed may be determined by a lumbar puncture: fluid is withdrawn from the spinal canal and tested. The test may also indicate which antibiotics will be best.

Meningitis patients almost always go into hospital for at least 48 hours for tests as soon as the disease is suspected. Patients with viral meningitis usually stay in the hospital for a shorter period than those with bacterial meningitis.

PRESCRIPTION DRUGS

Antibiotics are used in all cases of bacterial meningitis. (They are not used in viral meningitis, where they have no effect.) However, antibiotics may be used initially, regardless of diagnosis, until it is certain that the cause of the meningitis is viral.

The type of antibiotic used will depend on the type of bacteria causing the infection. Because delay in effective treatment may cause permanent brain damage, two or sometimes even three antibiotics are used in combination. They are usually given by injection, sometimes directly into the spine. To be effective, the dose has to be of a size which cannot be effectively administered by a pill. Duration of treatment is also longer than for most other infections, usually about ten days. The lumbar puncture is often repeated before the antibiotics are stopped, to make sure that the infection has completely cleared. Antibiotics may also be changed during the course of treatment if they are not working.

How they work: by killing bacteria responsible for the infection. They are discussed in more detail under ***pneumonia and pleurisy,*** *page 78.*

Anticonvulsants: Convulsions occur in some seriously ill meningitis patients, and these drugs may have to be used as a preventive measure.

How they work: *see* ***epilepsy,*** *page 110.*

Analgesics such as aspirin or acetaminophen will help to lower the temperature and ease the headache. In young children convulsions can occur if the temperature is high, and it can be difficult to know whether the fever or the meningitis is the cause.

How they work: *see* ***pain,*** *page 106.*

Intravenous fluids are usually given as a drip into a vein to correct dehydration.

With viral meningitis the patient is not usually very ill and the treatment is symptomatic. The temperature is controlled with analgesics and cool baths. Convulsions are uncommon. Recovery is usually complete.

QUESTIONS TO ASK THE DOCTOR

- Is hospital admission necessary?
- Is it likely to spread to other members of the family?
- Is it likely to cause permanent damage?

Not all of these questions can be answered immediately, but once the tests have been done, a doctor should be able to discuss these points.

SIDE EFFECTS

Antibiotics used for meningitis are stronger – because of the larger doses – than those used for most other infections. The side effects may be more marked and more varied, depending on which ones are used. They commonly include nausea, vomiting, diarrhea and allergy *(see* ***pneumonia and pleurisy,*** *page 78).* More rarely, they can affect the kidneys, ears and the blood. Tests for these complications are done while the patient is being treated. In each case, these very real disadvantages have to be weighed against the necessity of using antibiotics. Discuss the issue with your doctor.

Anticonvulsants: *See* ***epilepsy,*** *page 110.* Phenobarbital can cause drowsiness or irritability. Children over the age of two years are not usually given this drug as they can become very difficult and badly behaved. If treatment for convulsions has to be continued for any length of time, other drugs can be used. Diazepam causes drowsiness: it is not used in the long-term prevention of convulsions; *see* ***anxiety,*** *page 84.*

Analgesics/antipyretics: *see* ***common cold,*** *page 134.*

SELF-MANAGEMENT

Be aware of the symptoms of meningitis and report them to a doctor without delay.

PATIENT'S EXPERIENCE

"My little girl aged 11 months became ill with a high temperature and vomiting. Even when her temperature was back to normal, she screamed continually, arching her head backwards. She seemed to be in great pain when I tried to bend her head forwards. The doctor sent her to a hospital immediately, where a lumbar puncture was done. An I.V. was put into her arm and the doctor gave her fluids as she had become dehydrated from the vomiting. He also gave her an injection of phenobarbital to prevent convulsions. After that she slept a bit. Her fever had returned and the nurse sponged her down with cool water and set up a fan to blow cool air on to her. The infection was quite serious as it was caused by bacteria; she needed I.V. antibiotics. The doctor said that at this stage it was impossible to say whether there would be any permanent brain damage. However, as treatment had been started quickly, he was optimistic. The next few days were very difficult. Once she was a little better, she kept on trying to pull the I.V. out and although I spent as much time with her as I could, she cried dreadfully if I had to go. Luckily she did not have a convulsion and the phenobarbital was stopped after a few days. When she had completed the treatment with antibiotics, the lumbar puncture was repeated; apparently it was OK. She is now a year and a half, and completely normal, but she still has to go for special development assessments until she starts school."

Metabolic and endocrine disorders

Many complicated functions of the body such as body growth and development, sexual function, nutrient distribution and responses to stress are controlled by a series of glands that produce hormones. The pancreas in the abdomen produces insulin, the thyroid gland produces thyroxin and these as well as other glands are all controlled by the ''master gland'' – the pituitary gland at the base of the brain.

See also: *Infertility, page 174; drugs in pregnancy, page 184; period problems, page 190; problems of menopause, page 194.*

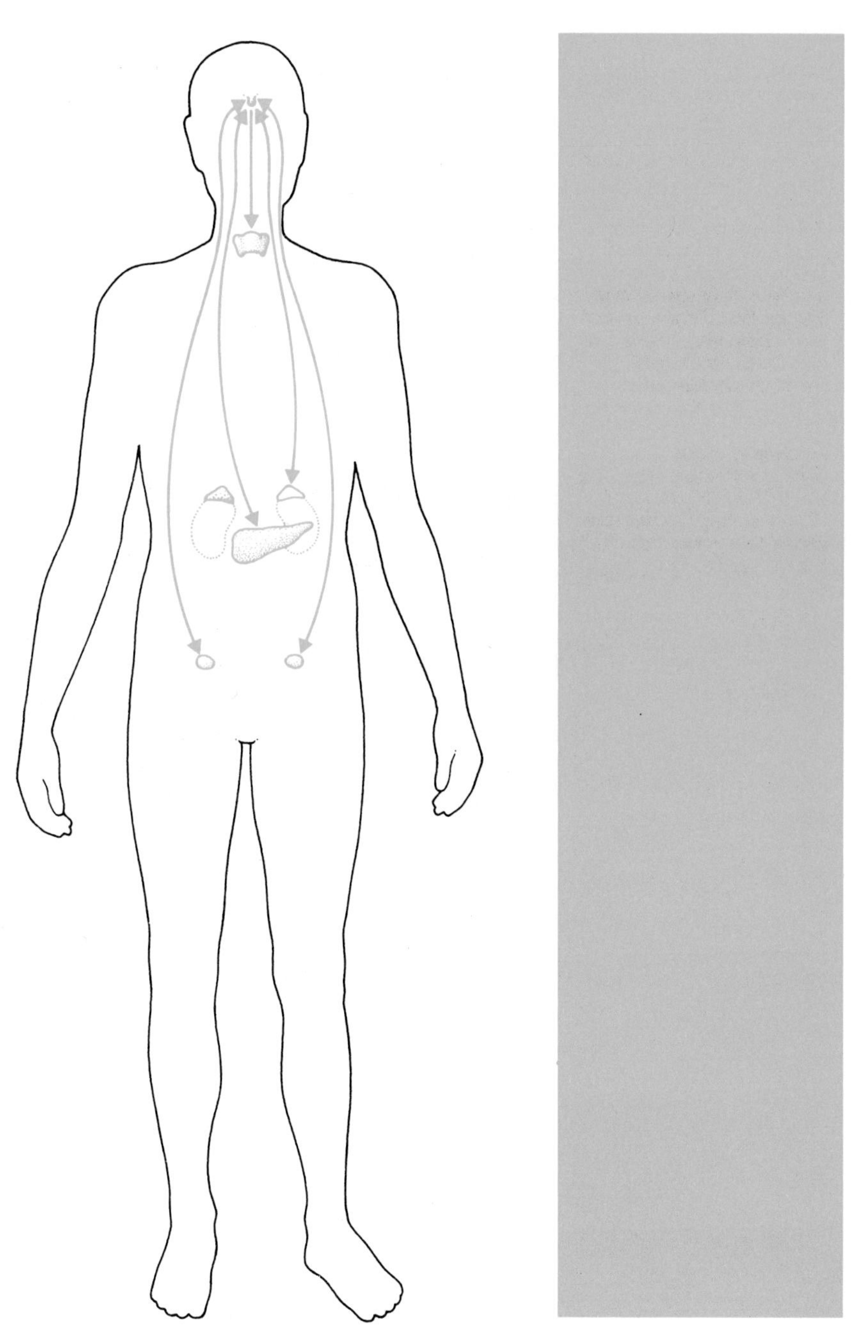

NAMES YOU WILL HEAR

Appetite suppressants
Generic name: diethylpropion hydrochloride; **trade names:** Tenuate, Tepanil, Apisate, Tenuate Dospan, Dietec, D.I.P., Nobensine-75, Regibon. **Generic name:** fenfluramine; **trade names:** Pondimin, Ponderax, Ponderax Pacaps, Ponderal. **Generic name:** mazindol; **trade names:** Mazanor, Sanorex, Teronac. **Generic name:** phentermine; **trade names:** Ionamin, Duromine, Fastin, Pronidin, Minobese. **Generic name:** benzphetamine; **trade name:** Didrex. **Generic name:** phendimetrazine; **trade names:** Bacarate, Plegine, Prelu-2, Statobex.

Bulk-forming agents
Generic name: methylcellulose; **trade names:** Celevac, Cellucon, Cologel, BFL, Cellulon, Nilstim. **Generic name:** sterculia; **trade names:** Normacol, Inolaxine, Karagum, Prefil.

WHAT IS OBESITY?

The word 'obese' means excessively fat, but what you understand by excessive depends on what you regard as normal. Doctors are divided in their understanding of what constitutes obesity. Most tables of 'ideal weight' are based on old statistics from a US insurance company. Their relevance is disputed. However, there is no doubt that very fat people suffer illness and may be at risk of premature death. These people are at least 30 per cent over average weight for height.

Doctors may still advise people thinner than this to lose weight because they have conditions such as high blood pressure or arthritis, where excess weight may worsen the problem, while not actually causing it. Apart from this, there is no evidence that mild obesity, say 10 per cent over 'ideal weight', affects health.

CAUSES Simply eating more than necessary. But why? Individual needs vary, but obese people cannot recognize when they have had enough; they do not respond in the normal way to feelings of hunger or satiation. They are influenced more than other people by the taste, smell and appearance of food. They have 'learned' to overeat. Once obese, you can remain so while eating no more than anyone else.

PRESCRIPTION DRUGS

Appetite suppressants play a very minor part. Those listed are only used under careful medical supervision.Their effect is short-lived, and there is a risk of dependency developing. Most obese patients will lose about 1 lb (0.5 kg) per week while taking these drugs, but the appetite, and the weight, usually return after stopping them. The drugs help with permanent weight reduction only when combined with a program of learning to eat less by recognizing the cues indicating one has had enough, and by ignoring those cues that lead to eating for pleasure.

How they work: probably by affecting the way the brain feels hunger, so suppressing the desire to eat.

Bulk-forming agents are available on prescription, but may also be bought without one. They are a means of supplementing the fiber content of the diet.

How they work: Everyone's diet should contain sufficient fiber, but the use of high-fiber, low-calorie supplements helps some people to feel satisfied on fewer calories. A high-fiber diet also leads to a reduction in blood cholesterol, which may lower the risk of coronary heart disease. *See **lipid disorders,** page 162.*

OVER-THE-COUNTER TREATMENTS

Many forms of diet foods and drinks are available. Advertisers' claims are carefully worded, but in reality these products are expensive low-calorie meals. You can create your own much more economically.

'Very low-calorie diets', containing less than 800 calories per day, are being marketed, usually through non-medical 'consultants'. They are effective, but their safety and long-term effectiveness are still being assessed. Crash diets can be very harmful, and may drastically alter the effect of certain drugs (eg warfarin).

QUESTIONS TO ASK THE DOCTOR

■ Do I really need to lose weight?

SIDE EFFECTS

Appetite suppressants: Diethylpropion and most other anorectic drugs (including fenfluramine) have a mild stimulant action, which can lead to dependence. While it may seem useful to take a drug that makes you feel less tired, the risk of addiction outweighs benefit.

Fenfluramine causes mild sedation, especially when first started; drowsiness and depression are the two most common reasons for stopping the drug. Sudden withdrawal can lead to severe depression. There is little risk of addiction.

Bulk-forming agents: Provided adequate fluid is taken, bulking agents are free from serious side effects, but people do find them unappetizing.

SELF-MANAGEMENT

Obesity is not a simple problem, nor are there easy answers. But since it has been estimated that more than a third of the population of most Western countries aged over 30 is more than 10 per cent overweight, some modification of eating habits would seem to make sense.

Fat is both the most concentrated form of calories, and the least obvious constituent of many processed ('junk') foods. It is associated with raised levels of cholesterol in the blood, and with the risk of heart disease. So reducing fat intake is worthwhile. Carbohydrates (sugar, starch) are converted by the body to fat if not needed as a source of energy. Sugar itself is also a common hidden ingredient in processed foods. A diet based on fresh vegetables, and bread, with meat, fish, eggs and cheese as sources of protein will provide fewer calories and more fiber than a diet composed mainly of processed food, sweets and cookies.

PATIENT'S EXPERIENCE

"I began to put on weight after having my first baby. I got to 150 lb (70 kg). As I am only 5ft 4 inches tall, I felt very fat. For three years I tried all sorts of diets, but couldn't lose weight. I felt really ugly. Then my doctor suggested I join a group run by the nutritionist. I carefully counted my calorie intake, and was surprised at how much I was eating. With the help of the group I found I could eat less. I started jogging, and began to feel more confident. I lost 30 lb (13 kg) in a year. My weight has remained around 130 lb, apart from after my second pregnancy."

EXERCISE

■ One hour's walking, or $\frac{3}{4}$ hour's cycling or $\frac{1}{4}$ hour's swimming every day should result in an extra two to four pounds' weight loss each month.

■ A useful target is 7 lb (3 kg) weight loss per month.

■ Regular exercise *combined* with a suitable diet, is the most effective way to lose weight. It can help lower serum cholesterol, too.

MORAL SUPPORT

Losing weight is difficult. Doing it alongside others with the same problem can be enormously helpful: don't dismiss joining a local Weight-Watchers' group which do much to encourage sensible eating habits.

Chart showing acceptable weight ranges: *see page 49.*

Insulin, oral hypoglycemic agents, guar, glucagon

NAMES YOU WILL HEAR

Short-acting insulin

Generic name: soluble or regular insulin; **trade names:** Insulin Insulin (beef), Hyparin Insulin (beef), Insulin Injection (beef). **Generic name:** neutral insulin; **trade names:** Neutral Insulin Injection (beef), Hypurin Neutral (beef), Neusulin (beef), Quicksol (beef), Velosulin (pork), Human Actrapid, Human Velosulin, Humulin S (human).

Intermediate and long-acting insulin

Generic name: insulin zinc suspension (amorphous); **trade names:** 125 Semilente (beef), Semitard MC (pork), IZS Semilente (beef), Regular Iletin. **Generic name:** insulin zinc suspension (crystalline); **trade names:** Ultralente (beef), Human Ultratard, Humulin Zn (human), Ultralente Iletin. **Generic name:** insulin zinc suspension (mixed crystalline and amorphous); **trade names:** IZS Lente (beef), Hypurin Lente (beef), Neulente (beef), Tempulin (beef), Lentard MC (pork), Human Monotard, Lente Iletin. **Generic name:** isophane insulin; **trade names:** Isophane Insulin Injection (beef), Hypurin Isophane (beef), Insulatard (pork), Monophane (beef), Neuphane (beef), Human Insulatard, Human Protaphane, Humulin I (human), NPH Iletin. **Generic name:** neutral and isophane mixed insulin; **trade names:** Initard (50% neutral: 50% isophane, pork), Mixtard (30% neutral: 70% isophane, pork), Human Actraphane (30% neutral: 70% isophane), Human Initard (50% neutral: 50% isophane), Human Mixtard (30% neutral: 70% isophane), Humulin M1 (10% neutral: 90% isophane, human), Humulin M2 (20& neutral: 80% isophane). **Generic name:** biphasic insulin injection; **trade name:** Rapitard MC (25% neutral pork: 75% crystalline beef insulin). **Generic name:** protamine zinc insulin; **trade name:** Hypurin Protamine Zinc. Insulins of beef and pork origin are gradually being replaced by human insulin.

continued on page 158

WHAT IS DIABETES?

A surprisingly common metabolic disorder, in most countries affecting one to two people in a hundred. Two types account for most cases:

Insulin-dependent diabetes; juvenile onset diabetes; Type I diabetes: tends to occur in children and young adults. There is a severe deficiency or absence of the hormone known as insulin, produced by the pancreas. This causes poor metabolism of carbohydrates, proteins and fats. Typical symptoms are loss of weight, despite a healthy appetite; thirst and passing large volumes of urine. There is also a tendency for ketones to accumulate in the blood. (Ketones are products of fat metabolism, and occur as increasing amounts of fat are metabolized to make up for the failure of carbohydrate metabolism caused by uncontrolled diabetes. They may be detected in the urine or smelled on the breath.) About 25 per cent of all diabetics have this form of the disease, which is fatal within a year unless treated with insulin.

Non insulin-dependent diabetes; adult onset diabetes; Type II diabetes: tends to occur in older people who are overweight. There is not such a severe shortage of insulin in older patients as in the insulin-dependent type, but the insulin which is produced does not work efficiently. A similar though less severe disruption of body metabolism is caused. Symptoms of thirst and passing large volumes of urine may occur, but often the disease comes on gradually and may only be recognized when the urine, which normally contains no sugar, is tested.

Diabetes can also occur during pregnancy, brought on by hormonal changes. This resolves immediately after the baby is born. It may also occur if the pancreas is badly damaged by pancreatits.

In diabetes the blood sugar (glucose) level rises because without insulin it can no longer be driven into the body's cells. When glucose in the blood reaches a certain level, it spills over into the urine. After several years of diabetes, damage to body organs may occur, particularly to the eyes, kidneys, blood vessels and nervous system. If the disease has been well controlled the risk is thought to be reduced.

CAUSES: In juvenile onset diabetes, the beta cells in the pancreas which make insulin are destroyed by the body's own immune system. Why this happens is not known, but it is thought that in susceptible people a stimulus, such as a virus, triggers the process. The cause of non insulin-dependent diabetes is not fully understood either, but there are many factors which increase the risk, including obesity, increasing age, and heredity.

PRESCRIPTION DRUGS

Insulin: obtained from the pancreas of cattle and pigs. It is not quite the same as human insulin which is now produced by or genetic engineering (bacteria are treated to produce insulin identical to the human variety). Insulin must be given by injection under the skin because it is a protein and would be digested and destroyed if taken by mouth. By combining it with retarding substances, the rate of absorption into the bloodstream can be delayed. Many insulin-dependent diabetics can control their diabetes with just two injections a day of a mixture of short- and longer-acting insulin, but the best control, allowing flexible meal times, is with three or more injections a day.

Using a pump, strapped to the body or hidden in clothing, it is possible to inject slowly over 24 hours, giving boosts when food is eaten. This can give excellent control of blood glucose, but is still experimental.

How it works: Injected insulin works in the same way as natural insulin, driving glucose into the body's cells and restoring fat and protein metabolism. The aim is to match the pattern produced by a normal pancreas, but even with a pump this can never be done exactly.

Oral hypoglycaemic agents: They are only useful in non-insulin dependent diabetes, and are prescribed when weight loss and dietary restrictions have failed to control the blood sugar. **Sulphonylureas** are particularly useful if diabetes has not been controlled by diet alone and the patient is not obese. Long-acting types are taken once daily before breakfast. Short-acting types may be taken before meals.

How they work: by stimulating the cells which produce insulin, and by increasing the effectiveness of insulin on peripheral tissues. They are therefore ineffective in patients whose insulin-producing cells have been destroyed.

Biguanides are useful in non insulin-dependent patients who are still obese.

How they work: by reducing absorption of carbohydrates from the gut. They may also increase uptake of glucose into cells and reduce the formation of glucose from glycogen (starch) in the liver. They are dependent on the presence of insulin for their action.

Guar: a naturally-occurring plant fiber (obtained from the

PATIENTS' EXPERIENCES

"I used to inject a mixture of soluble and isophane insulin before breakfast and before my evening meal, but I found that my early-morning blood sugars were high. I increased the number of units of isophane insulin before my evening meal to bring these sugars down. There was no improve-ment; some mornings my sugar was high and on others it was low; I also started sweating through the night. I decided to increase my isophane further, but was admitted to hospital with a very low blood sugar that night. The doctor explained that the second injection of isophane was acting most strongly in the early hours of the morning bringing my blood sugar very low; the high sugar before breakfast was my body's over-reaction to this. I now split my evening injection, and give the soluble before my bed-time snack. My blood sugars are now much better and I wake up in the morning feeling more refreshed."

NAMES YOU WILL HEAR

Oral hypoglycaemic agents

Sulphonylureas

Generic name: acetohexamide; **trade name:** Dimelor. **Generic name:** chlorpropamide; **trade names:** Diabinese, Promide, Chloromide, Chloronase, Novopropamide, Stabinol. **Generic name:** glibenclamide; **trade names:** Micronase, Daonil, Semi-Daonil, Euglucon, Libanil, Malix, Euglycon, Gutril, Diamicron. **Generic name:** gliclazide; **trade name:** Diamicron. **Generic name:** glipizide; **trade names:** Glucotrol, Glibenese, Minodiab. **Generic name:** gliquidone; **trade name:** Glurenorm. **Generic name:** glymidine; **trade names:** Gondafon, Lycanol. **Generic name:** tolazamide; **trade names:** Tolinase, Tolanase. **Generic name:** tolbutamide; **trade names:** Pramidex, Rastinon, Artosin, Chembutamide, Mellitol, Mobenol, Neo-Dibetic, Novobutamide, Oramide, Orinase, Tolbutase.

Guar

Generic name: guar gum; **trade names:** Glucotard, Guarem, Guarina, Lejguar.

Glucagon

Generic name: glucagon; **trade name:** Glucagon Novo, Glucagon Lilly.

cluster bean) which is not absorbed from the gut. It is available as granules or mini-tablets and is taken in a drink or, most effectively, when mixed with food.

How it works: by increasing the consistency of food in the gut, slowing the rate of carbohydrate absorption. It reduces surges in blood glucose after meals.

Glucagon: another naturally-occurring hormone produced in the pancreas. It is not affected by diabetes and is not used for treating diabetes itself, but it is very useful in treating patients whose blood glucose has fallen to very low levels. It must be given by injection either under the skin or into muscle.

How it works: it causes blood glucose to rise by converting glycogen in the liver to glucose; the opposite effect to insulin.

OVER-THE-COUNTER TREATMENTS

None.

QUESTIONS TO ASK THE DOCTOR

- How much weight should I aim to lose?
- How often and at what times of day should I test my blood glucose?
- Will I always need to take tablets/insulin?
- What will happen if I forget to inject my insulin? What should I do in this event?
- I am traveling by plane to another country; how should I adjust my insulin regime?
- Why should I monitor my diabetes with blood/urine tests even if I feel well?
- Can I have children and will they inherit diabetes?
- How can I reduce the risk of complications?
- How will I know if my blood sugar is too low?
- Can I continue to take beta-blocking drugs once I start treatment for diabetes?

SIDE EFFECTS

Insulin: Injecting too much insulin, not eating enough, and unaccustomed exercise without appropriate adjustment of diet or insulin dose can cause the blood glucose to fall too far (hypoglycemia). When this happens, the patient may first feel weak and hungry, then, as the blood glucose continues to fall, there is sweating, irritability, confusion, nervousness and dizziness; if this is not corrected, unconsciousness may follow. Not all diabetics experience identical symptoms from hypoglycemia. Minor allergic reactions can occur at the sites of injection but these soon settle; if they do not, a change to a purer form of insulin may help.

Sometimes the fat under the skin where insulin has been given decreases (atrophy) or increases (hypertrophy), leaving a lumpy appearance. If this should happen, change the site of your injection; a more purified insulin may also help.

Sulphonylureas can also lower the blood glucose too far if a meal is missed or with unaccustomed exercise. Some of these drugs can cause flushing of the face after drinking alcohol. There is a tendency to gain weight while taking these drugs, so it is especially important to keep to your diet. Occasionally the drugs cause skin rashes and very occasionally they reduce the production of blood cells.

Biguanides do not reduce blood glucose below normal, so 'hypos' do not occur. Patients who are obese often find it easier to lose weight while taking these drugs. They can reduce appetite and may cause an upset stomach; they are better taken with food. Diarrhea is a common side effect, but this usually settles in about ten days. Very rarely, a serious upset of the metabolism can occur, but this is almost exclusively in patients with poor kidney function.

Guar may cause flatulence and abdominal distension.

Glucagon is used to treat coma caused by low blood glucose. It may be given by a relative or friend, and works within ten minutes. If there is no response, an injection of glucose into a vein by a doctor is necessary. Occasionally, glucagon causes nausea and vomiting.

SELF-MANAGEMENT

Patients needing insulin treatment have to be their own doctor, nurse, dietician and laboratory technician. From time to time, the dose of insulin may need adjustment and it is preferable that you learn how to do this safely yourself.

■ Try not to let your diabetes interfere with work or hobbies. Discuss with your doctor/specialist.

■ Join a local or national diabetes group. You will meet others who have learnt to overcome most of your problems.

■ Dietary treatment is important in all forms of diabetes and in many cases may be the sole remedy. The main principles of diet are:

■ To maintain body weight appropriate to height.

- To avoid all forms of sugar (except during hypoglycemic attacks).
- To eat less fat.
- To eat more fiber.
- To eat regular meals.

PATIENTS' EXPERIENCES

"Before starting my family, I changed from one insulin injection a day to three, so that my blood sugars were all below 180. Once I knew that I was pregnant I let the hospital know and attended a clinic for diabetic mothers. I was seen every two weeks initially; and from 32 weeks in to the pregnancy, every week. I kept a careful record of my blood sugars as I needed to increase my insulin dose from time to time in order to keep my blood sugar below 100 before my meals. In the end I was taking nearly twice as much insulin as I had done previously. My obstetrician kept a careful check on the size of the baby, and since the baby was normal size, I was allowed to deliver naturally, which happened just three days before the expected date. I wanted to breast-feed my baby, so I took an extra 50 grams of carbohydrate in my diet and adjusted my dose of insulin. It was hard work coming to the hospital so many times, but it was well worth all the effort to have a normal healthy baby; and I've also learned that I can control my blood sugar much more easily."

Insulin, oral hypoglycemic agents, guar, glucagon

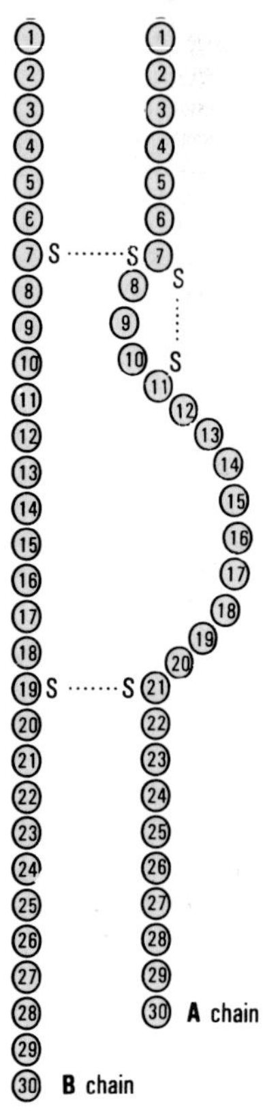

The structure of insulin: *Proteins, of which insulin is one, have large, complicated chemical structures built up from building blocks called amino acids, shown as numbered circles in the diagram. Different combinations of these amino acids, of which there are about 30, make up different proteins. Insulin is composed of two chains of amino acids linked by sulphur bridges (-S-S-). Beef insulin differs from human insulin in the amino acids in positions A8, A10 and B30. Pork insulin differs from human insulin only in the amino acid at B30. Insulin is not a flat structure as depicted in the diagram; the chains are coiled to produce a three-dimensional molecule.*

■ Monitor your diabetic control by measuring blood or urine glucose. If you are treated with insulin, blood tests are preferred. Blood glucose can be measured on a drop of blood from a finger prick using special reagent strips which are read in a meter or by observing a color change. Blood tests should be done before all meals at least two days a week. If you wake through the night for any reason, use the opportunity to check your blood glucose – the result may be surprising. For ideal control, blood glucose should be between 72 to 126 mg/d, but if you have frequent hypoglycemia you should not try to control your diabetes as tightly as this.

Insulin-dependent diabetes cannot be so well-controlled by testing urine for glucose.

■ Learn how to adjust your insulin according to blood glucose results, meals and exercise. If blood glucose is high at the same time on two successive days, you may increase the appropriate insulin dose by two to four units; similarly, if you have hypoglycemia regularly at the same time of day, you should reduce your insulin; eating a snack between meals can also prevent low blood sugar, and is necessary for most insulin-treated patients. Exercise will lower blood glucose, so take extra carbohydrate beforehand; you may also need to reduce your insulin.

■ Always carry glucose with you in case of a hypoglycemia attack.

■ Don't smoke. Risk of damage to blood vessels, eyes and kidneys is vastly increased in diabetic smokers.

■ The blood vessels and nerves in the feet are particularly vulnerable to damage in diabetics, so inspect your feet regularly and report any signs of damage to your doctor or podiatrist (including ulcers, black areas or blisters). Never walk barefoot. Always wear well-fitting shoes with soft uppers. Do not immerse your feet in water warmer than 110°F. Do not sit too close to fires or use heating pads on the feet.

■ If you wish to become pregnant it is important that your diabetes is well-controlled before you conceive. There is an increased risk of congenital abnormalities.

■ Even if you feel you are managing your diabetes well it is important to see your doctor regularly. He will be able to look for and treat complications which may not show symptoms until a late stage has developed.

SELF-HELP IN ATTACKS

Hypoglycemia (low blood glucose) As soon as you recognize an attack coming on, take some glucose or a glucose drink. Have a snack as soon as possible afterwards. If you are driving your car, stop, get out of the driving seat and take some glucose and a snack before continuing – preferably someone else should drive. If you are found unconscious, the paramedics should be called. A relative or friend may give an injection of glucagon, provided they have been trained in its use. When you recover you should have a glucose-containing drink to prevent another attack. It is a good idea to wear a 'Medic Alert' bracelet or carry a card saying you are diabetic, as delay in treating severe hypoglycemia can cause permanent brain damage.

Intercurrent illness: If a diabetic is taken ill with an infection or fever, or has been vomiting or eaten little, there is a temptation to reduce the insulin. This is a mistake owing to the stress of the current illness, the patient may need more insulin. Try to take the carbohydrate allowance in a more easily absorbed form such as glucose drinks if necessary. If you start to pass large volumes of urine, feel thirsty, start losing weight or show ketones in the urine, consult your doctor.

PATIENTS' EXPERIENCES

"I am 68 and have had diabetes for ten years. I was on diet and tablets for nine years, but my urine always showed two per cent glucose. I felt perfectly well (or so I thought), and was reluctant to go on insulin when the doctor suggested it. I was frightened of injecting myself and thought I was too old to learn about insulin. I was eventually persuaded, and was surprised to learn that I didn't have to go into hospital. A nurse practitioner in my doctor's office showed me how to draw up and inject the insulin. I now have two injections each day and realize that I was not as well as I thought while taking tablets; I feel much fitter now and don't mind the injections."

BLOOD GLUCOSE

Breakfast Lunch Dinner

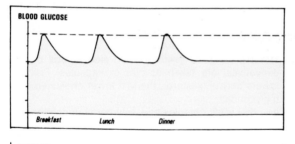

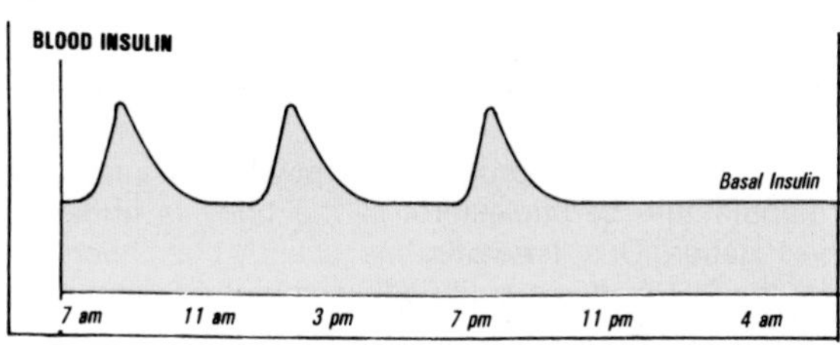

Blood glucose and insulin levels in non-diabetics taking three meals a day. *Insulin rises sharply with each meal to keep the blood glucose below 100 mg/dl. Insulin is present in the blood at all times, even if no food is eaten.*

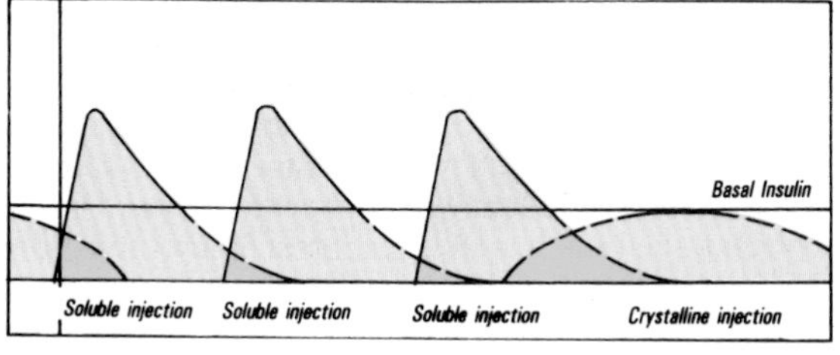

Blood insulin levels in a diabetic *injecting a crystalline insulin zinc suspension in the evening and three soluble insulin injections before the main meals. Note how this approximates to the pattern of blood insulin levels in non-diabetics in the graph above/below/opposite.*

Lipid-lowering drugs

NAMES YOU WILL HEAR
Generic name: cholestyramine; **trade name:** Questran. **Generic name:** colestipol; **trade name:** Colestid. **Generic name:** probucol; **trade names:** Lorelco, Lurselle. **Generic name:** clofibrate; **trade name:** Atromid-S. **Generic name:** bezafibrate; **trade name:** Bezalip. **Generic name:** gemfibrozil; **trade name:** Lopid. **Generic name:** omega-3-marine triglycerides; **trade name:** Mexepa.

WHAT ARE LIPIDS?

– A collective term for fatty substances such as cholesterol and triglycerides – which are essential for making cell membranes, bile acids and some hormones; or as a source of energy. If there is too much of them in the blood there is an increased risk of heart disease. *See **angina,** page 46* and ***myocardial infarction,** page 52.*

Cholesterol and triglycerides are derived partly from diet, and partly from the body, which makes them.

CAUSES of high blood fat levels: heredity, or life-style (mainly diet); or both.

PRESCRIPTION DRUGS

Cholestyramine and **colestipol** (latter not available in USA) are the first-line drug treatments for high-cholesterol, particularly in patients with a family history of hypercholesterolemia (too much cholesterol in the blood).
How they work: by binding to bile acids in the intestine, causing them to be lost in the stools. The body uses cholesterol to replace these bile acids and thus its supply of cholesterol is depleted. Note that these drugs are not absorbed by the body, but lost in the stools together with the bile acids.
Probucol, clofibrate, gemfibrozil and **nicotinic acid** plus its derivatives, are taken as pills or capsules. Probucol lowers only cholesterol; the rest lower cholesterol and triglycerides.
How they work: complex and only partly understood.
Marine triglycerides: fish oils. Eskimos, whose diet is rich in fish, do not get much coronary heart disease; on this principle, oils have been developed to lower blood lipids. See OVER-THE-COUNTER TREATMENTS.

A new group of drugs which powerfully inhibit the manufacture of cholesterol in the body is under investigation. One, **lovostatin,** has recently been approved by the F.D.A. It is a major advance in the treatment of high cholesterol.

OVER-THE-COUNTER TREATMENTS

Products such as garlic and lecithin are variously promoted as lowering blood fats and/or reducing the tendency of the blood to clot within blood vessels. Evidence on their effectiveness is controversial. Fish-oil concentrates are available on prescription and from pharmacists and health food shops. If used excessively they may cause failure of blood clotting.

QUESTIONS TO ASK THE DOCTOR

■ Why do I require drug treatment rather than a diet?
■ Is it safe to use this drug with others?

SIDE EFFECTS

The commonest side effects with **cholestyramine** and **colestipol** are constipation, nausea and bloating. Building up the dose gradually can help reduce these. A high roughage diet or a bulking agent should control constipation. **Probucol** is well tolerated but occasionally causes diarrhea. **Clofibrate** and **gemfibrozil** occasionally cause nausea, muscle pains or impotence. Clofibrate has been less widely used since it was suggested that it might be associated with an increase in unwanted side effects, such as gallstones, although it is still useful in certain patients. **Nicotinic acid** in large doses can cause nausea, flushing, itching and inflammation of the liver. Many of these will disappear spontaneously if the dose is increased gradually.

These drugs are not recommended during pregnancy or lactation; probucol is discontinued six months before pregnancy. As with most drugs, inform your doctor if you are trying to become pregnant. If you start an unplanned pregnancy while taking these drugs, stop the medication and get immediate medical advice.

SELF-MANAGEMENT

■ Diet, including weight reduction and exercise, is the first approach to lowering blood fats. If you can adhere to your diet, you may not need to take drugs at all. Even when taking drugs, such a program may reduce the dose or improve the result. Take advice from a dietician or doctor.

In many, however, the high fat level is inherited, and not due to poor diet. For these patients it is often impossible to lower blood fats without resorting to drugs.

Drugs for high lipid levels, like those for high blood pressure, only work while you are taking them. A prolonged reduction in lipid levels, and thus a reduction in risk of heart and blood vessel disease is only achieved if they are taken regularly and long-term.

■ If you think you are getting side effects from your drugs, seek medical advice.

■ Cholestyramine is likely to work best if taken with or close to meals. It may interfere with the absorption of other drugs, which should be taken an hour before.

■ If you are taking anticoagulants *(see page 62)*, let the clinic know of any change in your drug treatment in case it interferes with your lipid control.

PATIENT'S EXPERIENCE

"I had a heart attack when I was 36 years old and tests showed that the fats in my blood were higher than they should be. It is in the family: my brother died of a heart attack when he was only 40. I started on a low-fat diet – avoiding eggs, cheese, butter and other dairy products. After four months my doctor told me that the tests were better, but still not good enough. He started me on cholestyramine. I sprinkle the contents of a packet on my food at every meal; I can also mix them with a drink. The taste was a bit odd at first, but I am quite used to it now and the blood tests are almost normal."

NAMES YOU WILL HEAR
Generic name: propylthiouracil; **trade names:** Propylthiouracil, Propyl-Thyracil. **Generic name:** propranolol; **trade names:** Inderal, Angitol, Apsolol, Bedranol, Berkolol, Sloprolol, Cardinol. **Generic name:** carbimazole; **trade names:** Neo-Mercazole, Carbazole.

WHAT IS HYPERTHYROIDISM?

The thyroid gland controls the rate at which body cells use energy. If the gland is over-active, the skin becomes hot and sweaty, the heart rate increases even during sleep; sleep is very light, and the patient may become over-active during the day. The heart muscle becomes excitable, with a rapid pulse, and an irregular rhythm known as atrial fibrillation – *see* ***disorders of heart rhythm,*** *page 56*. In more extreme forms the condition is described as *thyrotoxicosis* and there is often marked weight loss. Menstruating women will find that their periods become lighter and scantier. Often, but not always, there may be swelling of the thyroid gland producing the condition known as *goitre*, and some patients develop protruberant eyes, a condition called *exophthalmus*. Thyrotoxicosis occurs in women eight times more commonly than in men; it can occur at any age group but is more difficult to detect in the elderly. In young people the onset is often sudden.

Thyrotoxicosis can often be confused with an anxiety state – *see page 84* – it really can be difficult to tell them apart. Diagnosis of hyperthyroidism is made by blood tests to measure the levels of the hormone in the body, but a thyroid scan may be needed prior to commencing any treatment.

CAUSE Usually, a so-called *auto-immune* reaction in which the body inadvertently reacts against its own cells.

TREATMENT

There are three options:

1 Drug treatment: This usually stops production of most of the thyroid hormone.

2 Surgery, in which most of the gland is cut away and the remaining portion thus produces less hormone. This is often necessary in young people who have failed to respond to drugs and also in those with a goitre that is pressing against the wind-pipe.

3 Radioactive iodine: Thyroid gland tissue is destroyed by giving radioactive iodine. This diminishes the amount of hormone produced. It is often the treatment of choice in patients past child-bearing age.

Propylthiouracil is a widely used anti-thyroid drug. Treatment usually lasts for two years, and is then stopped. About 50 per cent will relapse and need some form of further treatment.

A beta-blocker such as propranolol is often used for temporary control of symptoms prior to surgery or other treatments. With all treatments there is a long-term risk of developing an under-active thyroid (hypothyroidism); *see page 166*. Low-dose replacement therapy with thyroxine is given in these circumstances.

OVER-THE-COUNTER TREATMENTS

None.

QUESTIONS TO ASK THE DOCTOR

- Which treatment is best for me and why?
- How long will it take to work?
- What happens if the disease comes back after stopping treatment?
- How often do I need a blood test?
- How often do you need to see me?
- Is the treatment safe if I am pregnant or breast-feeding?

SIDE EFFECTS

If an anti-thyroid drug is working properly, the symptoms of thyrotoxicosis will recede within four to eight weeks. However, the gland may eventually become under-active *(see **hypothyroidism**, page 166)*, and replacement therapy with thyroxine will be needed. The thyroid gland itself may swell as a result of treatment, and a goitre may develop; or a pre-existing goitre may enlarge, making surgery necessary. Skin rashes are relatively common and the doctor may change drugs if this occurs. Rarer side effects include headaches, nausea, hair loss, jaundice and, perhaps most important, formation of white blood cells may cease. This makes the patient susceptible to infections. Any sore throat or other infection should be reported at once. As with all treatments for thyrotoxicosis, there is a long-term risk of the thyroid gland eventually becoming permanently underactive, in which case replacement therapy will be needed. Beta-blockers are usually free of serious side effects but some patients may develop a tight chest if they have a tendency towards asthma. Cold fingers and feet are common. A few patients get very tired; some have vivid dreams.

SELF-MANAGEMENT

- Take the drugs regularly.
- Report a sore throat or any other infection to your doctor without delay.

Once treatment is finished, have an annual check of thyroid function. If you enter hospital, or see another doctor, make it clear you have had thyroid treatment.

PATIENT'S EXPERIENCE

"Just because I had previously had trouble with my nerves, my family and my doctor thought that my symptoms were psychological. I was unable to sleep and felt sweaty and anxious. I lost weight and drugs like Valium made no difference. It was only when I developed a swelling in my neck that my doctor sent me to a specialist who put me on pills. After about two weeks I began to improve, and I felt almost back to normal within two months and my weight increased again. However, when the treatment stopped after two years, all the old symptoms came back again. I had to be referred to a surgeon who operated on my neck to remove part of my thyroid gland. I am fine now."

NAMES YOU WILL HEAR
Generic name: L-thyroxine; **trade names:** Choloxin, Synthroid, Euthroid, Levothroid, Eltroxin, Oroxine, Synthroid. **Generic name:** liothyronine (L-tri-iodothyronine); **trade names:** Tertroxin, Cytomel, Thyrolar.

WHAT IS HYPOTHYROIDISM?

The thyroid gland, one of a number of endocrine or hormonal glands, is in the front of the neck. It produces two hormones, the main one being thyroxine (T4), the other tri-iodothyronine (T3). These act on all the cells of the body to regulate the rate at which food is converted into energy. Iodine is essential for the manufacture of both the hormones. If the gland is not making the hormones, different illnesses result depending upon the age of the patient. **Cretinism** occurs in babies and young children. Body cells are starved of energy and are unable to develop; the infant is stunted and mentally handicapped. Treatment is usually undertaken in hospital. It is a very rare condition. **Myxedema** occurs in adults and is relatively common. It nearly always comes on very slowly and may go unrecognized by patient, relatives and doctor. It is at least ten times commoner in women than in men and usually occurs after the age of 45. The body temperature falls; the heart rate slows; weight increases; the skin becomes rough and coarse, the hair thins and the face and eyelids can become puffy. Brain activity can become sluggish, especially in the elderly. Menstruating women may have heavy periods. If suspected the condition can easily be diagnosed by a blood test. It is then simply a question of starting treatment. Further blood tests will be necessary to make sure that the dose of hormone given is correct.

CAUSE Both conditions are caused by the thyroid gland not working. In the past, and even today in developing countries, iodine deficiency caused the gland to swell; the swelling is known as a goitre. In developed countries the main causes of underactivity are inflammation in the gland, or as a consequence of previous treatment for ***hyperthyroidism*** – *see page 164*.

PRESCRIPTION DRUGS

L-thyroxine tablets are the usual treatment. Treatment is usually for life, in a once-a-day dose.
How it works: simply by replacing the substance that the body is unable to make.
L-tri-iodothyronine is rarely used except in severe cases when a rapid response to treatment is needed.
How it works: in the same way as L-thyroxine.

Replacing the hormone does not mean that a child with cretinism will grow normally, or be mentally normal; but it will prevent any further deterioration. In adults with myxedema, the majority of symptoms such as dry hair, coarse skin, cold intolerance and slowness

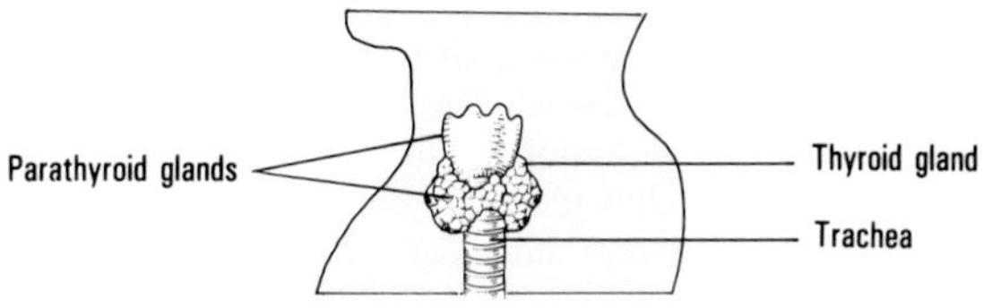

will slowly improve. However, it may be difficult to lose the weight that has been gained. A calorie-controlled diet, and considerable self-control, may be necessary.

OVER-THE-COUNTER TREATMENTS

None.

QUESTIONS TO ASK THE DOCTOR

- How do I know that I am on the correct dose?
- What should I do if I forget to take my pills for a few days?
- How often do I need to have a blood test?
- How often will you want to see me?
- Do I need to diet?

SIDE EFFECTS

Side effects in adults with myxedema are usually related to either under- or over-dosage. Too little **L-thyroxine,** and the symptoms will not disappear. Too much, and the patient may develop some of the signs and symptoms of ***thyrotoxicosis,*** *page 164*. These may include a rapid pulse with palpitations, an irregular pulse, excessive weight loss, inability to sleep, hot sweaty skin and restlessness. In the elderly, the replacement of the hormone is always done gradually, building up by small increases to the full replacement dose. This may take months; suddenly giving a full dose may unmask coronary artery narrowing by provoking angina as the heart's oxygen requirements increase. If you develop any chest pain or discomfort, or breathlessness when you are starting treatment, especially if you are elderly, see your doctor soon.

SELF-MANAGEMENT

Be especially careful to maintain the directed dose; don't miss the blood tests arranged by your doctor. Maintaining stable replacement is the key to successful treatment. You will need a full check-up at least once a year. If you go into the hospital or see a different doctor, don't forget to mention your thyroid condition, as it may affect treatment of other conditions.

PATIENT'S EXPERIENCE

"It was the new doctor who diagnosed it; he had just arrived in the practice and he wasn't as busy as the others. I went with a cold and mentioned that I was tired all the time. He asked me lots of questions about my skin, hair, weight, and whether I liked hot or cold weather. He sent me for a blood test and when he had the result, started me on some pills – just one a day. I now feel much better than I have done for the last five years and although I have not lost much weight, I have much more energy."

Hormone replacements, hormone suppression

NAMES YOU WILL HEAR

Generic names: hydrocortisone, cortisone acetate; **trade names:** Cortelan, Cortisyl, Cortate, Sterop, Cortemel. **Generic names:** thyroxine sodium, levothyroxine sodium (USP); **trade names:** Cytolen, Eltroxin, Oroxine, Thyroxinal. **Generic name:** ethinyl estradiol; **trade names:** Lynoral, Estinyl, Ovanon-E. **Generic name:** medroxyprogesterone acetate; **trade names:** Amen, Provera. **Generic name:** testosterone esters; **trade names:** Primoteston-Depot, Sustanon 100/250. **Generic name:** testosterone undecanoate; **trade name:** Restandol. **Generic name:** desmopressin; **trade name:** DDAVP. **Generic name:** bromocriptine; **trade name:** Parlodel.

THE PITUITARY GLAND AND ITS DISORDERS

The pituitary gland consists of two lobes, the anterior (front) and posterior (back). These are controlled by the hypothalamus – an important regulatory center in the brain – to which the gland is joined.

The most common diseases of the pituitary are benign tumours or adenomas of the anterior lobe. If these grow large, they may cause headaches and progressive loss of visual field on one or both sides because of compression of optic nerves. Large tumours may also cause decreased hormone secretion, characteristically affecting first the growth hormone (of minor consequence in adults) and also the gonadotrophins – the hormones which stimulate the testicles and ovaries. Thus sexual dysfunction is a symptom of pituitary disorder, eventually recognized by menstrual abnormality, or, in men, impotence and loss of libido.

Later, the production of hydrocortisone by the adrenal glands may be impaired, and this can have serious consequences: reduction of the ability to withstand such stresses as fevers, gastroenteritis, or trauma.

Thyroid deficiency is the other major consequence of pituitary tumor. Associated with it are lethargy, cold intolerance and modest obesity.

Some tumors of the pituitary overproduce certain hormones, such as prolactin, which interferes with function of the ovaries and testicles, and sometimes causes inappropriate milk production (galactorrhea). Others cause growth hormone excess, leading to excessive growth in children, and to enlargement of soft tissue and of certain bones: the condition known as acromegaly.

Pituitary overproduction of ACTH, the hormone which stimulates the production of hydrocortisone, is a rare but serious condition called Cushing's disease.

Pituitary tumors develop essentially only in the anterior lobe, and so do not directly affect the posterior lobe. But damage to the hypothalamus, which governs activity of both lobes, can cause not only all the features of anterior pituitary disease, but also loss of antidiuretic hormone (vasopressin). As a result, the kidney is unable to concentrate urine and the patient passes large amounts of dilute urine, a condition known as diabetes insipidus. This condition can now be controlled by taking artificial vasopressin.

PRESCRIPTION DRUGS

Hormone replacement therapy is designed to make good

the deficiencies described opposite.

Adrenal insufficiency is treated with hydro-cortisone (cortisol) tablets – the natural hormone – or cortisone acetate.

Thyroid under-activity is simply treated with thyroxine, or occasionally its precursor tri-iodothyronine.

Sex hormone deficiencies in women are treated with oestrogens and progesterone-type tablets in 21-day cycles with seven days off, either as separate tablets of ethinyl oestradiol throughout the cycle, with medroxyprogesterone acetate in the last half, or, more conveniently, as a low-estrogen contraceptive pill. Males are given injections of testosterone esters.

The management of growth hormone deficiency in children is usually confined to special centres.

Patients with diabetes insipidus have had their treatment revolutionized by the use of a synthetic form of ADH, desmopressin, which is taken as snuff, absorbed through the nose.

Suppression of excessive hormone production: Irrespective of the cause, excessive levels of prolactin can usually be suppressed, often to normal, by the drug **bromocriptine;** it also gives control of galactorrhea, and restoration of potency, menstruation and fertility.

OVER-THE-COUNTER TREATMENTS

None.

QUESTIONS TO ASK THE DOCTOR

■ Is it safe to continue hormone replacement therapy if I get another illness?

SIDE EFFECTS

The doses of **hormones** used as replacement therapy *do not* cause side effects. **Bromocriptine** can cause nausea, giddiness and indigestion which, though not dangerous, can be severe, even disabling. It is therefore all the more important to lessen the chances of these side effects by building up the dose slowly, starting with half a tablet last thing at night in the middle of a snack, and aiming eventually to take tablets during the three main meals.

SELF-MANAGEMENT

See **QUESTIONS TO ASK THE DOCTOR.** It is important to understand that steroid dose should be increased under certain circumstances – for example stress from another illness. DISCUSS THIS WITH YOUR DOCTOR.

PATIENT'S EXPERIENCE

"After suffering from headaches for years, I eventually consulted my doctor. I wasn't surprised to find I had high blood pressure, but I was when I was told this was not the cause of the headaches and they were probably due to a disease of the pituitary gland called acromegaly. He referred me to a specialist in hormone disorders who surprised me even more by revealing how long I must have had the condition, judging from old photographs. At first I was upset by his talk of a pituitary tumor and by the delving into my sex life, which had been non-existent. But I was assured that tumor in this context meant swelling, not cancer. Treatment was with tablets of bromocriptine at first, and later a remarkably minor operation which left no scar as it was done through the nose from behind the upper lip. My skin soon became less greasy, followed by quite a marked reduction in the soft tissues in my face, hands and feet – while I also experienced a return of my libido and potency, which I had presumed had gone forever."

Obstetrics, gynecology, urinary and children

The genito-urinary system has evolved for the dual functions of reproduction and excretion. Disorders can be hormonal, infective, or structural – and many are still poorly understood.

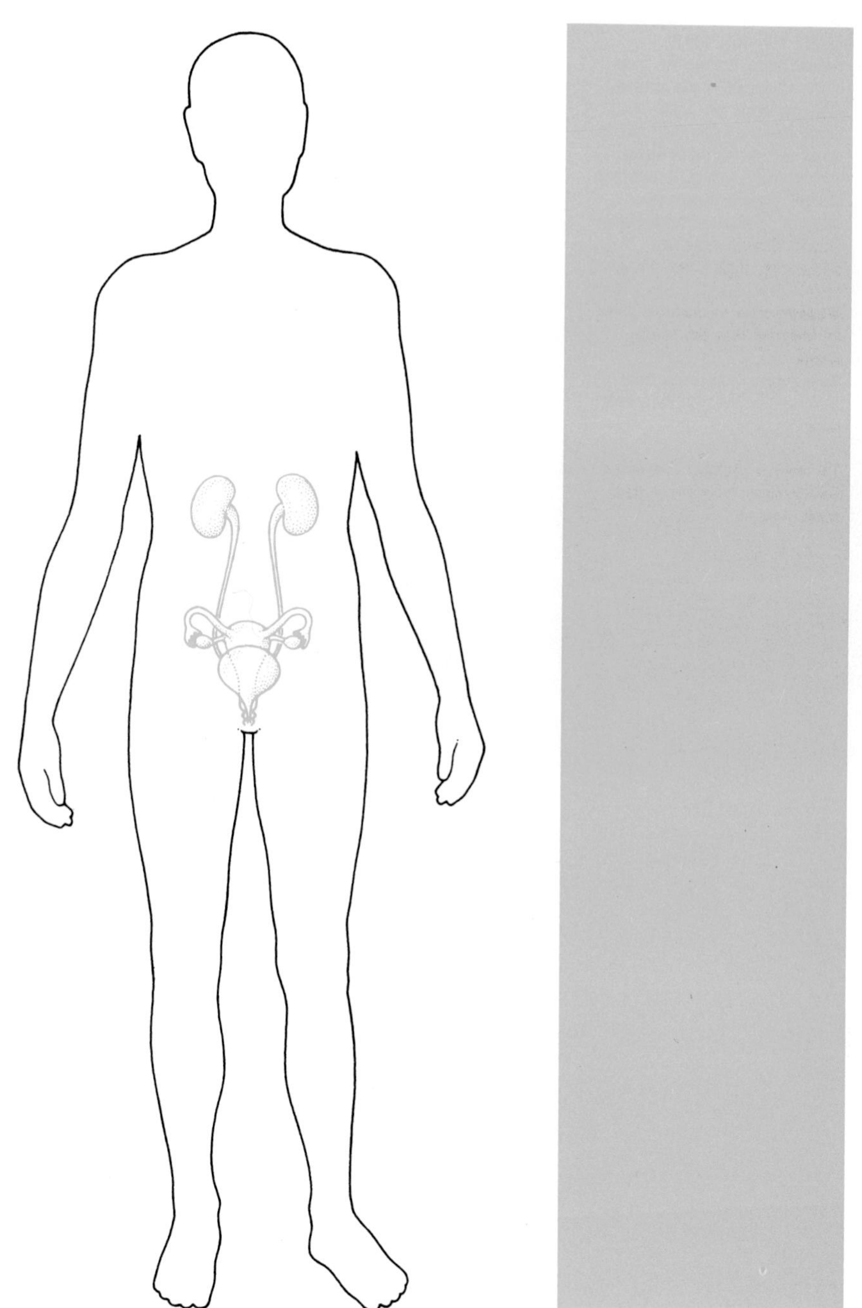

NAMES YOU WILL HEAR
Generic name: testosterone (male hormone) injection; **trade names:** Sustanon, Biosterone, Primoteston Depot, Malogex, Virormone. **Generic name:** testosterone subcutaneous implants; **trade names:** Testosterone, Malogen. **Generic name:** oral sublingual testosterone; **trade name:** Testoral. **Generic name:** oral testosterone; **trade name:** Restandol.

Intracorporeal vasodilator given by injection into the penile tissue
Generic name: papaverine; **trade name:** usually prescribed by generic name.

To reverse prolonged erection
Generic name: metaraminol; **trade name:** Aramine.

WHAT IS IMPOTENCE?

– A failure to obtain or maintain an erection for satisfactory sexual intercourse. This includes premature ejaculation and failure of pleasurable ejaculation.

CAUSES Either psychological, physical, or a combination of both. In order to have an erection, men need an adequate nerve and blood supply to the penis; male hormones are also necessary but their role in creating libido – sexual appetite – is more important. Poor blood supply is caused by: blockage of the lower aorta, as may happen with ***atherosclerosis,*** *page 44;* or by blocked small blood vessels as may may happen with ***diabetes,*** *page 156.* Poor nerve supply can have a multitude of causes: diabetes mellitus; alcohol; spinal injury; antihypertensive drugs, especially beta-blockers and methyldopa; diseases such as multiple sclerosis and ageing. The underlying causes of psychological impotence are of course complex, but it is probably fair to summarize them as fear of failure; anxiety; inexperience; communication problems with sexual partner; depression; drug treatment for depression, paradoxically; and deep rooted fears related to sex.

WHAT THE DOCTOR WILL ASK YOU

How long has it been a problem? Was the onset gradual or sudden? Is it related to some work or family problem? What was intercourse like before? What is the attitude of your present partner(s)? Do you wake with erections in the morning? Can you get an erection at all? Do you ejaculate, get a sensation of orgasm? Do you masturbate?

TREATMENT

Counselling of both partners is the usual recourse for psychological impotence. This may be undertaken by a GP, a psychologist, a psychosexual clinic, or marriage guidance counsellors.

If the cause is not obviously psychological, the patient may need blood tests for hormone and blood sugar levels. If hospital investigations are considered necessary, penile tumescence (swelling) studies and penile rigidity measurements, often performed overnight, can confirm absence or presence of erections while asleep. If they are present, the problem is probably psychological. Injection of **vasodilator** drugs directly into the penile tissue will re-establish erections in most patients if the penile blood supply is adequate. This can be self-taught.

Penile implants (semi-rigid or inflatable) are another option in irreversible impotence. The implant is inserted inside the penile tissue. Semi-rigid implants give a semi-permanent erection, and, depending on one's style of clothes, can be more or less obvious.

Testosterone is only prescribed when the level of this hormone is low, typically as a result of removal of testes. In such cases it will restore performance.

QUESTIONS TO ASK THE DOCTOR

- Why have I become impotent?
- Am I too old to be treated?
- If my partner is no longer interested, will I be treated?
- Would guidance counselling help me?

SIDE EFFECTS

Intracorporeal **vasodilators** do have drawbacks which make them unsuitable in the long term: bruising and scarring of the penile tissue can occur or a painful, prolonged erection. Penile implants have a low failure rate. The main problem is infection, but this is uncommon if antibiotics are given at the time of operation and the surgery is done carefully.

Testosterone can cause jaundice: regular liver function tests are required. If there is evidence of liver damage, the treatment is stopped. The hormone also increases the individual's level of aggression.

SELF-HELP (PSYCHOLOGICAL IMPOTENCE)

Admit to yourself that impotence is a problem and see a doctor. This creates a situation in which the problem can be discussed between the man, his partner and the doctor in a relatively rational manner. Also, frankly discuss with your partner aspects of each other's behavior that you like or dislike, if this seems to cause problems. Try a return to petting without necessarily having sexual intercourse. Many counsellors advise a ban on intercourse at the beginning of treatment – to get rid of the large component of fear of failure.

PATIENT'S EXPERIENCE

"I'm in my early forties – and I have multiple sclerosis. As if this isn't enough, I started going impotent six months back, as a result of the disease. My wife always said she wouldn't mind – the doctor warned us it might happen – but when it came to it, she did mind. She said it was the final blow on top of all the other problems with my disease; I was annoyed because I thought she should be more understanding.

The atmosphere between us got so bad that I really thought our marriage was threatened. So I told my doctor. He immediately suggested initial treatment with intracorporeal Papaverine: I had to inject myself just before making love – and it worked beautifully. Unfortunately, my doctor said I shouldn't use the drug long-term; but he did say I was a suitable patient for a penile prosthesis."

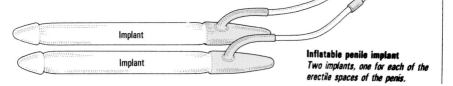

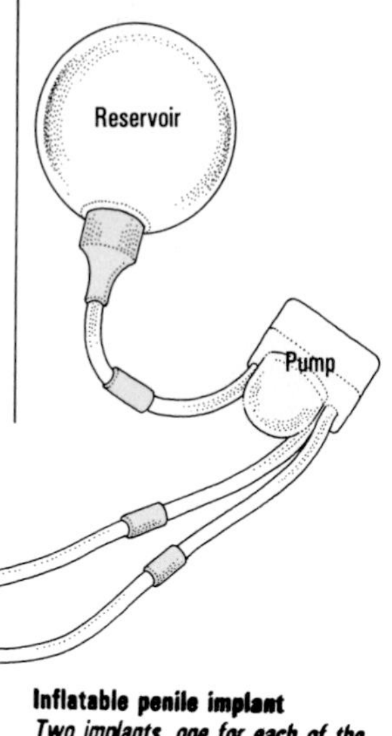

Inflatable penile implant
Two implants, one for each of the erectile spaces of the penis.

Ovulation inducers

NAMES YOU WILL HEAR
Ovulation inducers
Generic name: cyclofenil; **trade name:** Rehibin. **Generic name:** clomiphene citrate; **trade names:** Clomid, Serophene. **Generic name:** chorionic gonadotrophin HCG; **trade names:** Pregnyl, Profasi, Gonadtrophon LH. **Generic name:** follicle stimulating hormone (FSH); **trade names:** Metrodin, Pergonal, Gonadotraphon FSH, Profasi. **Generic name:** bromocryptine; **trade name:** Parlodel.

WHAT IS INFERTILITY?

The practical definition is when the female has failed to conceive after two years of normal sexual relations. If pregnancy has occurred, but the outcome has been unsuccessful, the couple are considered to be subfertile, a condition outside the scope of this section.

If pregnancy is to occur without medical assistance, it usually does so in the first year; however, about a quarter of pregnancies do occur in the second year. Estimates of the true level of infertility vary in different societies and social groups; however, it is generally agreed that at least ten per cent of couples are infertile and recent studies indicate that the real prevalence is nearer 20 per cent.

Of those who have investigation and treatment, between 30 per cent and 60 per cent will eventually produce a live baby. Sadly, however, there remains a large group who will never be able to produce a child of their own. Modern treatments are certainly offering hope, but this too can bring problems. Having hopes raised, only to be dashed, can only prolong the agony of facing up to, and dealing with, childlessness. Couples faced with the possibility of infertility need more than average patience and realism.

CAUSES The most common factor remains disorders of ovulation. These can be detected in over 40 per cent of infertile women. Abnormalities of the male partner's semen are discovered in 30 per cent. Blocked or damaged Fallopian tubes and scarring also involving the ovaries are also common, being found in 20 per cent of women.

Problems with the neck of the womb and immunological factors are rare causes.

Less than four per cent of couples have unexplained infertility – that is to say all the tests are normal. Many of these couples do eventually conceive.

In about ten per cent, abnormalities in both partners are detected. This does not mean pregnancy cannot occur; treatment of both partners should take place simultaneously.

TREATMENT

The treatment of infertility depends, of course, on the cause.

Disorders of ovulation are complex and involve the use of a wide range of drugs.

Many of the problems with the Fallopian tubes, and often with the ovaries, are caused by previous infection. Usually this has been silent and symptomless, but where a diagnosis of salpingitis (infection in the tubes), has been made, drug treatment should be intensive and active: see below. Sometimes endometriosis is the cause of infertility, or associated with it, and here drug therapy is sometimes combined with surgery *(see **period problems,** page 190)*.

If the Fallopian tubes and/or ovaries are physically damaged, rather than infected, microsurgery is the first line of treatment. Success rate varies from 20 per cent to 80 per cent, depending on the nature of the problem. The next option is IVF (*in vitro* fertilization) – a ''test tube pregnancy'', which usually involves the use of drugs to produce superovulation. The overall success rate of IVF remains low, probably less than ten per cent, but as the technique is refined, success rates may well rise as high as 30 per cent.

New techniques using drugs to produce superovulation are currently being researched.

When the only problem identified is with the husband's semen, the first-line treatment is surgical; drug therapy may also be used; both tend to be unrewarding.

PRESCRIPTION DRUGS

To understand specific drug treatment of infertility, it is essential to appreciate the biochemical events of the female reproductive cycle: read what follows in association with the diagram and caption on page 176.

Steroids have been used to treat cervical and immunological problems in the woman and also to treat the male. The treatment is not without risk or side effects and conception rates are no higher than those that occur naturally.

How they work: by suppressing antibodies that sometimes interfere with normal sperm movement.

A variety of drugs including **estrogens, progestogens** and **clomiphene** have been used to treat those with unexplained infertility. One study showed a 50 per cent success rate using a six-month treatment program. The first two months of treatment involved no drugs, blood tests and continual emotional support and encouragement of the female partner. The following four months involved a variety of different drug combinations to induce ovulation. One of the patients who successfully conceived had been trying to have a child for 12 months, and she conceived during the first two months of the program.

PATIENTS' EXPERIENCES

"We travelled clear across the state to see the specialist. I had been infertile for seven years. All the tests were normal, and then I had a laparoscopy. The doctor told me afterwards the ovaries were rather cystic and he had pricked them both with a needle.

I conceived the next month. Three years later I went back and eventually persuaded him to relaparoscope me – and to give the ovaries another prick. He did, but I didn't get pregnant. He says my getting pregnant the first time had nothing to do with the laparoscopy.

I've got to accept that things haven't worked out the way we planned: hard, because we both come from large families and feel that that is the only way a family should be."

Ovulation inducers: Choice depends on the cause of ovulatory failure. The commonest problem is oversensitive feedback with suppression of the pituitary production of FSH by circulating estrogen. Clomiphene citrate blocks the estrogen receptor sites in the brain, thus resetting the mechanism. Where this does not work on its own, chlorionic gonadotropin or menopausal gonadotropin may be added. These act as a substitute for the LH surge, to stimulate ovulation. The injections of both FSH and LH can be used to mimic the natural production by the pituitary.

More recent techniques involve suppressing or down-regulating natural production of LH/FSH to get better control with injected hormones.

Other sophisticated techniques act even more radically, and involve hormones produced in the brain which actually release LH and FSH. A special pump may be used to inject gradually the gonadotrophin-releasing hormone. Combinations of these drugs are used in the IVF regime. Bromocriptine can be used to lower the level of prolactin, thus allowing FSH and LH to stimulate the ovaries.

OVER-THE-COUNTER TREATMENTS

None.

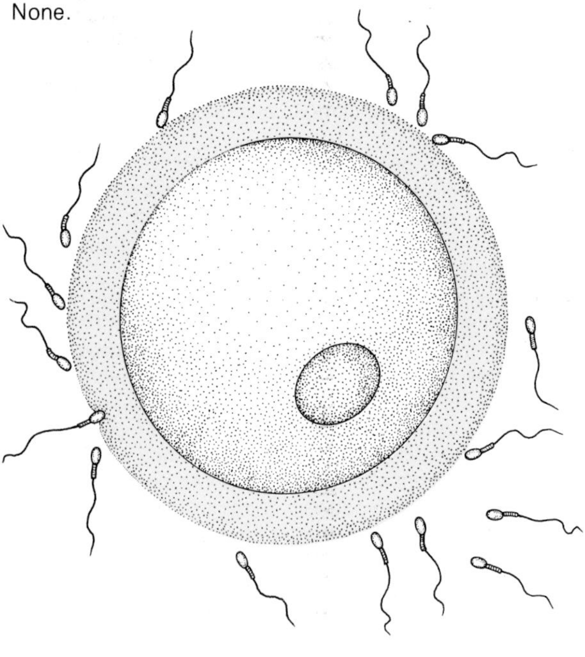

The moment of conception – *in a test tube. The technique involves removing a number of eggs from the ovaries and culturing them with sperm. Four days later, a few of the successfully fertilized eggs are returned to the womb.*

QUESTIONS TO ASK THE DOCTOR

- At what time of the month am I most fertile?
- What is the success rate with this (these) drugs?
- Are there any special problems I am likely to run into when taking drugs, like having multiple births, for example?
- If my husband's sperm count is low, are there any simple measures that may improve it?
- If all the tests are normal, is there anything else we can do?

SIDE EFFECTS

The milder **ovulation inducer,** clomiphene citrate, produces fairly minor side effects such as flushes, sometimes breast tenderness, irritability, mid-cycle pain and feeling bloated. Occasionally, particularly with higher doses, over-stimulation of the ovaries occurs, with pain and cyst formation. Up to 10 per cent of clomiphene-induced pregnancies result in multiple births.

More complex regimes of ovulation treatment require careful monitoring of hormone levels to reduce the risk of over-stimulation of the ovaries. Such complex treatment is not available in all hospitals. Bromocriptine commonly produces side effects and the dose has to be built up slowly. It should always be taken with meals to avoid nausea and vomiting. A general feeling of malaise, headaches and dizziness are also common. **Steroids** can produce severe side effects *(see **anemia,** page 224)* but in short courses these are unusual.

SELF-MANAGEMENT

- Don't let your life revolve around the presence or absence of the next menstrual cycle. Don't blame yourself, your partner or your doctor for your failure to conceive. Cultivate interests other than your desire for a child.
- The period of maximum fertility starts 19 days before a woman's next period is due and lasts about five days.
- If the sperm count is low, it may be improved by wearing loose fitting underpants and trousers.
- Let neither partner get so obsessed about sexual intercourse and its frequency that the other begins to wonder whether their role has been down-graded to that of baby-producer.
- Keep hopeful, but be realistic. If success eludes you, accept that you may never have a child. Pregnancy would be a bonus rather than a likelihood.

PATIENT'S EXPERIENCE

"I'm a school teacher. I don't know why I bothered with those tests or operations. Hospitals are so inefficient, it takes months. They told me I had Stein Leventhal syndrome and treated me for it. Being a teacher – rather a forceful person – made the whole thing intolerable. I remember a day my doctor wasn't there and in my anger, I tore into his assistant. I should have written to her and apologized. Instead I turned my face to the wall, and gave up. I had had drugs; I had had tubal microsurgery; and I only had the one side left. I didn't keep my follow-up appointments and the doctor wrote to me sending a prescription for more fertility drugs. I tore the prescription up. I telephoned the hospital a month later. I was three months pregnant. After the first child, a daughter, I had a second – another girl."

NAMES YOU WILL HEAR
Generic names: combined contraceptive pills contain ethinyl estradiol in varying doses and a progestogen. Progestogen-only pills (in italics) contain just progestogen.
Trade names: Trinordiol, Logynon, Trinovum, Marvelon, Neocon, Norimin, Ovysmen, Brevinor, Microgynon 30, Ovranette, Eugynon 50, Minilyn, Norinyl-1, Anovlar, Gynovlar, *Femulen, Micronor, Microval,* Triphasil, Biphasil, Nordette, Eugynon, Ortho-Novum 1/50, *Microlut,* Triquilar, Marvelon, Brevinor-1, Lyndiol, *Femulen, Noriday,* Orthonovum 777, Ortho-Novum 1/35, Brevicon, Min-Ovral, Ovral, Norinyl 1 & 50, Trinordiol, Trinovum, Nordiol, *Micronovum, Mocroval.*

WHAT IS CONTRACEPTION?

– The prevention of pregnancy. This can be achieved by using hormones, barriers, IUD's or Intrauterine Devices or, more permanently, by sterilization. The ideal contraceptive, one that is one hundred per cent effective and one hundred per cent safe does not exist, so couples must decide which method is most appropriate. Means of prevention divide into two broad types: hormonal (this page, and pages 179-180); and 'others' (pages 180-183). 'Others' comprise barriers, coils and sterilization.

PRESCRIPTION DRUGS

The combined pill: This is the most popular hormonal method. Many different brands are available, but they all contain two hormones: estrogen and a progestin.
How it works: by stopping the woman's ovaries releasing an egg each month. It also makes the womb less receptive to the egg, and makes it harder for sperm to swim into the womb. It should be taken regularly for 21, 22 or 28 days depending on which type you have. If it is taken for 21 or 22 days, bleeding usually occurs in the seven or six days when the pill is not taken. If a 28-day packet is taken, bleeding usually occurs in the last few days of taking the pill.
The progestin-only pill (POP): This pill is little-used in the USA. Many brands are available, but they all contain one hormone called progestogen. It is taken every day without a break, and should be taken at the same time of day every day.
How it works: Although it may prevent the normal release of eggs, it mainly works by making it harder for sperm to swim into the womb. It also makes the womb less receptive to the egg.
The 'morning after' pill: An emergency-only measure. It is mis-named: you can take it up to 72 hours after unprotected intercourse. It consists of a strong dose of estrogen and progestogen (usually given as two tablets) followed by another dose 12 hours later.
How it works: either by stopping the egg being released, or, if this has already occurred, it can prevent the egg settling in the womb. (Not available in the USA.)
Injectables: A large dose of one hormone, progestogen, by injection every three months.
How it works: prevents the egg being released; also makes it harder for the sperm to swim into the womb.

OVER-THE-COUNTER TREATMENTS

None.

QUESTIONS TO ASK THE DOCTOR

- Why is it so important to start taking the pill at the right time of my menstrual cycle?
- What should I do if I am sick or have diarrhea while on the pill?
- Can other medicines interfere with taking the pill?

SIDE EFFECTS

The combined pill is nearly one hundred per cent effective in preventing pregnancy, provided it is taken regularly. It has beneficial effects such as making periods regular, lighter and less painful. Problems such as sickness and breast tenderness usually settle in a couple of months. However, taking the pill does carry some serious, albeit rare, risks. These include the formation of blood clots (which may cause strokes and heart attacks) and, in a few people, increased blood pressure. Studies of the risk of cancer of the neck of the womb, and of breast cancer, are conflicting. Some have found an apparent link between breast cancer and the use of this pill at a young age (less than 25), or before the birth of the first baby. Other studies have completely failed to find any such link. Until further evidence is available, the experts feel there should be no change in prescribing policy. If concerned, discuss this with your doctor.

The progestin-only pill is not as effective as the combined pill, especially in younger women. It may be taken by women for whom the estrogen-containing pill is unsuitable – breast-feeding mothers, heavy smokers and diabetics. The major problem is irregular bleeding: some women have no periods, others bleed much of the time. Some women develop depression. It is not suitable for women who have had a Fallopian tube pregnancy.

The 'morning-after' pill: Many women suffer sickness after taking these pills. Their next period may be early or delayed. It is not suitable for women who have had a blood clot. It may not work in one in 50 of those treated. (Not available in the USA.)

Injectables: Some women have heavy bleeding after the injection, and the injection cannot, like a pill, be stopped once given. It takes some women longer to become pregnant once they have stopped using this method, compared with the other hormonal methods.

SELF-MANAGEMENT AND SELF-HELP

- When asking for the pill, be honest with your doctor about any health problems, your own or among close blood relatives. The pill may not be suitable if there is a

PATIENT'S EXPERIENCE OF STERILISATION

"I got pregnant when I was 25. I had stopped taking the pill because I was worried about what it was doing to my body, and I smoked. When I had had the baby, the question of contraception was naturally raised again at the hospital. I'd already had three children; I didn't want to take the pill, and I didn't like any of the other methods so I was sterilized. I wished they'd told me how tired you'd feel after the operation. I noticed that my periods were heavier, too; however, the doctor said that was because I'd stopped taking the pill.

That was seven years ago. My husband left me four years ago and my new boyfriend has no children. He wants me to have his children – which of course I can't. Now I'm worried he won't marry me because of this. The decision to be sterilized is one of the most difficult a woman can ever take."

family history of cardio-vascular disease.

■ Stop smoking. This dramatically reduces the risk of any of the serious problems associated with taking the combined pill.

■ Remember to take the pill. If you forget a combined pill (and anything longer than 12 hours is a forgotten pill) you must use additional precautions for the rest of the cycle. If less than a week from the end of the cycle, you must take two packets consecutively – do not have a break that month.

If you take the POP you have only three hours to remember your pill. If forgotten you must use additional precautions for 48 hours.

■ If you bleed while taking your pills, do not worry; carry on taking the pill and mention it to your doctor at your next visit.

■ If you have heavy bleeding after the injection, see your doctor, who may give you some tablets that will help with the problem.

■ If you miss a period with any of these methods, carry on taking the pill and arrange to see your doctor.

■ See your doctor immediately if you: develop pain or swelling of the legs; develop pain in the chest or stomach; develop breathlessness or cough up blood; have a bad fainting attack or collapse; develop an unusual headache, blurred vision or difficulty with speech; develop numbness or weakness of an arm or leg; notice your skin or eyes have become yellow.

BARRIERS, IUD'S, STERILIZATION BARRIERS

These comprise caps, diaphragms, the condom and the contraceptive sponge; all require enthusiasm from the couple if they are to be effective.

Caps and diaphragms should be used with a spermicide to ensure maximum effectiveness. They are not as effective as the hormonal methods in preventing pregnancy. They may be inserted into the vagina several hours before intercourse; however, if intercourse does not occur within three hours, additional spermicide is required. They need initial fitting by a specially-trained nurse or doctor and require practice before they can be fitted reliably by the user.

Condoms are male-only and can have a high failure rate, especially when used by less experienced couples. They may protect against many sexually transmitted diseases.

The contraceptive sponge is, like the condom, available over-the-counter. It should be moistened prior to use. Insert it into the vagina several hours before intercourse, but do not remove once intercourse has occurred for at least six hours. Unfortunately it has a high failure rate – approximately one in five users become pregnant during 12 months' use.

SELF-MANAGEMENT AND SELF-HELP

- If using a cap or diaphragm, check every time that the cervix is properly covered.
- Ensure that the condom covers the penis before *any* genital contact occurs.
- Withdraw the penis before it becomes too soft. Hold the base of the condom during withdrawal so as not to spill any semen.
- Use each condom once only.
- If the condom should break or come off, or if you find the cap or diaphragm was not in the correct place, see your doctor who may prescribe the 'morning after' pill.

INTERUTERINE DEVICES IUD'S (COILS)

An IUD coil is a solid object placed in the womb to prevent pregnancy. There are three varieties: inert, copper-bearing and hormone-releasing. Only the latter type is now marketed in the USA. The device is usually inserted immediately after a period. It may also be used to prevent pregnancy if unprotected intercourse has occurred and hormonal treatment cannot be given. It may be used up to five days after the egg was released.

EFFECTS AND SIDE EFFECTS

The main effect is to stop the fused egg and sperm attaching to the womb. The hormone-releasing IUDs may also prevent sperms swimming into the womb.

Most IUDs cause periods to become heavier and longer than normal; periods may also become more painful than usual. They also appear to increase the risk of pelvic infection. (Infection in the Fallopian tubes – a serious matter which may prevent a future pregnancy.) Because of this, many doctors have stopped using these devices. IUDs are not the ideal method for women who have never had

IUDs prevent pregnancy first and foremost inside the womb, so if pregnancy occurs in a woman using a coil it is likely to be in a Fallopian tube. IUDs should not be used by women who have had tubal pregnancies.

SELF-HELP AND SELF-MANAGEMENT

- Since the IUD may increase the risk of pelvic infection, think very carefully before using one if you have already had an infection.

PATIENT'S EXPERIENCE OF THE COMBINED PILL

"I started taking the pill when I was 18 because I had heavy, painful periods; it helped a lot. My breasts were sore for the first few months, but this eventually improved.

After taking the same pill for a few years, I started bleeding at odd times during the month. My doctor changed the pill I was taking but warned me to give the new one at least three months to 'settle down'. For the first two months, I had the same bleeding troubles; but it now suits me fine."

■ If you have more than one partner (or at the time of changing a partner), use a condom as well as a IUD to help prevent infection.

■ Your doctor will leave the threads attached to your IUD so you can feel them by the neck of your womb. Check for these threads after your period. If you cannot feel them, use additional contraception and see your doctor.

■ See your doctor immediately if you miss a period, develop bad stomach pains, get pains during intercourse or develop a heavy vaginal discharge.

QUESTIONS TO ASK THE DOCTOR

■ What type of coil should I have?

■ How long can the coil remain in the womb?

Different types of coil can be left different lengths of time.

STERILIZATION

This is the most effective form of contraception of all and very difficult to reverse. Either partner may be sterilized. Technically, the procedure is easier in the male. However it may not always be appropriate for the male to be sterilized – men are fertile for most of their lives, whereas women are only fertile for 30 to 40 years. A woman can often be sure she never wants children even if she was with a new partner, whereas a man cannot be so sure what any future, possibly younger, partner might want. The procedure is straightforward in either sex. However, counselling is most important. Both partners must be certain they want no further children, whatever may happen. Sterilization is not a solution to sexual problems, a failing marriage or contraceptive problems.

SIDE EFFECTS

In the male, the operation – a vasectomy – is usually performed under out-patient conditions under local anaesthetic. The tubes that carry the sperm from the testes to the penis are cut and tied or cauterized. This does not interfere with subsequent sexual performance. The operation takes a few weeks to become effective.

In a woman the operation is usually performed under general anesthetic, although local anesthetic can be used. The Fallopian tubes which carry the eggs to the womb are either cut, cauterized or blocked with clips or rings. The abdominal wall has to be opened surgically to gain access.

QUESTIONS TO ASK THE DOCTOR

- How is the operation performed?
- Is a vasectomy painful when the anesthetic has worn off?
- How much time off work is required?
- How long after the operation is it effective?

STERILIZATION

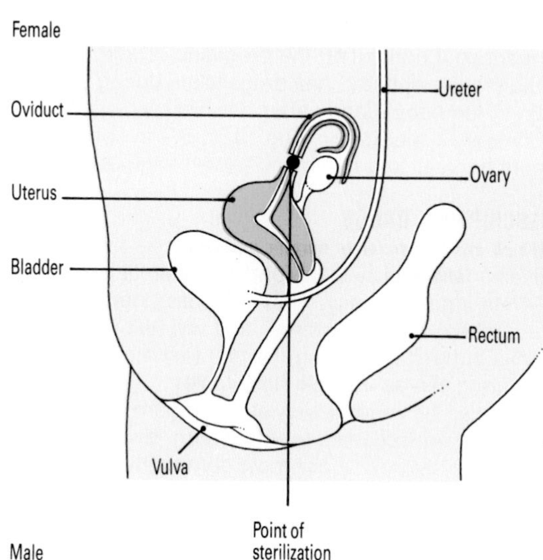

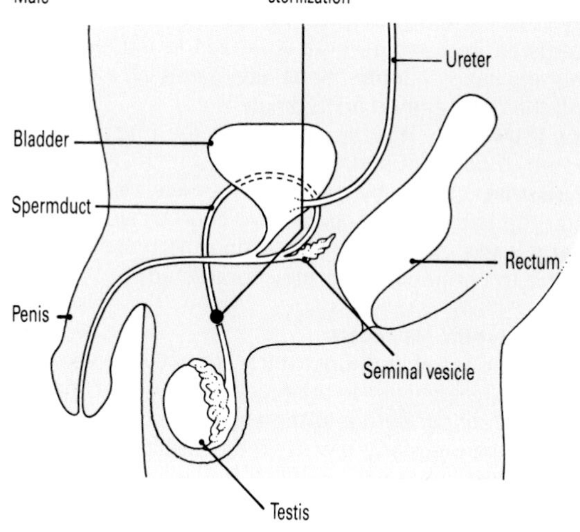

DOCTOR'S EXPERIENCE OF THE COMBINED PILL

"A 23 year-old woman consulted me recently, complaining of acne, a dry vagina and low sex drive. She was taking Norimin – a combined contraceptive pill. I thought her problems were caused by the pill, and so changed it to another type which is intended to be better for those with skin problems. I mentioned that her dryness might be caused by thrush, and prescribed some treatment.

Three to four weeks later, she returned and said she felt no better. I told her to persevere with the new pill. However, as she was leaving, she burst into tears and said she thought her husband was having an affair – and that she'd driven him to it as she had gone off sex – although it used to be fine.

Of course, I thought again. She had, after all, been taking Norimin for three years. If it was really causing adverse effects, wouldn't she have come sooner. Perhaps the problem was not the drug, but the relationship; possibly even her dryness was really a sign of lack of arousal. I should have suspected this earlier instead of just reaching for the prescription pad."

NAMES YOU WILL HEAR
Generic name: rubella vaccine; **trade names:** Meruvax, Almevax. **Generic name:** ferrous fumarate and folic acid; **trade names:** Cevi-Fer, Chromagen, Feostat, Ferancee, Ircon FA, Natalins, Prenate, Pregaday, Bramiron, Hematon, Filabon.

Analgesics during labour
Generic name: nitrous oxide and oxygen; **trade name:** Entonox. **Generic name:** lignocaine hydrochloride, lidocaine hydrochloride with adrenalin injection; **trade names:** Xylocaine, Lignocaine and Adrenalin Injection.

Oxytocics
Generic name: oxytocin; **trade names:** Syntocinon, Pitocin. **Generic name:** ergometrine maleate and oxytocin; **trade name:** Ergometrine and Oxytocin Injection. **Generic name:** ritodrine; **trade name:** Yutopar.

Antacids – *see* ***peptic ulcer,*** *page 26.*

Beta-stimulants – *see* ***asthma,*** *page 74.*

Anti-emetics – *see* ***dizziness,*** *page 96.*

Antibiotics – *see* ***pneumonia*** *and* ***pleurisy,*** *page 78.*

Antihypertensive drugs – *see* ***hypertension,*** *page 48.*

Laxatives – *see* ***constipation,*** *page 30.*

Antihistamines – *see* ***hay fever,*** *page 260.*

PREGNANCY

During the first three months after conception, most of a baby's organs are being formed. This is the most vulnerable time for the developing fetus: any illness in the mother, or drugs taken during this period, has the potential to cause abnormalities or deformities in the baby (the fetus). After the first three months, the fetus is almost completely formed; it continues to grow, and the organs to mature. Any drugs taken during this period, or indeed illness in the mother, are unlikely to cause abnormality, but may affect growth of the fetus.

Labor usually starts spontaneously, but may have to be induced if continuing the pregnancy could be a risk to the mother or baby. Any drugs taken during labor remain in the baby's body after delivery.

Generally speaking, drug therapy in pregnancy should be kept to a minimum – even when essential.

PRESCRIPTION DRUGS

– Which are beneficial to mother and child:

Iron and **folic acid** help to prevent anemia *(see page 224)* during pregnancy. They will pass from mother to fetus, where they are stored, and will help to prevent anemia in the baby during the first few months of life. They are given as a single daily tablet.

Antacids can be used to alleviate heartburn, which may occur late in pregnancy. Aluminum hydroxide and magnesium hydroxide are most commonly used.

Beta-stimulants are given to inhibit premature labor, initially by injection into a vein; the dose may be continued in tablet form.

Oxytocin is given by drip to improve contraction of the uterus (womb) when there is a need to induce or encourage labor. Contractions are carefully monitored and the dose altered accordingly.

How it works: by directly stimulating the muscle of the womb to contract and then to relax.

Ergometrine is given by injection to reduce bleeding just after the baby and placenta have been delivered.

How it works: by directly stimulating the muscle of the womb to contract and to stay contracted.

– Which benefit the mother:

Whenever possible, drugs which are known to be safe for the fetus are given in preference to new and improved preparations. Before taking any drugs when you are or could be pregnant, discuss the possible effects with your doctor.

Antiemetics (promethazine and meclizine) should only be

used as a last resort for persistent vomiting and not for nausea. See SIDE EFFECTS.

Certain **antibiotics** are safe in pregnancy, including penicillins and erythromycin. It is seldom necessary to use one which causes problems. Those to avoid include sulfonamides, tetracyclines, aminoglycosides and cotrimoxazole.

Antiasthmatic preparations can be safely used during pregnancy. Some, such as salbutamol, are beta-stimulants and can delay the onset of labor; treatment may have to be changed just before the baby is due.

In some women hypertension (high blood pressure) is a complication of pregnancy; it requires treatment as it can decrease the blood supply to the fetus and retard growth. Not all **antihypertensives** are safe during pregnancy, but methyldopa is commonly used.

Antidiabetic preparations: Young diabetics are usually on insulin, and the dose will probably have to be adjusted during pregnancy. Proper control of diabetes during pregnancy is vital, otherwise there is risk to the fetus.

Antiepileptics must be continued during pregnancy if a patient is subject to fits. Unfortunately, some anti-epileptic drugs can affect the fetus, so if you are an epileptic, discuss this with your doctor *before* getting pregnant. He may be able to recommend a more suitable drug.

Many **analgesics,** including aspirin and indomethacin, are better not used during pregnancy. A few, such as ibuprofen, are relatively safe. Discuss with your doctor.

Epidural anesthesia is an injection of local anesthetic (lidocaine) into the spine. It suppresses all pain stimuli from nerves in the lower half of the body, and can be used for normal deliveries, forceps-assisted deliveries and even Cesarian section operations. The mother is fully conscious, but pain-free. It is the best form of pain control in labor.

Pain relief during labor: Meperidine is a strong analgesic which can be given by injection during labor, but if given near the time of delivery, it may depress breathing in the newborn.

In some countries, but not typically in the USA, nitrous oxide and oxyen mixture is used to ease the discomfort of contractions without loss of consciousness. It is usually inhaled through a mask which the mother can use herself as and when necessary.

X-RAYS

X-rays may be a risk during pregnancy, depending on whether they are of the abdomen, and the dose.

OVER-THE-COUNTER TREATMENTS

Many commonly-used drugs may affect the fetus. Before taking anything, think whether it is absolutely necessary and safe. Drugs you can take include acetaminophen and laxatives which work by increasing the bulk of the stool. Drugs to avoid include: aspirin, laxatives which stimulate the bowel, antihistamines, cough mixtures containing iodine, cigarettes, alcohol and drugs of addiction. See SIDE EFFECTS.

QUESTIONS TO ASK THE DOCTOR

- Are you sure this drug is safe during pregnancy?
- What kind of sedation can I have during labor?

SIDE EFFECTS

Iron and **folic acid:** *See **anemia,** page 224.*
Oxytocin can cause excessive uterine contractions which in turn may affect blood supply to the fetus. It can also cause hypertension and fluid retention in the mother: these tend to be dose-related, and are thus usually controlled. **Ergometrine** cannot be used until after delivery as it causes marked and sustained uterine contraction.
Beta stimulants: *See **asthma,** page 74.* Some **antiemetics** have been used for many years with no adverse effects, but they have also been associated with fetal abnormalities. **Tetracyclines** can discolor the teeth of the child, **sulfonamides** can damage the red blood cells and cause anemia; **co-trimoxazole** can, in theory, cause fetal abnormalities.
Methyldopa has no specific side effects in pregnancy, likewise insulin in the correct dose. **Anti-epileptic drugs** which may cause fetal abnormalities include sodium valproate, phenytoin and phenobarbital. Substitutes can sometimes be found, but if one of the above drugs is the only one which adequately controls the fits, its benefit will outweigh the risk to the fetus. *See **epilepsy,** page 110.* **Aspirin** causes abnormalities of blood clotting in the fetus and may lead to hemorrhage. Many of the **anti-inflammatory analgesics** can cause heart problems in the fetus and prolonged labor. Ibuprofen can however be used: for side effects *see **rheumatoid arthritis,** page 242.*
Meperidine, may suppress uterine contractions (prolonging labor) but this is not usually significant. Epidural anesthetic may cause headache and a fall in blood pressure. Sometimes the anesthetic fails to reach all nerve fibers, and pain is not suppressed.
Laxatives like senna which work by increasing the con-

tractions of the bowel may also stimulate uterine contraction and precipitate labor; in large doses, they may also cause diarrhea. **Antihistamines** may cause abnormalities in the fetus. Cough mixtures containing iodine may produce a goiter in the fetus. **Nicotine** inhaled with cigarette smoke constricts the blood vessels and can thus reduce blood supply to the fetus, resulting in a small baby and an increased risk of mental retardation and other abnormalities. **Alcohol** taken even in moderate amounts is implicated in higher incidence of fetal abnormality, including mental retardation. **Drugs of addiction** can cause fetal abnormalities, and if present in the mother at the time of birth, can cause irritability and withdrawal symptoms in the newborn.

SELF-MANAGEMENT

Before pregnancy, ensure that you are fit by:

■ Maintaining a healthy diet; try not to be overweight at the start of the pregnancy.

■ Giving up smoking.

During pregnancy:

■ Prenatal examinations really are important for enabling doctors to detect early signs of complications such as hypertension.

■ Report any unusual symptoms to your doctor.

■ Avoid taking any drug unless it is absolutely necessary.

■ Guard against excessive weight gain. Don't attempt to 'eat for two': small, frequent meals tend to be best. Keep active: boredom can be a cause of weight gain.

■ Don't curtail normal activities unless advised by a doctor: if working, you can usually continue quite late into pregnancy. ■ Minimize constipation by using a high-fiber diet. *See* ***constipation,*** *page 30.* ■ Lessen the nausea of early pregnancy, and later heartburn, by eating small meals, frequently. ■ Minimize backache with a firm bed, sound posture and a regular daily rest.

■ Go to prenatal classes: the exercises they teach will help deal with labor pains.

Labor:

■ Air your feelings about how much pain relief you want. Discuss it with your doctor well before childbirth.

■ If you have a Cesarian section, consider the possibility of an epidural, and so remain conscious during the whole procedure. Many mothers prefer this, and most doctors feel that it improves bonding.

PATIENTS' EXPERIENCE

"I was 12 weeks pregnant with my first baby when I developed a high temperature, vomiting and pain on passing urine. I had stopped smoking a few months before I became pregnant and had been quite well. I was afraid to take any medicines and went straight to my doctor. He sent a specimen of urine to the laboratory and started me on an antibiotic which he said was safe in pregnancy. He said that I could take acetaminophen for the pain, but that he would not give me anything for the vomiting unless it was very severe. The symptoms improved quite quickly and I was well for the rest of my pregnancy."

"My doctor told me that because I am quite small, I would probably need a Cesarian section instead of normal delivery. I asked him if I could have it under epidural anesthetic and he said that it would probably be possible and explained the procedure. I was given the epidural quite soon after contractions started: I could feel my abdomen and legs going numb. They wheeled me into the operating room and draped sterile sheets over me ready to do the Cesarian. I couldn't see where the doctors were cutting because I was lying flat, and I couldn't feel a thing. The doctor told me that he was taking the baby out and then I heard her cry. The nurse wrapped her in a towel and gave her to me immediately. My husband and I were thrilled – he had been with me the whole time. I was able to get up and about much quicker than other mothers who had had general anesthetics."

URINARY INCONTINENCE

Imipramine. propantheline, emepronium, terodiline

NAMES YOU WILL HEAR
Generic name: amitriptyline; **trade names:** Elavil, Limbitrol, Tryptizol, Lentizol, Domical, Laroxyl, Tryptanol, Saroten, Amiline, Deprex, Levate, Meravil, Novotriptyn, Amilent, Trepiline, Tryptanol. **Generic name:** imipramine; **trade names:** Tofranil, Imiprin, Tramil, Melipramine, Prodepress, Simipra, Impril, Novopramine, Panpramine. **Generic name:** propantheline bromide; **trade name:** Pro-Banthine. **Generic name:** emepronium bromide; **trade name:** Cetiprin. **Generic name:** terodiline; **trade name:** Terolin.

IN THE ELDERLY
The cause of the incontinence should be sought and treated appropriately. Loss of bladder control in old people should not be regarded as "normal".

General measures to assist old people include: enabling them to be as mobile as possible; advising against restrictive clothing; moving the bedroom closer to the bathroom, and/or providing the old-fashioned expedient of a commode; minimizing use of tranquillizers and sleeping tablets – they can make incontinence worse; reminders to go to the bathroom may be helpful, particularly in mildly confused patients. ■ Diuretic therapy, see page 52, can cause incontinence. It may be possible to adjust the timing of tablets to fit in with the patient's daily activity. If possible, diuretics should not be taken after 4 pm. Discuss with the doctor. ■ Poor motivation makes incontinence more likely: give plenty of encouragement. ■ Any acute illness or move to unfamiliar surroundings can precipitate incontinence, which may then clear up of its own accord when conditions have stabilized.

WHAT IS URINARY INCONTINENCE?

– The involuntary passing of urine. There may be no sensation that the bladder is full or that urine is being passed. It may be impossible to prevent the flow of urine, even with effort – it ''comes away'' regardless. ''Double incontinence'' refers to loss of control over both bowel and bladder emptying.

CAUSES ■ Infants normally acquire bladder control at about two years. Incontinence at night can last until five or six years. Some children will have the occasional ''accident'' much later than this. ■ Stress/urgency incontinence which usually occurs in middle-aged women is due to laxity of the pelvic muscles (especially after childbirth). The pelvic muscles support the bladder and when they are stretched some degree of bladder control is lost. ■ Following damage to the nerves of the bladder (for example in paraplegia and certain nerve diseases), there is no sensation that the bladder is full and no control over the passage of urine. ■ In the elderly, incontinence is the commonest consequence of nerve damage (as in ***stroke,*** *page 58,* or ***senile dementia,*** *page 124);* poor pelvic muscle tone in women; prostatic enlargement in men.

PRESCRIPTION DRUGS

Drugs are not particularly effective and they have a high incidence of side effects.

Imipramine and **amitriptyline** are used to treat urinary incontinence at night in the young and the old, if drugs are considered necessary. In children, the first line of treatment is usually behavioral, with bell alarms and a reward system.

How they work: by causing retention of urine. It depresses nervous impulses to the bladder, and allows it to dilate. Also, children sleep less deeply and thus recognize the sensation of an enlarging bladder.

Propantheline can help the patient urinate less frequently.

How they work: by decreasing contraction of the bladder muscles, so increasing bladder capacity.

Physiotherapy can provide exercises for the pelvic floor muscles to improve bladder support.

OVER-THE-COUNTER TREATMENTS

None with any proven value. However, barrier creams are useful in dealing with the redness, and the damage to the skin of the buttocks which is a secondary result of incontinence. Disposable sheets backed with plastic help to save laundry, as do absorbent pads worn inside underwear.

QUESTIONS TO ASK THE DOCTOR

■ Is my child's bed-wetting severe enough to justify drug treatment, or would a buzzer system be better?
■ Is the incontinence reversible?
■ Is it necessary to test the urine for infection?

SIDE EFFECTS

Imipramine can cause a dry mouth, blurring of vision and constipation. It can also reduce blood pressure, and cause dizziness or fainting, convulsions and irregularities in heartbeat.
Propantheline can cause a dry mouth, blurring of vision, constipation and a rapid heartbeat. It can precipitate glaucoma and heart failure. Urinary retention may occur.

SELF-MANAGEMENT

Children:
■ Tensions associated with toilet training can have long-lasting effects, and the same applies to being dry at night. ■ Don't take a toddler out of diapers if he or she is likely to wet the bed. ■ Routine measures including limiting fluid intake after 4 pm; getting the child up to urinate after three or four hours' sleep (this need not involve waking the child completely); and using a reward system for dry nights. ■ Don't put undue stress on being dry and don't show anger over wet sheets. A child is not in control of the bladder when asleep. ■ Family tension may be a cause. If bed-wetting continues beyond five, consult your doctor.
After nerve damage:
This can cause total loss of bladder control. ■ If a man has sufficient penile length, a condom ''catheter'' attached to a bag may be helpful. Otherwise absorbent pads and plastic-backed sheets are the only other relatively simple options. ■ The skin must be kept clean and dry to reduce the risk of bed sores. Apply barrier cream after cleaning. ■ Catheters are only used in selected cases: they can cause bladder infection.
Sudden onset:
Sudden urinary incontinence in any age group should be investigated by a doctor for the possibility of bladder infection. This will mean sending a specimen of urine to a laboratory. It is very important to provide a clean ''mid-stream'' specimen – the urine should go straight into a sterile container.

PATIENT'S EXPERIENCE
"My mother, aged 83, was becoming more and more senile. When the doctor put her on a diuretic for her heart, she suddenly became incontinent. He said I should remind her to go to the bathroom every half-hour after taking a pill. He also said that the second pill of the day could be taken at 4 pm, to give it a chance to work before bedtime.

Things went well enough until she developed arthritis in her knees. She just could not reach the bathroom in time. I persuaded her to wear an absorbent pad which made her less apprehensive of accidents."

Hormone therapy

NAMES YOU WILL HEAR

Estrogens
Generic name: ethinylestradiol; **trade names:** Brevicon, Demulen, Levlen, Feminone, Lynoral, Estinyl. **Generic name:** estradiol; **trade names:** Estrace, E-cypionate, Progynova. **Generic name:** oestriol; **trade name:** Ovestin.

Progesterones
Generic name: medroxyprogesterone acetate; **trade names:** Amen, Curretab, Depo-Provera, Provera. **Generic name:** noresthisterone; **trade name:** Primolut-N. **Generic name:** progesterone; **trade names:** Progestasert, Cyclogest. **Generic name:** dydrogesterone; **trade name:** Gynorest.

Combined contraceptive pills
*see **contraception,** page 178.*

Danazol
Generic name: danazol; **trade names:** Danocrine, Danol.

Antifibrinolytic drugs
Generic name: aminocaproic acid; **trade names:** Amicar, Epsikapron. **Generic name:** ethamsylate; **trade name:** Dicynene. **Generic name:** tranexamic acid; **trade name:** Cyclokapron.

Antispasmodics
Generic name: alverine citrate; **trade name:** Spasmonal. **Generic name:** hyoscine butyl bromide; **trade name:** Buscopan.

Analgesics
Generic name: aspirin; **trade names:** Ascriptin, Ecotrin, Measurin, Aspirin, Astrin, Bi-Prin. **Generic name:** mefenamic acid; **trade names:** Ponstan, Ponstan Forte. Many non-steroidal anti-inflammatory drugs also used – *see **pain,** page 106 and **rheumatoid arthritis,** page 242.*

Vitamin B6
Generic name: pyridoxine hydrochloride; **trade names:** Beelith, Eldertonic, Mega-B, Senilezol, Vicon-C.

WHAT ARE PERIOD PROBLEMS?

– Several different and distressingly common conditions including: **heavy periods; frequent periods; infrequent** or **absent periods** (amenorrhea); **painful periods** (dysmenorrhea); **bleeding between periods** (intermenstrual bleeding) and **premenstrual tension/syndrome** (PMT/PMS). The last is a complex of symptoms including fluid retention, bloating and irritability prior to periods. These are the commonest complaints; a less common problem is endometriosis, an abnormality in the growth and location of the lining of the womb which gives rise to painful periods.

CAUSES Generally, it is thought that the most usual cause of period problems is an imbalance in the levels of hormones – estrogen and progesterone. Very rarely there may be a more serious underlying cause. In particular:

Heavy periods (menorrhagia) are often "normal" periods which simply become heavier as a woman grows older. Other (rarer) causes include having a coil (IUD) in place; fibroids; an underactive thyroid gland, *see **hypothyroidism,** page 166;* and blood clotting disorders.

Painful periods (dysmenorrhea) can start soon after puberty (primary dysmenorrhea) and are caused by hormone imbalances which cause high levels of prostaglandins to be present in the uterus. These are believed to cause uterine contractions/cramps. Period pain which starts later on in life (secondary dysmenorrhea) can be due to endometriosis or to chronic pelvic infection (pelvic inflammatory disease or salpingitis).

Bleeding between periods can be due to miscarriage (abortion), tubal (ectopic) pregnancies, the progesterone-only pill (POP) *(see **contraception,** page 28),* the coil, cervical erosion, polyps and cancer (of the cervix, ovary or uterus).

Lack of periods (amenorrhea) can be due to pregnancy, severe weight loss (***anorexia,*** *page 220*), ***stress*** *(page 88),* and, very rarely, ***tumors of the pituitary gland*** *(page 168)* or an underactive thyroid gland – *see **hypothyroidism,** page 166.*

The cause of PMT/PMS is not fully understood, but hormone imbalances are thought to be implicated.

PRESCRIPTION DRUGS

Hormones help relieve the symptoms of period disorders. They don't usually "cure" the condition and their effects tend to wear off soon after stopping them. Progesterone is often used on a cyclical basis (for example one to three weeks in a month) to help reduce imbalances in the levels of estrogen and progesterone. The treatment can stop or reduce the amount of bleeding. Estrogen can be used on its own to induce an artificial period, but is more often used in combination with progesterone in the combined oral contraceptive pill. This is usually taken for three weeks in every month and as well as acting as a contraceptive (by inhibiting ovulation) it helps regularize periods and reduces pain and bleeding.

Danazol is a hormone which inhibits the production of hormones from the pituitary gland, the master gland in the brain which controls all hormones. It is useful in the treatment of endometriosis and is also used to reduce heavy bleeding. It is a particularly expensive drug.

Antispasmodic drugs can relieve painful periods.

How they work: by relaxing the muscle in the wall of the uterus. *See **irritable bowel syndrome,** page 32.*

Prostaglandin inhibitors such as mefenamic acid are used for reducing heavy and painful periods.

How they work: by blocking prostaglandin production. *See **pain,** page 106.*

Antifibrinolytic drugs also reduce bleeding and are quite useful in treating heavy periods.

How they work: by acting on the blood clotting system.

Vitamin B6 (pyridoxine) is very helpful in the treatment of PMT. Its action is not understood.

Mild diuretics are also useful in PMT as a remedy for water retention. They are often taken on a cyclical basis, for example one or two weeks prior to a period.

How they work: *see page 52.*

A dilation and curettage (D & C) is a relatively simple procedure in which most of the lining of the womb is scraped away. It then re-grows, with new, healthier tissue, possibly less likely to give rise to period problems.

OVER-THE-COUNTER TREATMENTS

Simple painkillers such as acetaminophen, aspirin and ibuprofen will help relieve mild period pains. Self-treatment is perfectly appropriate. Many over-the-counter preparations contain combinations of simple painkillers, anti-spasmodics and caffeine (which acts as a stimulant). These are more expensive than simple painkillers, and probably no more effective. If period pain does not respond to simple painkillers, see your doctor. Hormone treatments, including the pill are not available over-the-counter.

PATIENT'S EXPERIENCE

"I started having period pains on the very first day of my first period when I was 12 years old. For many years while I was at school I was told period pains were normal and to carry on as usual. I rarely took anything for the pain and occasionally had to be sent home from school because I felt so awful. When I first went on the pill I was pleasantly surprised to find my periods were less heavy and painful. After coming off the pill I found it took almost a year for the pain to recur. I then asked my doctor if I could try something else. He suggested mefenamic acid pills three times a day from the moment my period started, continuing for two days. I still have some pain, but I find that by taking the pills I can at least manage to carry on with work. Some people say period pains lessen as you get into your early 20s, but I'm 28 now and they are just the same as when I was 12 years old. Others say that they improve after having a baby – I suppose that is something to look forward to."

Hormone therapy

QUESTIONS TO ASK THE DOCTOR

- How many days in each month should I take any drugs?
- How long should I continue the treatment?
- What will happen to my periods?
- Do the drugs have a contraceptive effect?
- Is the treatment curative, or for symptom relief only?
- Would a D & C be helpful?

SIDE EFFECTS

Estrogen: nausea, vomiting, weight gain and fluid retention. Rare, and adverse, side effects include liver problems, rashes, depression, headache, blood thrombosis and cancer of the uterus. Withdrawal bleeding occurs two to four days after stopping estrogen treatment.

Progesterone: the main side effect is a withdrawal bleed on reducing the dose or stopping the drug. Others include headache, depression and, rarely, liver problems.

Antifibrinolytic drugs: principally nausea.

Antispasmodics: dry mouth, blurred vision, palpitations, difficulty passing urine and constipation. *See **irritable bowel syndrome,** page 32.*

Prostaglandin inhibitors: drowsiness, dizziness, nausea, diarrhea and stomach ulceration.

SELF-MANAGEMENT

Because of the close relationship of the brain to the pituitary gland, any illness which has an effect on the brain can affect the menstrual cycle. This applies to many physical illnesses as well as psychological problems such as stress. It follows that avoidance of stress can be of help in avoiding period problems. Maintaining a normal body weight is also important for regular periods.

SELF-HELP

- If the problem is really severe, rest in bed with a heating pad over the lower abdomen. A hot bath may also help. Take regular analgesics. Change sanitary towels or tampons regularly. With persistently heavy/painful periods, try and organize your life so that you have a lighter than normal day or two when your period first starts. Take regular aspirin or mefenamic acid as soon as the period starts, before the pain comes on. Consider going on the pill if you are in need of contraception. For inexplicable bleeding between periods or bleeding after the menopause, always consult a doctor.

The Menstrual Cycle
Numerals refer to days from start of menstrual cycle

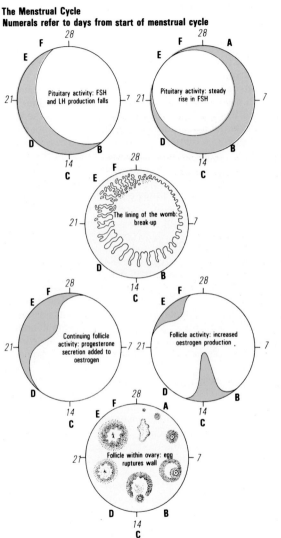

The ovaries are controlled by a small gland in the brain called the pituitary. It secretes several hormones, three of which affect the ovaries. Two of them, follicle stimulating hormone (FSH) and luteinizing hormone (LH) are actually responsible for ovulation.

A In the first half of the menstrual cycle, there is a steady rise of FSH: it stimulates the ovarian follicles which contain the eggs.

B As the follicles approach the moment for releasing the eggs, they produce increasing amounts of the hormone oestrogen. It is discharged into the bloodstream and carried through the body, in particular to the lining of the womb which it stimulates and enriches in preparation for the fertilized egg.

Hormone replacement therapy

NAMES YOU WILL HEAR
Generic name: conjugated estrogen; **trade name:** Premarin. **Generic name:** ethinyl estradiol; **trade names:** Estinyl, Feminone. **Generic name:** diethylstilbestrol (DES); trade name: Stilphostrol. **Generic name:** progesterone; **trade name:** prescribed by generic name. **Generic name:** MPA; **trade names:** Amen, Curretab, Depo-provera, Provera.

WHAT IS THE MENOPAUSE?

– Strictly speaking, the date of the last menstrual period, usually around the age of 50. A 'surgical' menopause occurs in younger women who have the uterus (womb) or ovaries removed; if only the womb is removed and the ovaries are left behind, the periods stop, but the changes in hormone balance which occur with the menopause do not take place until later.

All women experience these changes. As menstrual periods get less frequent and cease, the ovaries make less estrogen (female hormone) and this may cause hot flashes. Some get dryness or soreness in the vagina. The bones get thinner, and this increases the risk of fractures later in life. For some, these changes can be lived with; for others they are unendurable. The worst affected will want to consider estrogen hormone replacement therapy (HRT).

PRESCRIPTION DRUGS

Estrogen can be given in several different ways.

1 Women who have had a hysterectomy can take estrogen tablets continuously, use a vaginal cream, or stick slow release patches on the skin. The treatment offers some interesting benefits: it prevents flashes and sweats; prevents vaginal dryness; prevents thinning of the bones and thus the risk of fractures later in life; prevents premature ageing and changes in vagina and urethra.

2 Women who have a uterus run a slight risk that its lining will be stimulated to form cancer if they take estrogen on its own. In order to take estrogen safely, they must take an additional hormone, progestin, for at least ten days every month. When the progestin is stopped, the lining of the womb may be shed, as in a normal period. These monthly withdrawal bleeds are necessary to remove the risk of cancer and do not mean that the woman has become fertile again. If these drawbacks can be tolerated, replacement therapy will prevent flashes and sweats; prevent vaginal dryness; prevent ageing changes in vagina and urethra and the 'urethral syndrome'.

3 Estrogen cream can be used to prevent dryness and soreness in the vulva and vagina. This may be a problem during intercourse and the treatment is simple and effective. It should be used for about two weeks initially, then every few days as often as necessary.

OVER-THE-COUNTER TREATMENTS

Calcium pills are widely available, and are used to prevent osteoporosis – thinning of the bones. They are not as effective as estrogen for this purpose, but they may be useful to women on diets low in calcium. Hormone treatments such as estrogen are not available without a prescription.

QUESTIONS TO ASK THE DOCTOR

■ Are you sure that hormone therapy really will help my menopause problem?
■ What are the side effects?
■ How long should I take HRT? Should I have estrogen alone, or estrogen with progestin?

SIDE EFFECTS

Because of the risks of taking **estrogen,** a doctor should ask the menopausal patient about major past illnesses such as breast cancer. Make sure the doctor takes your blood pressure, does a breast examination and a Pap smear. Hormone replacement therapy can then be started unless something needs further investigation. Before taking the final decision to start HRT, doctor and patient have to weigh, against the advantages listed under **PRESCRIPTION DRUGS,** the following disadvantages:

If a woman has a uterus: possible monthly bleeding; supervision by doctor; unknown long-term risk of breast cancer and coronary heart disease; also of dependency on estrogen.
If a woman has had a hysterectomy: medical supervision is required, but only for heart and blood pressure; unknown long-term risk of breast cancer. Estrogen alone probably lessens risk of heart disease unless the patient has had a thrombosis; possible dependency on estrogen. All these risks are very slight and long-term results with patients on HRT are reassuring.

COMMONSENSE MEASURES TO MAINTAIN HEALTH AFTER THE MENOPAUSE

■ **Exercise:** Energetic walking or aerobics improve the bones, heart and lungs. ■ **Sunshine:** Even a few minutes out of doors every day will increase the Vitamin D content of the body. This helps with the absorption of calcium. ■ **Diet:** Calcium in the form of low-fat dairy products, and mineral supplements, in canned fish and green vegetables, helps the bones to stay healthy. ■ **Don't smoke,** and don't drink heavily. These poisons harm your bones, liver and heart. ■ **Regular sex** (with a lubricant if necessary) keeps the vagina healthy.

PATIENT'S EXPERIENCE

"My periods stopped when I was 51. I soon experienced hot flashes; they kept me awake at night. Sex was less enjoyable: my vagina became dry and sore. A lubricant jelly only partially helped this problem. Eventually, my doctor suggested hormone treatment; but I had to accept that this would cause bleeding every month. The flashes have now stopped and our sex life is fine; I also feel more relaxed and less negative about life and am sleeping much better. I am not sure how long to go on taking hormones but the doctor says it is OK if we discuss it at my next check-up."

DURATION OF HRT

As long as side effects do not develop, HRT can continue for many years after the menopause if necessary. Even a few years' treatment can mean significantly lesser risk of bone fractures in old age. If you think you want to stop taking the pills, discuss with your doctor taking a few months off HRT – you can always start again if your menopausal symptoms return.

Antibiotics, anti-worm preparations, fluoride preparations

NAMES YOU WILL HEAR

Antibiotics

Generic name: amoxycillin sodium; **trade names:** Augmentin, Polymox, Triniox, Wymox, Amoxil, Moxacin, Moxilean, Novamoxin, Penamox. **Generic name:** co-trimoxazole; **trade names:** Septra, Bactrim, Fectrim, Nodilon, Septrim. **Generic name:** erythromycin; **trade names:** Benzamycin, Erymax, Ilotycin, Pediazole, Erythrocin, Erythromid, EpMycin, Erostin, Emu-V, Ethryn, Eromel, Ilocap, Ilosone, Rythrocaps.

Anti-worm preparations

Generic name: mebendazole; **trade name:** Vermox. **Generic name:** piperazine salts; **trade names:** Antepar, Pripsen.

Analgesics/antipyretics

Generic name: acetaminophen; **trade names:** Phenaphon, Panadol, Tempra, Tylenol, Pamol, Calpol, Tylenon, Paracin, Parmol, Panado, Ceetamol, Atosol, Exctol, Ennagesic, Ilvamol. **Generic name:** aspirin; **trade names:** Ascriptin, Ecotrin, Measurin, Aspirin, Astrin, Bi-Prin. *See also **pain**, page 106.*

Fluoride preparations

Generic name: sodium fluoride; **trade names:** Adeflor, Fluoritab, Luride, Mulvidren, Pediaflor, En-De-Kay, Fluor-a-day Lac, Zymafluor, Floran, Zymafluor.

Many illnesses covered in this book occur in children; their drug therapy is discussed under the relevant section. There are, however, some illnesses, and specialized applications of drugs, which occur almost exclusively in childhood. Some of the most important general issues are covered here, but see particularly comments on children's problems under diarrhea, *page 28;* asthma, *page 74;* insomnia, *page 92;* pain, *page 106;* common cold, *page 134;* eczema, *page 278.*

PRESCRIPTION DRUGS

Antibiotics are frequently prescribed for children. The most common illnesses in childhood are due to viral infections and include the common cold, many of the ear infections and diarrhea. Antibiotics have no effect against viruses, but bacteria may cause a secondary infection and it is often difficult to tell whether the illness is viral or bacterial. Parents are naturally eager for their child to recover as quickly as possible and some are reluctant to "wait and see" – which is all that is needed for viral infections. So the pressure is on the doctor to prescribe an antibiotic at the start of an illness.

At the same time, parents have reason to be anxious about the excessive use of antibiotics. Side effects may occur; they are usually mild, but they can be severe. Diarrhea is a particularly common one; thrush is another. Tetracycline given to young children may discolor the adult teeth. Bacteria can become resistant to the commonly used antibiotics *(see **pneumonia and pleurisy,** page 78),* and then they will not work when they are really needed. A second treatment with the same antibiotic within three months is inadvisable.

If needed, however, repeated treatments with antibiotics will not weaken or damage your child's body. If you are concerned, raise the issue with your doctor.

If a child has a recurrent runny nose and cough, and seems to go from one antibiotic to the next, and if in addition there is a family history of hay fever, eczema or asthma, discuss the possibility of allergy with your doctor. Many children whose problems are really due to allergies like hay fever are treated with antibiotics on the assumption that they have an infection. The presence of fever helps to discriminate: allergies rarely cause fever, but infections often do.

How they work: *see **pneumonia and pleurisy,** page 78.*

Anti-worm preparations: Children get worms from accidentally swallowing the eggs of worms, which are present in, for example, sandboxes or parks and gardens. Several different types of worm are involved,

the most common being thread worms and whip worms. These, and most others, can be treated with a single dose of mebendazole. Another common anti-worm drug is piperazine.
How they work: by inhibiting the metabolism of the worm. The worm is paralyzed, allowing it to be excreted from the bowel.

OVER-THE-COUNTER TREATMENTS

No drug should be used in children without specific reason. Some, including acetaminophen, aspirin and iron can cause severe illness in overdose. Analgesics/antipyretics are commonly used to treat pain and fever. Acetaminophen is safe in the correct dose for age, and may be used even in babies as early as three to six months for the treatment of colic, fever and teething. Dose should be four to six hourly. Aspirin should not be given to children under 12 because of the risk of Reye's syndrome *(see **common cold,** page 134).*
Fluoride preparations, taken regularly, can significantly reduce the amount of decay in developing teeth, and is recommended where there is not sufficient fluoride in the drinking water (ask your local dentist). It can be started at a few months old and should be continued until at least ten years. It is given as a single daily dose. The value of giving fluoride during pregnancy has not been established.
How they work: by making the dentine and enamel of teeth more resistant to acid.

QUESTIONS TO ASK THE DOCTOR

■ Is an antibiotic absolutely necessary, or could we

PATIENT'S EXPERIENCE
"My little boy had been at nursery school for a few months when I noticed that he was frequently scratching his bottom. I took him to the doctor who thought that it was worms. I asked him where he thought that my son had picked it up, and he said it was most likely he had swallowed some sand with worm eggs in it, either at nursery school or in the park. He gave me a prescription for some medicine which lasted a few days and told me to go back within a few weeks if the symptoms had not disappeared."

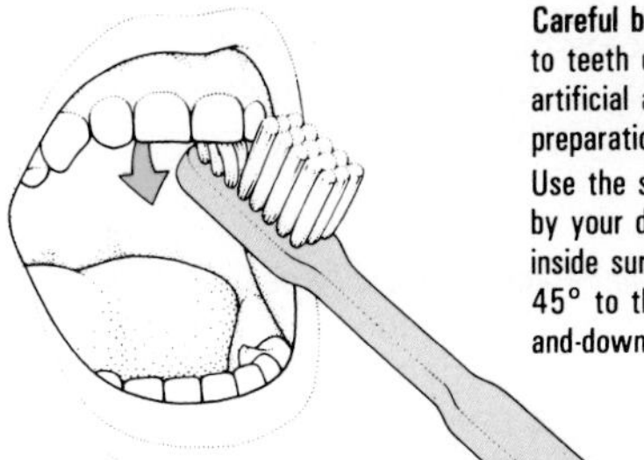

Careful brushing is as essential to teeth care in the young as any artificial assistance from fluoride preparations
Use the size of brush recommended by your dentist. Begin brushing the inside surfaces. Keep the bristles at 45° to the teeth and use an up-and-down movement.

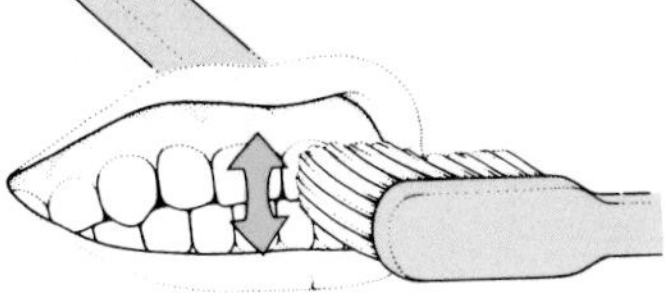

After brushing the inside surfaces, *brush the chewing surfaces; then the outside surfaces. Encourage a child to adopt this sequence as a routine.*

A fever strip: *easy to use for a quick indication; get an accurate reading with a thermometer*

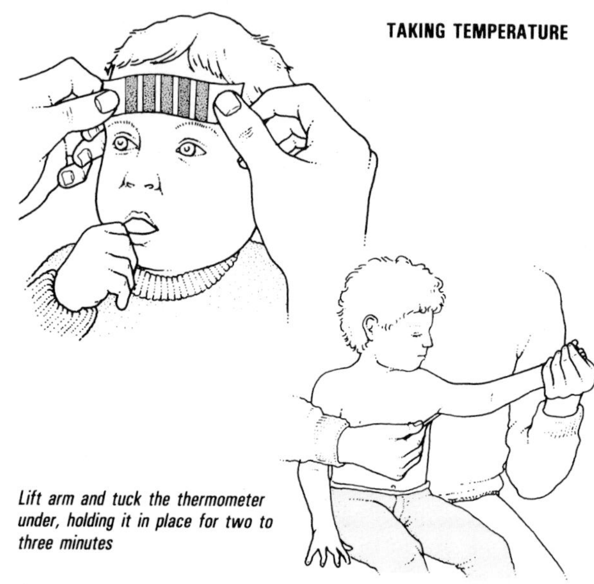

TAKING TEMPERATURE

Lift arm and tuck the thermometer under, holding it in place for two to three minutes

wait and see if she gets better without it?

- Is it ever necessary to repeat worm treatment?
- What can I give my baby for teething?

SIDE EFFECTS

Antibiotics: *see* ***pneumonia and pleurisy,*** *page 78.* Mebendazole rarely causes side effects, though headache, abdominal pain and diarrhea have been reported. It should not be used during pregnancy.

Analgesics/antipyretics: *see* ***common cold,*** *page 134.*

Fluoride can, in chronic overdose, cause discoloration of the teeth. If a large number of pills are taken, nausea, vomiting, abdominal pain, diarrhea and paralysis can occur.

SELF-MANAGEMENT

- Use only drugs which are absolutely necessary, and double check that the dose is correct.
- If a child has a reaction to a drug, contact your doctor immediately.
- Some drugs pass to the baby in breast milk. Many prescription and non-prescription drugs can adversely affect a baby, so always check with your doctor first. The common ones to avoid while breast-feeding include aspirin, indomethacin, tetracyclines, some antimigraine preparations and antidepressants. Many other

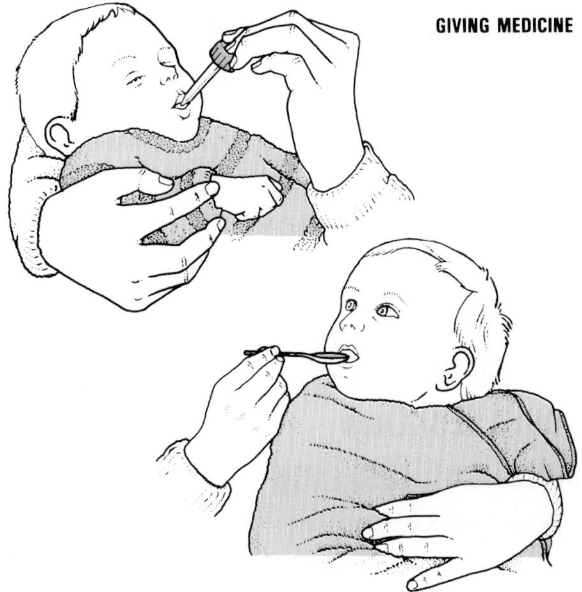

GIVING MEDICINE

A dropper *makes a useful tool for giving a baby medicine; whatever the method used, wrapping a child in a towel will help to prevent struggling and resulting spillage*

drugs are not known to be safe, so don't take any drug unless it is absolutely necessary.

■ Dosage: Drug dose in children is most accurately calculated by the child's weight, whereas the recommended dose on the bottle is often given by age group. If your child is underweight or overweight for his or her age, this must be taken into account.

■ Children under a year old are particularly sensitive to drugs. Always check that the drug is recommended for that age or weight range. In children under three months, the liver and kidneys may be immature, and drugs that are broken down in the liver or excreted by the kidneys will need to be used in reduced doses.

■ Worms: Treatment for worms must be accompanied by washing hands and nails regularly. The worm lays eggs around the anus. This causes itching and eggs deposited under the nails while scratching are transferred to the mouth, perpetuating the infection.

■ Many liquid medicines contain sugar, which causes tooth decay. If medicines have to be taken for a long period, sugar-free preparations or pills may be available; or give the child a drink of water afterwards.

■ Teething is often difficult to diagnose with certainty, and can be distressing. If a baby really appears to be in pain, a dose of acetaminophen can be used safely; if it appears to ease the pain, use it every four hours.

Malignant disease and the immune system

For many people, the words cancer or leukemia imply an automatic death sentence, but this is certainly not true today. In several types of malignant disease treatments have progressed a long way: cures are not uncommon, and the majority can hope for effective long-term control of their disease.

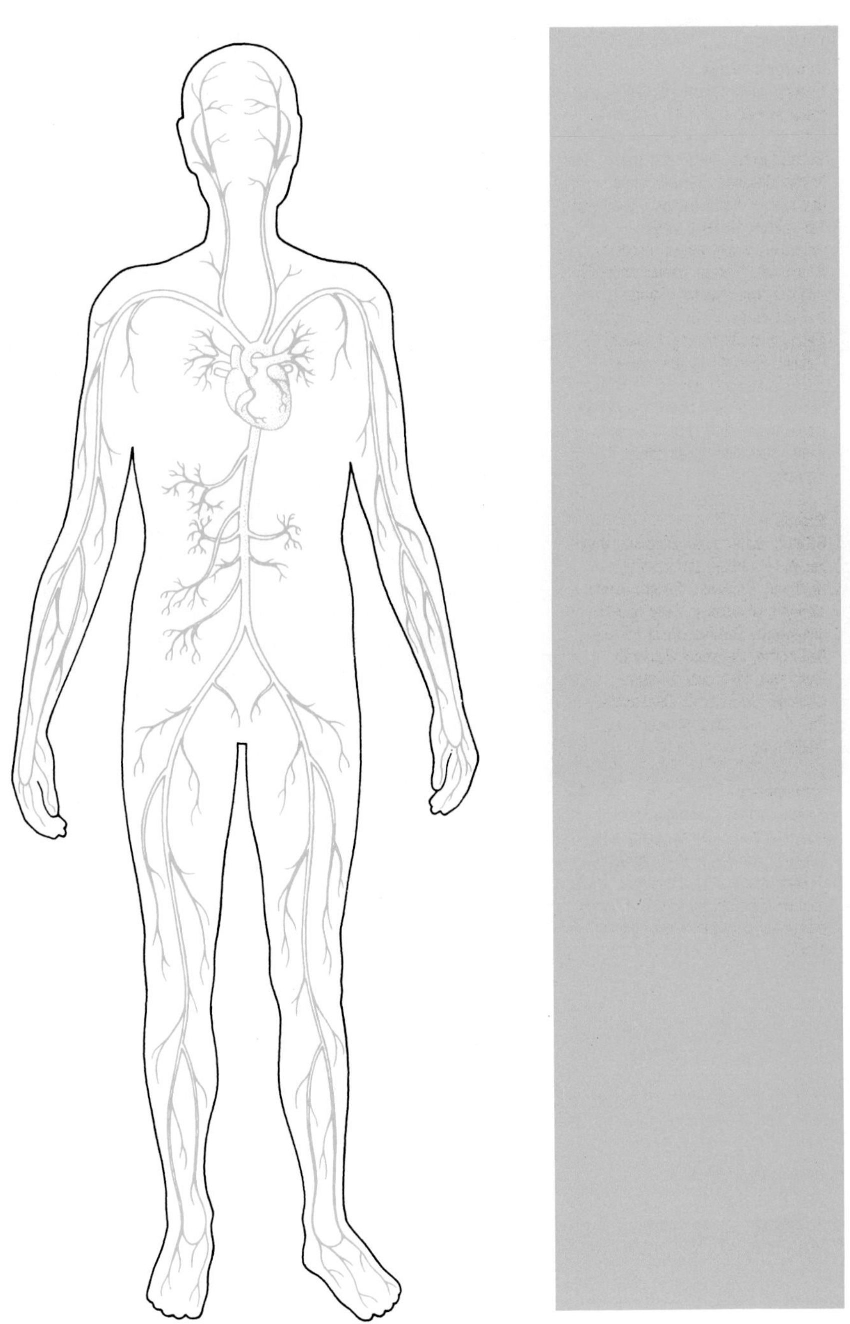

NAMES YOU WILL HEAR

Cytotoxic drugs
Generic name: cyclophosphamide; **trade names:** Endoxana, Endoxan-Asta, Cytoxan, Procytox, Endoxan. **Generic name:** ifosfamide; **trade name:** Mitoxana. **Generic name:** doxorubicin; **trade names:** Adriamycin, Adriblastina. **Generic name:** vincristine; **trade names:** Oncovin, Pericristine. **Generic name:** vindesine sulphate; **trade name:** Eldisine. **Generic name:** cis-diammino-dichloro-platinum; **trade names:** Cisplatin, Platinol, Platinol. **Generic name:** carboplatin; **trade names:** Paraplatin, Paraplatin. **Generic name:** mitomycin; **trade name:** Mitomycin-C. **Generic name:** etoposide; **trade name:** Vepesid.

Steroids
Generic name: dexamethasone; **trade names:** Decadron, Dexacortisyl, Oradexon, Oradexon. **Generic name:** methyl prednisolone; **trade names:** Solumedrol, Codelsol, Delta Phoricol, Deltacortril, Deltalone, Deltastab, Precortisyl, Prednesol, Sintisone, Nisolone, Delta-Cortef, Deltasolone, Prelone, Lenisolone, Meticortilone, Predeltilone.

Antiemetics
Generic name: prochlorperazine mesylate; **trade names:** Compazine, Stemetil, Anti-Naus, Mitil, Vertigon. **Generic name:** metoclopramide; **trade names:** Maxolon, Primperan. **Generic name:** domperidone; **trade names:** Motilium.

WHAT IS LUNG CANCER?

– Malignant or invasive cell growth in the lungs. There are four main types, classified by part of the lung or bronchi from which the cancer cells originate. The abnormal cells can grow either in the lung itself, giving rise to shortness of breath, wheezing, pain and coughing up blood; or they can spread to other areas of the body such as the bones, liver or the brain, in which case a variety of symptoms may arise from these sites.

The cancers known collectively as non-small cell may remain localized for many years, and are frequently amenable to local treatment by surgical resection or radiation therapy. Others are of quite a different type, termed small cell. These can spread rapidly, but they are often remarkably sensitive to the anti-cancer drugs.

A particular problem of lung cancer can occur when the tumor presses on the large blood vessels just above the heart. The face and arms become swollen, a condition known as superior mediastinal obstruction (SMO). The central nervous system can also be involved if a tumor invades the brain or spinal cord.

The outlook with this disease is better than commonly supposed. Perhaps 25 per cent of patients may survive several years. Control of symptoms such as pain and nausea are much improved.

CAUSES The two proven causes of lung cancer are cigarette smoking, particularly those brands with a high tar content; and exposure to asbestos, for example in building workers or dock laborers. Up to 80 per cent of cases are attributable to smoking; otherwise (leaving aside asbestos involvement) the cause is unknown.

PRESCRIPTION DRUGS

Cytotoxic drugs: These can be given either alone or in combination, and while usually given by injection, some are available in tablet form.

How they work: By killing the cancer cells giving rise to the tumor. However, some normal cells are often damaged in the process, and this causes side effects. At some point the cancer cells may become resistant to the drug or drugs used. A change may have to be made, either to different drugs or by introducing a different type of treatment such as radiotherapy (radioactive rays are beamed at the cancer to kill the cells). *See also **breast cancer**, page 206.*

Corticosteroids: If SMO is present, or there is tumor spread to the brain or other parts of the central nervous system, corticosteroids can improve the symptoms

dramatically though often temporary.
How they work: by reducing the swelling around the tumor and relieving the pressure on the nerve cells.
Antiemetics: Most of the cytotoxic drugs cause some degree of nausea, and this can usually be controlled by oral or rectal administration of antiemetics. Occasionally an intravenous infusion of a higher dose of antiemetic may be required.
How they work: by acting on the centre in the brain responsible for the stimulus to vomit.
For **analgesics** and **antibiotics,** *see pages 106 and 78.*

OVER-THE-COUNTER TREATMENTS

None.

QUESTIONS TO ASK THE DOCTOR

- How long will the course last?
- What side effects will I get?
- What if any of these become particularly severe?
- How do I get further supplies of the tablets?
- Which pills are part of the treatment and which are to control side effects?
- How often do I need to have a blood test?
- How long will it be before you know if the treatment is working?
- What should I eat and drink?

SIDE EFFECTS

Cytotoxic drugs are usually given by injection every three to four weeks or in tablet form daily for seven to 14 days, in which case the side effects may be less marked, but more prolonged. The principal side effects are nausea, with or without associated vomiting, loss of hair, and damage to the normal cells produced by the bone marrow. The normal cells of the lung, kidney or heart can be affected, but this is rare.

Nausea may be due to either a local effect on the stomach, or directly on a 'trigger zone' in the brain.

Hair loss is due to damage to the follicles by the cytotoxic drugs and is nearly always temporary. Cooling of the scalp at the time of drug administration can occasionally prevent this occurring.

The effects on the bone marrow are more complicated and potentially serious: if the red cells are affected, anamia may occur and blood transfusion may be required. If a cytotoxic drug affects the platelets, which are important for blood clotting, bleeding can occur from the nose, intestine or into the skin and appear as a rash. However, the white blood cells are most

PATIENT'S EXPERIENCE

"I had smoked on and off for many years, but never really very heavily, and suddenly I just didn't feel like it any more. Then I began to notice a pain on the right side of my chest, particularly when I breathed deeply or ran. The doctor diagnosed pleurisy, and with a course of antibiotics things cleared up at first. But then I became worse again a week or two later. An X-ray showed a shadow on the lung and I had to have a bronchoscopy to inspect the breathing tubes. A thin tube was passed into my airways under anesthetic – not as unpleasant as it sounds. A sample of a suspicious area showed lung cancer of the small cell type and I was started on a course of injections every three weeks. It was pretty awful: I felt sick, and my hair came out in handfuls over the next few weeks. However, my chest improved rapidly, the pain went and my appetite and breathing returned to normal. The doctors gave me the all-clear after almost six months, but I still have to attend regularly for check-ups. I am realistic enough to know the tumor can recur; but I know that if that does happen it will be picked up in good time."

commonly affected; when their number falls below a critical level, there is a high risk of infection which may urgently require antibiotics. Often there is no obvious site for this infection, and a sore throat, fever, or general malaise are the only signs.

Other less common side effects are mouth ulcers, diarrhea, a skin rash and nerve damage. *See also* ***breast cancer,*** *page 206.*

Steroids can cause a range of side effects, including some serious ones, but as the drugs are usually given only short-term for lung cancer, increased appetite, retention of fluid with weight gain and change of mood are the only side effects commonly seen. Patients with high blood pressure associated with diabetes have to be monitored carefully when on steroids.

Antiemetics are unfortunately not without side effects themselves: they may cause drowsiness, skin rash and in some cases where high doses are used, muscle weakness, tremor or twitching of the limbs: these may be disconcerting, but are usually temporary.

SELF-MANAGEMENT

When taking anti-cancer drugs, moderation in one's habits without withdrawing from normal social activity is the best approach.

■ Try to continue to eat a balanced diet, avoiding spicy or fatty food which may upset you. If you do not feel like eating, at least keep drinking to keep your fluid intake and output high. Small quantities of alcohol, avoiding undiluted liquor, are unlikely to be harmful.

■ Continue moderate activity along the lines you are used to, whether that is swimming, walking, housekeeping or golf, but do stop when you are tired, and get plenty of rest.

■ Get a wig, do go outdoors, meet friends or invite them over to see you. Try and maintain your self-esteem as much as possible and confide in your close family and friends – they can prove understanding and helpful.

■ Organize your house to minimize the amount of routine work or movement you have to do: for example, move the bedroom downstairs, or put in a downstairs bathroom.

■ While infection is a risk, most of the organisms involved come from within your own body; however, it is best to avoid children with chickenpox.

■ Take advantage of any counselling services available through your doctor's office as well as the cancer nurse specialists.

SELF-HELP

■ Keep your doctor appointments and have blood tests on time – the results can help to give advance warning of complications.

■ Take the tablets only for the prescribed time. You may have a mixture of cytotoxic drug tablets and painkillers. If in doubt, write the names and frequency down, and check it over with your doctor.

■ Infection: If you have a fever, sweating or shivering, contact your doctor or hospital immediately for advice.

■ Bleeding: For a nose bleed, sit quietly with a cold compress over the bridge of your nose and your head slightly forwards. If bleeding does not stop in 15-20 minutes, contact your doctor. Coughing up blood may be disconcerting, but is rarely serious.

■ Breathing difficulties: Sitting up and leaning forward often helps; use several pillows. Remain calm. If your breathing suddenly becomes worse, seek medical advice.

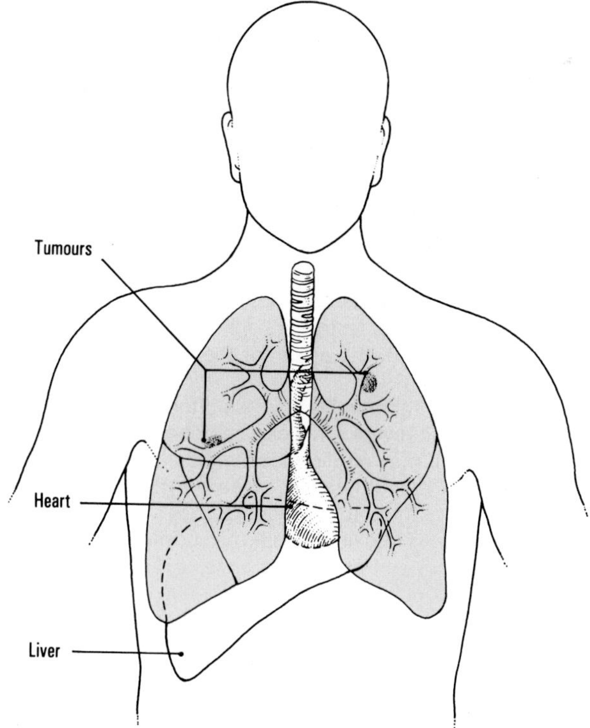

Lung cancer *often begins in the bronchi or breathing tubes which join together in the centre to form the trachea. Symptoms arise when the cancer cells grow inwards blocking the tube, often collapsing part of the lung. If there is a raw edge or ulcer, bleeding may occur and specks of blood will appear in the sputum. The cancer can spread locally to the rest of the lung, by the lymph glands and channels to the centre of the chest, and by the bloodstream to the bones, liver or brain.*

NAMES YOU WILL HEAR

Hormonal treatments

Generic name: tamoxifen; **trade names:** Nolvadex, Tamofen, Kessar, Noltam. **Generic name:** aminoglutethimide; **trade names:** Cytadren, Orimeten. **Generic name:** medroxyprogesterone acetate; **trade names:** Amen, Curretab, Depoprovera, Provera, Farlutal. **Generic name:** megestrol acetate; **trade name:** Megace. **Generic name:** stilbestrol; **trade name:** Tampovagan. **Generic name:** ethinylestradiol; **trade names:** Feminone, Lynoral, Edrol, Estigyn, Estinyl, Primogyn. **Generic name:** drostanolone propionate; **trade name:** Drolban, Masteril. **Generic name:** nandrolone; **trade names:** Androlone, Nandrolin, Durabolin, Deca Durabolin.

Cytotoxic drugs

Generic name: doxorubicin; **trade names:** Adriamycin, Adriblastina. **Generic name:** epirubicin; **trade name:** Pharmorubicin. **Generic name:** mitoxantrone; **trade name:** Novantrone. **Generic name:** vincristine sulfate; **trade names:** Oncovin, Pericristine. **Generic name:** cyclophosphamide; **trade names:** Cytoxan, Neosar, Endoxana, Endoxan-Asta, Procytox, Endoxan. **Generic name:** fluorouracil; **trade names:** Adrucil, Fluorouracil, Fluoroplex. **Generic name:** methotrexate; **trade names:** Folex, Mexate, Emtexate, Maxtrex.

WHAT IS BREAST CANCER?

– Malignant growth of cells originating in the breast. Most lumps in the breast are minor abnormalities of fatty tissue and are benign. They do, however, need medical assessment in order that the minority of lumps due to breast cancer can be detected.

Early breast cancer is treated by surgery often combined with radiotherapy. The intention is to remove every malignant cell and thus to effect a complete cure. Surgeons used to remove the whole breast (radical mastectomy), but nowadays this is only done in advanced cases. Whenever possible, only the lump is removed, with the object of restoring body shape to near-normal. But since the disease may be present in microscopic form, surgery cannot be a guarantee against recurrence in another site.

When breast cancers do give rise to tumors in other sites, they are known as secondary cancers or metastases. Drugs have an important role in the treatment of overt symptomatic metastases; they can also be used to eliminate undetectable ones. This is known as adjuvant treatment and is given to patients when there is a possibility of ''secondaries'' being present and developing later. Radiotherapy may be used instead of, or in addition to drugs.

Improvements in treatment mean that the outlook for breast cancer gets better and better. This is a form of cancer which can be cured, provided treatment is started early enough.

PRESCRIPTION DRUGS

Hormonal (endocrine) treatments: usually given as pills, although some are administered as injections one to three times a week.

How they work: A substantial proportion (50 to 60 per cent) of breast cancers are known to depend on hormones (in particular estrogen) for their growth. The drugs interfere with the action of the hormone on the cancer cells.

Cytotoxic drugs (''chemotherapy'') is often administered by injection into a vein. This can be done on an outpatient basis, but may require hospital admission for one or two days. Chemotherapy is given in cycles of one to five days every three to four weeks.

How they work: Cytotoxic drugs are all poisons: they affect normal as well as abnormal cells. The recovery powers of normal cells are greater than those of the cancer cells and provided that the drug is given intermittently, the normal cells will recover between doses while the abnormal ones may not. The dose of cytotoxics which can be given is limited by the amount of damage which the normal tissues can stand.

Antiemetics may be used to treat the side effects of cytotoxic drugs: *see* ***lung cancer,*** *page 202.*

QUESTIONS TO ASK THE DOCTOR

- Is the treatment chemotherapy or hormone therapy?
- What side effects can I expect?
- What can I do to lessen the side effects?
- How will I know the treatment is working?

SIDE EFFECTS

Hormonal treatments are associated with mild side effects. The commonest is probably nausea, but this is usually transitory and does not require stopping the drug. Tamoxifen given to pre-menopausal women may produce disturbances of menstruation and hot flashes. In post-menopausal women it causes almost no side effect. Sedation and fleeting skin rashes are common with amino-glutethimide. Androgens are associated with the growth of unwanted hair and deepening of the voice. Estrogens give rise to vaginal bleeding. The latter two groups of drugs are rarely used.

Chemotherapy side effects range from the unpleasant to the seriously adverse. The latter may not give rise to any symptoms until very advanced and may only be detected by monitoring the patient.

The common side effects are nausea, vomiting and alopecia (hair loss). Hair always grows again. Some drugs may give rise to unpleasant tingling sensations. Prolonged tiredness may also occur, and a feeling of weakness. The serious side effects are changes to the bone marrow resulting in increased susceptibility to infection and likelihood of abnormal bruising and bleeding. These will usually be found by the doctor before they become a problem, but sore throat, mouth ulcers or bruising may be the first signs of trouble and should be reported immediately. *See also* ***lung cancer,*** *page 203.*

SELF-MANAGEMENT

- Prevention: regular, monthly self-examination of the breasts is important. Ask your doctor to teach you the technique. Mammography (breast X-ray) will detect cancer before you can feel it. ASK YOUR DOCTOR. The earlier the cancer is detected, the better, in general, is the outlook.
- Self-help groups can give invaluable moral support.

PATIENT'S EXPERIENCE

"When I first went to my doctor with a blotchy rash which had suddenly appeared I had no idea that I was suffering from breast cancer. I was referred to a skin specialist who biopsied the rash and discovered that it was due to secondaries from breast cancer. She referred me to a specialist who found a lump in my breast and removed it. They confirmed that it was breast cancer. Because of the widespread rash, I was told that mastectomy or other local treatments were not suitable and I was told I would need chemotherapy.

For the first treatment I went into the hospital for three days, but since then I have attended as an out-patient. Whenever I arrive at the hospital, my blood is taken for tests and I have to wait for the results. So far the results have always been satisfactory. They put an I.V. in my arm and then give the injections. There have been no unpleasant sensations during the injections, but afterwards I feel sick until the following day. Three weeks later I go back for another treatment. After two treatments the rash started to disappear and nine months after I started chemotherapy there is no rash and I feel well. I have continued my office job throughout this time."

NAMES YOU WILL HEAR
Cytoxic drugs
Generic name: busulfan; **trade name:** Myleran. **Generic name:** chlorambucil; **trade name:** Leukeran. **Generic name:** cytarabine; **trade names:** Ara-C, Cytostar-U, Cytosar, Alexan. **Generic name:** daunorubicin hydrochloride; **trade names:** Cerubidine, Cerubidin. **Generic name:** doxorubicin; **trade names:** Adriamycin, Adriblastina. **Generic name:** etoposide; **trade name:** Vepesid. **Generic name:** mitoxantrone; **trade name:** Novantrone. **Generic name:** thioguanine; **trade name:** prescribed by generic name in USA; elsewhere Lanvis. **Generic name:** vincristine sulfate; **trade names:** Oncovin, Vincasar, Pericristine.

WHAT IS ADULT LEUKEMIA?

– A malignant blood disorder which, in adults, is divided into acute and chronic forms. There is further division into myeloid and lymphoid sub-types, depending on the type of white blood cell involved. Diagnosis is established by examination of the blood and bone marrow.

Acute leukemia in adults, in contrast to that in children, is usually of the myeloid type, although acute lymphoblastic leukemia may occur in adults of any age. The first symptoms reported to a doctor are usually related to anemia (tiredness and breathlessness) or bleeding (particularly from the gums, nose and into the skin), or infection (again particularly in the mouth, skin and chest). These problems arise because of a lack of normal red cells, platelets and white cells.

Chronic leukemias in adults are again of two types. Chronic myeloid leukemia, also known as chronic granulocytic leukemia, is most common in middle age. Symptoms include fever, tiredness and malaise. Enlargement of the spleen and liver may cause swelling of the abdomen. Chronic lymphatic leukemia is a more indolent condition often occurring in older age groups. This may be discovered during a routine blood count, or may present with anemia, bleeding or infection. Enlargement of the lymph glands, particularly in the neck, under the arms and in the groin, is another common feature. Enlargement of the spleen may produce abdominal swelling and a feeling of fullness in the abdomen.

CAUSES In most cases unknown, but exposure to certain chemicals, and to radiation, may be responsible for a small percentage of cases.

PRESCRIPTION DRUGS

Cytotoxic drugs are given by pills or injection to control the growth of the abnormal white blood cells. The chronic leukemias usually respond well to less intensive treatment with pills, while the acute leukemias are treated with intensive combinations of drugs given both orally and by injection.

Acute myeloid leukemia in adults is treated using intermittent intensive combinations of drugs with "rest" periods to allow the normal bone marrow to recover. Acute lymphoblastic leukemia in adults is treated with similar regimes to those used in children.

Chronic myeloid leukemia is, in the early stages, usually readily controlled by drug treatment. Control may become more difficult after one or two years, and in some cases the disease changes its character and acute leukemia develops. Bone marrow transplantation may be the preferred treatment, once the disease is under control, for some cases of acute leukemia and also for some cases of chronic myeloid leukemia. Chronic lymphatic leukemia is usually only treated, particularly in older people, if it is causing problems, and indeed no treatment may be required for long periods. Troublesome swelling of the lymph glands or anemia are usually treatable.

Drug treatment forms only a part of the total care of a person with leukemia, and transfusions of blood (to correct anemia) and platelets (to correct bleeding) are commonly required. Antibiotics are given to control and treat infections.

How the drugs work: *see **lung cancer,** page 202.*

QUESTIONS TO ASK THE DOCTOR

- What sort of leukemia do I have?
- How long will treatment last?

OVER-THE-COUNTER TREATMENTS

None.

SIDE EFFECTS

Cytotoxic drugs are all poisons. They may thus damage healthy cells as well as leukemic cells. Damage to healthy tissues may produce loss of hair, soreness of the mouth and diarrhea. Damage to normal bone marrow cells may produce anemia, bleeding problems and a temporary increase in susceptibility to infection. Some cytotoxic drugs may cause nausea and vomiting and antiemetic drugs are often given routinely to prevent this. Some of the drugs used to treat the diarrhea may damage heart, lungs and liver. All these potential side effects are closely monitored during treatment and doses are modified to minimize the problems.

SELF-HELP

- Pay close attention to personal hygiene, especially in the mouth.
- Report to your doctor immediately if you feel ill in any way, but especially with fevers or other signs of infection, particularly when your white blood cell count is low.
- Avoid unnecessary exposure to people with obvious infections, especially when your white blood cell count is low.

PATIENT'S EXPERIENCE

"I went to my doctor because I was unusually tired and had noticed I was breathless on climbing the stairs. I had noticed I was bruising easily and that my gums bled excessively when I cleaned my teeth. My doctor sent me for a blood count and this was abnormal. I then had a bone marrow test which showed I had acute myeloblastic leukemia.

I had to go into the hospital for several weeks to receive cytotoxic drugs. I also had blood and platelet transfusions and treatment with antibiotics for a severe chest infection. It was ghastly, but the doctors tell me the disease has been completely cleared. I am going on with a further program of cytotoxic drugs, which, I hope, will prevent the leukemia recurring."

CHILDHOOD LEUKEMIA

Cytotoxic drugs, antibiotics, acyclovir

NAMES YOU WILL HEAR

Cytotoxic drugs

Generic name: vincristine sulfate; **trade names:** Oncovin, Vincasar, Pericristine. **Generic name:** daunorubicin hydrochloride; **trade names:** Cerubidine, Cerubidin. **Generic name:** mercaptopurine; **trade name:** Puri-Nethol. **Generic name:** methotrexate; **trade names:** Emtexate, Maxtrex. **Generic name:** colaspase; **trade names:** Erwinase, Leunase, Kidrolase, Laspar. **Generic name:** methyl prednisolone; **trade names:** Solumedrol, Codelsol, Delta Phorical, Deltacortril, Deltalone, Precortisyl, Prednesol, Sintisone, Nisolone, Delta-Cortef, Deltasolone, Prelone, Lenisolone, Meticortilone, Predeltilone.

Antibiotics

Generic name: co-trimoxazole; **trade names:** Bactrim, Bactrim DS, Septra, Fectrim, Nodilon, Septrim. Other antibiotics may be given to treat individual infections.

Anti-viral agent

Generic name: acyclovir; **trade name:** Zovirax.

WHAT IS LEUKEMIA?

– A malignant condition involving the white blood cells: normal blood production is affected leading to anemia, infection and bleeding. There may be enlarged lymph nodes in the neck, armpits and groin and an increase in the size of the liver and spleen. Bone pain, especially in the back and knees, may occur. Leukemia afflicts one in 2,000 children. Eighty per cent have acute lymphoblastic leukemia (ALL); these days, 60 per cent are cured. A small number have myeloid leukemia, which responds less well to treatment. This disease is similar to that in adults. Both are diagnosed by examination of the blood count and of the bone marrow.

CAUSES No cause can be found in most children. But it can be caused by excessive radiation, and it does occur in association with some other rare childhood diseases. Certain animal leukemias are transmitted by viruses, but no such virus has been identified in man.

PRESCRIPTION DRUGS

Cytotoxic drugs ('chemotherapy'): the mainstay of treatment. Some of the drugs can be taken as pills or liquids, others have to be given by injection, usually directly into a vein. Treatment for ALL is administered as a program usually lasting two years or more. Initial intensive drug treatment is given to obtain a remission, when the disease is no longer detectable in blood or bone marrow. Local X-ray treatment to the head is then applied to reduce the risk of nervous system involvement. Further treatment, mainly oral, is continued to maintain remission until treatment is completed. Acute myeloid leukemia is treated more intensively and for a shorter period with a different combination of cytotoxic drugs. Certain cases may best be treated after initial therapy by a bone marrow transplant.

How they work: cytotoxic drugs are cell poisons, and act by killing leukemia cells. Once the bone marrow is cleared of these cells, normal blood production will resume.

Antibiotics: Co-trimoxazole is given three days a week throughout treatment to reduce the risk of serious lung infection. Other antibiotics may be given to treat specific infections.

How they work: by killing the bacteria responsible.

Acyclovir: an anti-viral agent given to prevent or treat chicken pox, shingles or cold sores, which can occur more readily in a leukemia patient, or while on treatment for the disease.

OVER-THE-COUNTER TREATMENTS

None.

QUESTIONS TO ASK THE DOCTOR

■ What time of day should my child take the drugs? Should they be taken before or after food?
■ What should I do if my child vomits the drug?
■ What will happen if I forget my child's treatment for a day or two?
■ How long are the medicines stable?

SIDE EFFECTS

Cytotoxic drugs: Besides killing leukemic cells, cytotoxics also damage healthy body tissues. Injury to the hair follicles is likely, and leads to hair loss; it always regrows. Damage to the lining of the mouth is also common, and causes local pain and ulceration. Normal blood cell production is affected. Effective treatment always leads to some periods of reduction in the white blood cell count, with a depression of immunity and a risk of infection. Some infections, especially measles and chicken pox, may prove very serious to children being treated for leukemia. The administration of some intravenous drugs causes vomiting. Leakage from the vein during an injection may cause a local painful chemical burn.
Antibiotics: Co-trimoxazole's side effects are rare, but skin rashes may occur. For further information on antibiotics, *see* ***pneumonia,*** *page 78.*
Acyclovir's side effects are very rare in children, but doctors will monitor kidney function.

HOW PARENTS CAN HELP

Treatment requires continuous expert supervision, including regular blood counts, but you can help:

■ Hygiene, particularly the care of teeth and gums.
■ Ask school teachers and friends to warn you if your child is likely to come into contact with chicken pox or measles. Inform your doctor promptly: preventive treatment is available.
■ Avoid unnecessary crowds at times when the blood count is very low, but encourage the child to attend school and other normal activities whenever possible.
■ Don't have a child immunized while on treatment.
■ Do not over-indulge your child, despite the serious nature of the illness.
■ Keep yourself well informed about the frequent developments in treatment.

A PARENT'S EXPERIENCE

"My child started to bruise easily and became pale and unwell. He was diagnosed as having acute lymphoblastic leukemia; he started treatment with intravenous drugs and a blood transfusion. He improved, but had to have further treatment that made him very ill. Later he had a series of X-rays to his head. After about three months he began to get back to normal life, but continued to take regular pills and attend for check-ups every two weeks. Now, after two years, the treatment has stopped. We hope he is cured."

NAMES YOU WILL HEAR
Generic name: bleomycin; **trade name:** Blenoxane. **Generic name:** cyclophosphamide; **trade names:** Cytoxan, Neosar, Endoxana, Endoxan-Asta, Procytox, Endoxan. **Generic name:** dacarbazine; **trade name:** DTIC-Dome. **Generic name:** doxorubicin; **trade names:** Adriamycin, Adriblastina. **Generic name:** nitrogen mustard; **trade names:** Mustargen, Mustine. **Generic name:** methyl prednisolone; **trade names:** Solumedrol, Codelsol, Delta Phorical, Deltacortril, Deltalone, Precortisyl, Prednesol, Sintisone, Nisolone, Delta-Cortef, Deltasolone, Prelone, Lenisolone, Meticortilone, Predeltilone. **Generic name:** procarbazine; **trade name:** Matulane, Natulan. **Generic name:** vincristine sulfate; **trade names:** Oncovin, Vincasar, Pericristine. Combinations for Hodgkin's lymphoma: MOPP, MVPP and ABVD. For Non-Hodgkin's lymphoma: COP, CVP and CHOP. Each letter represents a drug listed above. It usually corresponds with the generic name but sometimes the trade name.

WHAT ARE LYMPHOMAS?

– Tumors affecting the body's immune system. They usually develop first in the lymph glands, but can also start in, and spread to, spleen, liver, bone marrow, bowel and sometimes other organs. Several types exist, including Hodgkin's lymphoma and non-Hodgkin's lymphomas. Common symptoms are enlarged neck glands, weight loss, fever and sweats. Diagnosis is confirmed by biopsy – removing a lymph gland or other tissue and examining it under a microscope. The extent or stage of the disease is found by X-ray tests, body-scan or sometimes by an abdominal operation. The disease is lethal without treatment; however life expectancy can be as high as 20 years given diagnosis at an early stage, and good response to treatment. Indeed some cases are cured.

CAUSE Unknown. The disease is not infectious.

TREATMENT

Most lymphomas respond well to drugs and radiotherapy. Radiotherapy alone may be used if only neck glands are involved and it cures some cases.

Combinations: The disease will respond to treatment with a single drug, but it does tend to recur. For this reason a combination of drugs is used as the chances of the tumor developing resistance to all the drugs are extremely small. A typical combination is **nitrogen mustard, vincristine** (Oncovin), **prednisolone** and **procarbazine** – MOPP for short – widely used in treating Hodgkin's disease. Two week's treatment including injections might be given to start with, followed by a break, then the next course. At least six treatments are given.

New combinations are frequently being tested, and often these lead to improvements in treatment.

How they work: by killing tumour cells. Normal body cells can also be damaged in the process, but this can be minimized by using the appropriate dose and by having rest periods between treatments.

OVER-THE-COUNTER TREATMENTS

None.

QUESTIONS TO ASK THE DOCTOR

- What sort of lymphoma have I got?
- How far has it spread?
- Will it respond to treatment?
- What will be the side effects of the treatment?
- Can I continue at work?

SIDE EFFECTS

Patients receiving **combination** treatment have to allow for: reduction in the blood cell count – needs to be detected early by regular blood tests; mouth ulcers, nausea and diarrhea – may be prevented or treated; scalp hair loss, and sometimes body hair loss – the hair always regrows; cessation of menstrual periods; sterility in men; proneness to infection. **Vincristine** additionally causes tingling or burning in the hands and feet; **bleomycin** and **doxorubicin** cause breathlessness. Most of the side effects are distressing but manageable; fever, rash, bleeding, persistent headache and breathlessness should be reported to a doctor without delay.

SELF-MANAGEMENT

Get treated at a specialized clinic: these have the necessary experience to give the best results. Try to accept that you may have a massive emotional reaction as well as lymphoma. Doctors can help you with both: try to accept help. Keep up your interest in your work, family and friends. Do something that you really enjoy every day. Live within your capabilities; think of ways of doing things easily. If hair loss bothers you, get a wig matched and fitted, sooner rather than later. If you are male and might want children, consider storing sperm before chemotherapy. You may find a self-help support group useful.

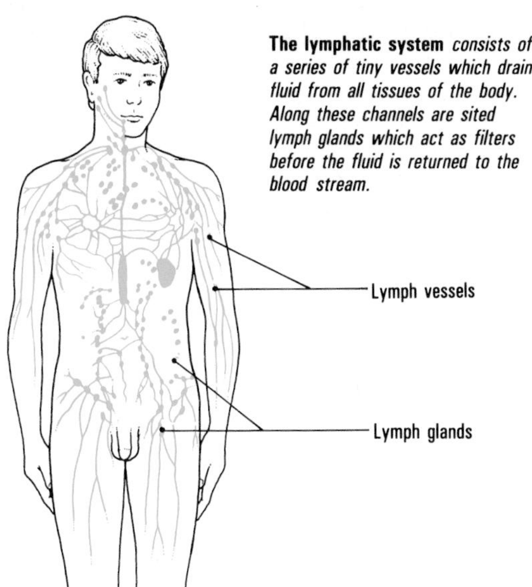

The lymphatic system *consists of a series of tiny vessels which drain fluid from all tissues of the body. Along these channels are sited lymph glands which act as filters before the fluid is returned to the blood stream.*

PATIENT'S EXPERIENCE

"When I was told I had a lymphoma I was absolutely shattered. However, after a few weeks I started to get back on my feet again – but I wouldn't say I'd recovered. That was more gradual: knowing more about my disease and realizing that I was responding to effective treatment gave me hope. Now I look upon it as a condition needing long-term treatment – like diabetes."

NAMES YOU WILL HEAR
Anti viral agent
Generic name: zyclovucline; **trade name:** Retrovir.

Antibiotic
Generic name: co-trimoxazole; **trade names:** Septra, Bactrim, Fectrim, Nodilon, Septrim.

Cytotoxic drugs
Generic name: vincristine sulfate; **trade names:** Oncovin, Vincasar, Pericristine. **Generic name:** etoposide; **trade name:** Vepesid.

AIDS (Acquired Immune Deficiency Syndrome)
– The disease develops when the body's defense against infection – the immune system – is badly damaged by the human immunodeficiency virus (HIV). A variety of serious infections may develop affecting the lungs, brain, digestive system and skin. An unusual tumor (Kaposi's sarcoma) may also develop.

Most AIDS sufferers are infected without being initially aware of symptoms. After a highly variable period of time (possibly many years) swollen glands may develop, particularly in the neck and armpits. Later, other symptoms may develop, including fever and night sweats, loss of appetite, weight loss, profound fatigue, prolonged diarrhea and skin rashes. Full-blown AIDS may eventually develop in perhaps 35 per cent of infected people: but the final percentage is not known, because the disease has only recently spread to developed countries.

AIDS patients often first go to their doctor with a form of pneumonia (caused by the organism Pneumocystis carinii), complaining of shortness of breath, dry cough and fever. Kaposi's sarcoma may also develop: pinkish-purple blotches – firm to the touch – on any part of the body.

If you are worried, see your doctor soon, or attend a clinic which specializes in AIDS.

CAUSE HIV infects white blood cells (lymphocytes), which have a key role in defense against infection. Their numbers are severely reduced, leaving the body open to attack by various micro-organisms to produce opportunistic infections.

There is no cure for AIDS as yet; nor is there a protective vaccine. Attempts to develop one are underway, but the virus changes its form (mutates) so frequently that it may never be possible to develop one.

PRESCRIPTION DRUGS
Antiviral drugs have a role: they can prevent the virus from multiplying and infecting other cells in the blood.
Zyclovucline may be prescribed in patients who have AIDS or related conditions but has to be taken six times daily to be effective. Treatment must be continued indefinitely to hold the virus in check.
How it works: by selectively blocking the metabolism of the virus, and preventing it from multiplying.
Antibiotics – many different types – may be used, both to treat acute infections and to prevent recurrences.
Cotrimoxazole is often used to treat pneumocystic

pneumonia, and is usually injected into a vein at the hospital.

How they work: by killing the bacteria responsible.

Cytotoxic drugs such as etoposide or vincristine are sometimes used in the treatment of severe Kaposi's sarcoma.

How they work: cytotoxics are all poisons: they rely on healthy cells' ability to recover from their effect, while malignant or abnormal cells are completely destroyed.

QUESTIONS TO ASK THE DOCTOR

■ How can I be certain I am infected?

■ What are the advantages and disadvantages of getting tested for HIV infection?

■ Whom should I tell?

■ Could I infect others?

■ What is "safe sex"?

■ Is it safe to have vaccinations?

SIDE EFFECTS

Zyclovucline sometimes affects cells in the bone marrow, causing anemia: patients have to be regularly monitored. The antibiotic **cotrimoxazole** commonly produces skin rashes in AIDS patients: inform your doctor at once if this occurs.

Cytotoxic drugs: *see **lung cancer**, page 202.* Etoposide may produce hair loss, but the hair usually regrows when the drug is stopped.

SELF-MANAGEMENT

■ Take care of yourself: see your doctor for regular checks: get plenty of rest when you need it and aim for at least eight hours' sleep at night.

■ Regular exercise is beneficial, but don't overdo it. A local AIDS support group can advise you on this and other issues.

■ Meals should be well-balanced and include plenty of fresh fruit and vegetables.

■ Stop or considerably cut down on smoking: it makes you especially prone to chest infection.

■ Don't get pregnant: there may be a 50 per cent chance of infecting your baby, and pregnancy may accelerate the development of AIDS.

■ Never share items likely to be contaminated by blood. These include tooth brushes, razors and body brushes. It follows that acupuncture, tattooing, ear-piercing and electroysis should be avoided because of blood-contaminated equipment. Don't allow a barber to shave you. See also in margin.

PATIENT'S EXPERIENCE

"My doctor informed me that I was antibody-positive some months ago. I had felt ill for some time, but was too frightened to seek advice. I had lost weight, and had had appalling diarrhea and a sore mouth; the doctor sent me to a special clinic and they sent me to a hospital, where I was quickly diagnosed as having full-blown AIDS. Treatment started immediately. I was really quite surprised by the kindness and honesty of the staff. When I was discharged, I had gained nearly 14 lb in weight.

AIDS is mostly transmitted through sexual contact, and is commonest among male homosexuals. The greater the number of partners the greater the risk. It may also be transmitted by heterosexual intercourse. Transmission may occur if an uninfected person is exposed to body fluids in other ways (blood and blood products, although these are now carefully screened), shared needles contaminated with blood, possibly also saliva and tears. The question of air borne transmission is not finally resolved, and as the incubation period may be as long as 15 years, it will be a long time before we really know.

FURTHER SAFETY PRECAUTIONS

■ Don't donate blood, milk or semen or any body organ. Don't carry a kidney donor card.

■ Cover cuts with water-proof band-aids until healed.

■ Be honest about your present and past sexual activities with your partner and practise safe sex: a local self-help group or doctor will advise you.

■ Drug misusers must stop taking drugs, or if this is impossible, don't inject.

■ Spills of blood or body fluid: cover with paper tissues and carefully apply diluted bleach – one part of chlorine bleach to nine parts water. If possible, leave in contact for 30 minutes before wiping up and flushing down the toilet. Wear rubber gloves for this.

Immunosuppressives

NAMES YOU WILL HEAR
Generic name: aluminum hydroxide; **trade names:** Alu Caps, Aludrox, Amphojel, Mylanta, Alu-cap. **Generic name:** alphahydroxycholecal-ciferol; **trade name:** Alpha Calciferol, 1 Alpha. **Generic name:** cyclosporin A; **trade name:** Sandimmune. **Generic name:** azathioprine; **trade names:** Imuran, Azathioprine Tablets. **Generic name:** methyl prednisolone; **trade names:** Solumedrol, Codelsol, Delta Phorical, Deltacortril, Deltalone, Deltastab, Precortisyl, Prednesol, Sintisone, Nisolone, Delta-Cortef, Deltasolone, Prelone, Lenisolone, Meticortilone, Predeltilone. **Generic name:** cimetidine; **trade name:** Tagamet. **Generic name:** ranitidine; **trade name:** Zantac. **Generic name:** magnesium trisilicate, iron, vitamin supplements; **trade name:** Fefol Vit. **Generic name:** furosemide; **trade names:** Lasix, Burinex.

Antibiotics are also commonly given after transplant operations to fight infection. Choice depends on the nature of the problem.

Sodium bicarbonate is also commonly used: see under **PRESCRIPTION DRUGS.**

THE NEW TRANSPLANT

A transplanted organ, unless taken from an identical twin, is bound to be regarded by the body as foreign. Rejecting it is the body's natural response; from the day of the operation this tendency has to be countered by use of sophisticated drugs, some developed specially for the purpose. Although this section is relevant mainly to kidney transplants, much of the information also applies to heart and lung transplants.

PRESCRIPTION DRUGS

The typical first choice of immunosuppressive is actually to give two together: azathioprine and the steroid prednisolone are commonly used.

How they work: Azathioprine stops blood cells dividing: when given in the right dose, it has a selective effect on lymphocytes, thus inhibiting rejection. Prednisolone, as a steroid, suppresses inflammation and therefore rejection. Cyclosporin, often given with prednisolone, is a more efficient immunosuppressive than azathioprine-with-prednisolone, and it carries less risk of infection; however it has the major drawback of causing kidney damage and the dose has to be adjusted to exactly the right level for the individual and it must be re-checked frequently. There is a risk of developing tumors after prolonged use of this drug.

Other drugs given to correct complications of kidney disease include **antihypertensives,** *see page 46*. Because patients on immunosuppressives are very vulnerable to infection, antibiotics are also likely to be given.

SIDE EFFECTS

Immunosuppressives decrease the body's tendency to reject a foreign organ; they also undermine its natural ability to combat bacteria, viruses and fungi. The specialist's main concern is therefore to adjust the dose so that it is just enough to prevent rejection and no more. The other major problem is kidney damage with cyclosporin: if the drug is given, patients have to be very carefully monitored. Cyclosporin also has the minor side effects of increased body hair and gum overgrowth. Azathioprine may suppress the bone marrow with risk of infections, and it may cause nausea and vomiting. Prolonged use may lead to the development of tumors. For side effects of **antihypertensives** and **antibiotics,** *see pages 46, 44 and 78.*

OVER-THE-COUNTER TREATMENTS

None.

DRUG INTERACTIONS

Cyclosporine is broken down in the liver. Other drugs may alter the rate at which this happens, leaving to organ rejection or cyclosporine toxicity. Similar risks exist for azathioprine.

QUESTIONS TO ASK THE DOCTOR

■ For how long do I have to take each drug?
■ What are the symptoms of deterioration in graft function?
■ Are there any drugs or immunizations which are unsafe in combination with immunosuppressives?
■ What happens if I forget a dose?
■ Are there any foreign countries where I run particular risk of infection?

SELF-MANAGEMENT

■ Never stcp taking immunosuppressives unless specifically told by the specialist: if you do, the transplant may be acutely rejected.
■ Have an adequate supply of the drugs at all times.
■ Be vigilant for signs of infection: fever, boils, pain in the chest, cough, pain on passing urine.
■ Assist your doctor by accurately reporting side effects; co-operate with all routines to check the level of immunosuppressives in the blood. This will include self-monitoring of blood pressure (twice a day with a sphygmomanometer); taking the temperature once a day; collecting urine sample.
■ Keep a list of telephone numbers of your specialist and hospital by you at all times.
■ Remember, it takes team work to keep a transplant going well.

PATIENT'S EXPERIENCE

"The difference between dialysis and transplantation is like chalk and cheese: being dependent on an artificial kidney machine wrecked my life and destroyed my work. The limited sex life and restricted diet made me depressed and I lost my self-respect. After three years, everything seemed to be drawing to an end; then I had the kidney transplant. I am now back at work, and although the first few months were hard, I am now as good as I was five years ago. It's made me into a crusader for organ donation."

DRUG INTERACTIONS

Cyclosporine is broken down in the liver. Other drugs may alter the rate at which this happens, leaving to organ rejection or cyclosporine toxicity. Similar risks exist for azathioprine.

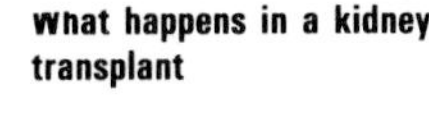
wnat happens in a kidney transplant

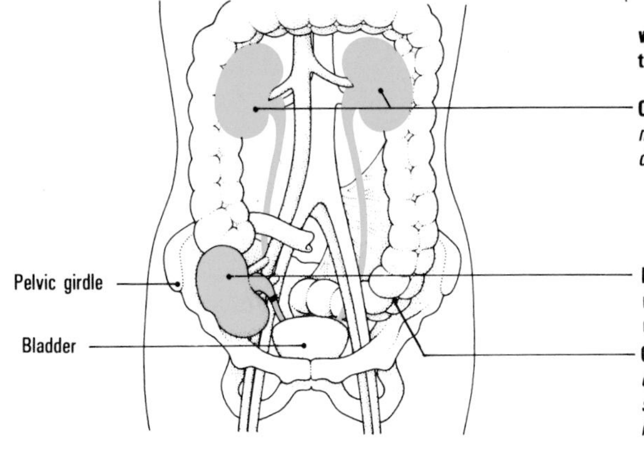

Old (non-functioning) kidneys *may or may not be removed depending on their condition.*

New kidney, *with its artery and vein joined to the iliac artery and vein.*

Colon and blood vessels *serving colon fill the avilable space this side, so the transplant is always installed on the other side.*

Blood and nutritional

Nutrition involves everything from eating a diet containing suitable foods to the way the individual cells are reached by the bloodstream. Psychological, dietary and hormonal factors are all relevant to nutritional disorders.

See also: *Malabsorption, page 36; alcoholism, page 94; fatigue, page 90; lipid disorders, page 162; obesity, page 154; diabetes, page 156; hyper- and hypothyroidism, pages 164-167; adult leukemia, page 208; childhood leukemia, page 210.*

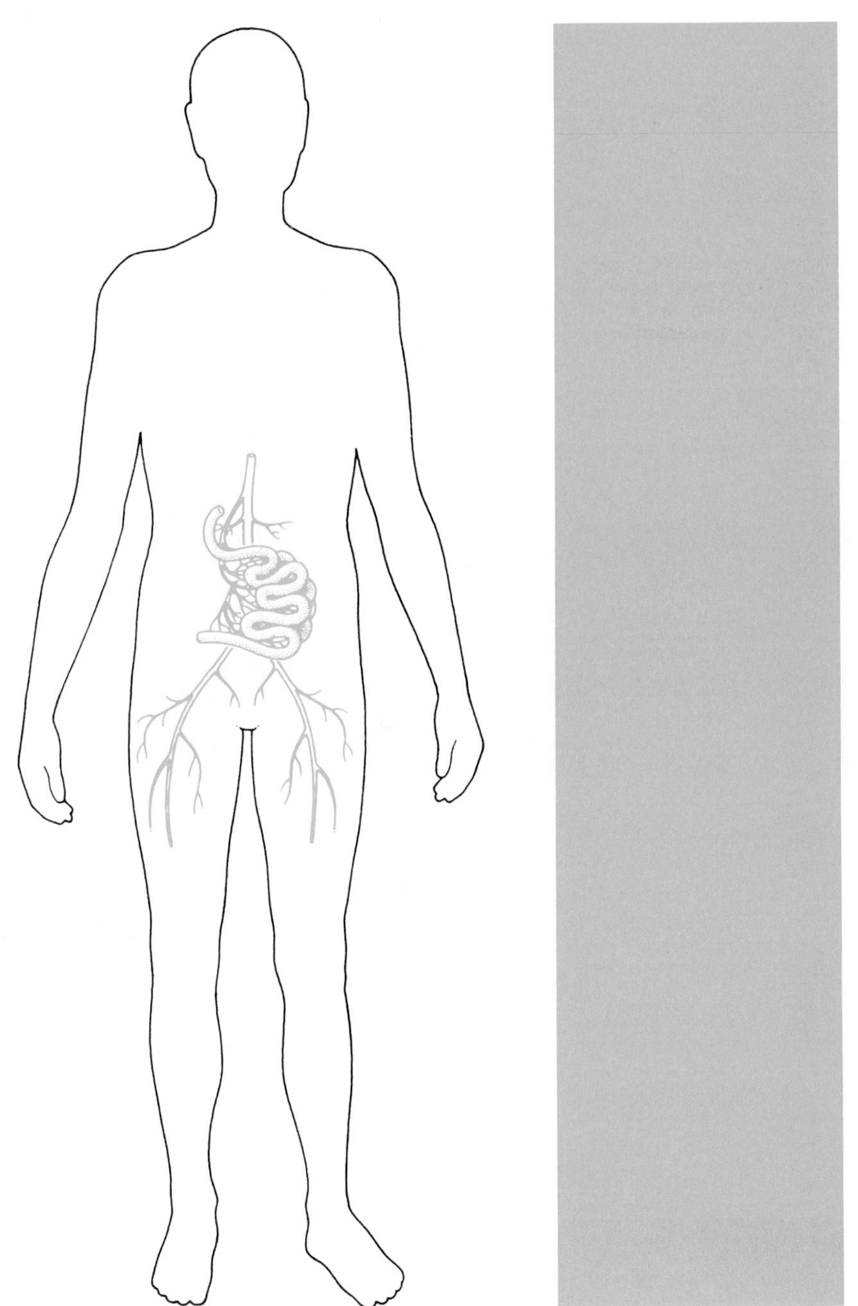

NAMES YOU WILL HEAR
Tranquillizers
Generic name: diazepam; **trade names:** Valium, Alupram, Atensine, Evacalm, Solis, Tensium, Valrelease; see also anxiety, page 84.

Antidepressants
Generic name: amitriptyline; **trade names:** Elavil, Tryptizol, Lentizol, Domical, Laroxyl, Tryptanol, Saroten, Amiline, Deprex, Levate, Meravil, Novotriptyn, Amilent, Trepiline, Tryptanol; *see also* ***depression,*** *page 116.*

ANOREXIA NERVOSA AND BULIMIA

– These are the technical terms for the two commonest disorders of eating. Anorexia is voluntary starvation accompanied by substantial weight loss and malnutrition. Bulimia is overindulgence in food followed by self-induced vomiting or use of large doses of laxatives, causing diarrhea. Bulimia develops into anorexia, or alternates with it. Some patients with bulimia have a history of obesity. The problems are most common in adolescent girls, although they may occur at any age. Men are rarely affected.

The anorectic is obsessed with food, weight and diets. There is excessive fear of becoming fat, and a loss of judgement regarding food requirements and body image: the anorectic often believes she is overweight when in fact she is extremely thin.

Other common symptoms of both conditions include amenorrhea (interruption of normal menstrual bleeding); loss of scalp hair; increase in the fine hair on the face and arms; obsessional commitment to physical exercise and a general restless activity. In patients who regularly vomit after meals, acid from the stomach can cause rapid tooth decay.

CAUSES Ultimately unknown, though it appears that a number of complex factors come together to cause both conditions: ■ There is often conflict within the family, including a poor mother-daughter relationship, sibling rivalry and alcoholism in parents. Families (and especially mothers) must not be thought of as the sole cause, but they are involved in the problem. ■ The typical anorectic is often an 'easy' child, insecure and eager to please her parents. Until adolescence she does not challenge their expectations; then, she finds she has her own ideas of how she wants to develop. Anorexia seems – almost literally – to be the embodiment of this conflict. ■ Social pressure: slimness as a mark of female attractiveness is of course a goal for many adolescent girls. ■ Hormonal changes do occur, but they are thought to be a result of the malnutrition, rather than a cause of it. ■ Brain mechanisms: poorly understood as yet.

PRESCRIPTION DRUGS

The basic aims of treatment are **1** to restore a safe weight on a balanced diet: this is not the solution to the problem but may be necessary for survival – and it can be impossible for a therapist to work with a patient whose thinking is impaired by gross malnutrition; **2** to help the patient to readjust psychologically. Severe cases of anorexia are treated in psychiatric units; many specialists would argue that drugs play a minor role in the treatment of eating disorders. However, **tranquillizers** can help decrease the anxiety which the patient feels when she does eat. The most commonly used are the benzodiazepine group.

How they work: *See* ***anxiety****, page 84.*

Antidepressants may be used, too, but they are relatively ineffective. The most commonly used group are the tricyclic antidepressants.

How they work: *see* ***depression****, page 116.*

It is essential for doctors, patients and anyone else concerned to understand that giving drugs and enforcing weight gain without tackling the root cause are ineffective, even dangerous.

OVER-THE-COUNTER TREATMENT

Appetite stimulants and food supplements may seem appropriate to friends and family, but the anorectic self has no use for them and they don't work.

SIDE EFFECTS

Tranquillizers should be used for the shortest time and in the lowest possible dose because of the risk of dependence. *See* ***anxiety****, page 84.*

Tricyclic antidepressants: *see* **depression,** *page 116.*

QUESTIONS TO ASK THE DOCTOR

- Are the drugs really necessary?
- What can the family do to help?
- Can the family obtain outside support if necessary?

SELF-MANAGEMENT

First of all, understand that:

- Doctors are anxious not to over-diagnose anorexia. Many teenagers have food fads; doctors tend not to act unless weight is ten per cent below the average for age and height. Then danger to health is significant.
- It is natural for parents to react with anger, guilt and despair; it is difficult for them to cope with the way the anorectic appears to reject their love and care.
- The patient's behavior is driven by fear of lack of control over life. A constructive approach, of understanding, support and working together often requires the help of a psychologist working in a hospital setting to bring about step-by-step changes in behavior. Doctors and therapists will attempt to explore family problems, many of which parents may feel they have

PATIENT'S EXPERIENCE

"I started anorexia at the age of 17. I did well at school and was never really fat, but I had put on some weight over Christmas and I was also concerned about the approaching exams. My parents wanted me to go to college to study medicine. They were both doctors, so it was more or less taken for granted. My mother kept going on about how many more opportunities there were for women doctors these days, compared with when she was young. I wanted to do what they said, but I was just not sure. At first the dieting was hard, but as I lost more weight I had a real sense of achievement. I still wanted to eat, but it felt good to say 'no'.

My parents were worried, but soon they realized that they were fighting a losing battle. They took me to see a psychiatrist. I didn't want to speak to him, not because I was afraid that he might think me crazy, but because I just didn't trust myself. I was afraid that I would lose control of the situation, that he might be able to break down my resistance to eating and I was desperately afraid of that. He was very gentle and we just talked. He seemed to understand my fear and did not once mention food. We talked about my parents and their careers, my younger sister and life in general.

Over a period he helped me to draw my own conclusions about what had happened. I came to realize that my life was being planned for me by my parents, and because I loved them, I did not want to disappoint them. The control over my diet gave me security: it showed me that I could make my own decisions about myself. My parents were very understanding. They had believed that I really did want to do medicine and that they were just helping. I decided that I would take the rest of the year off and work in a nursery school. Next year I will think about going to college and then who knows? But this time I will decide."

handled successfully. This is a threatening experience, but airing the problems *can* help.

IF YOU SUSPECT ANOREXIA OR BULIMIA:

■ Don't delay in seeking help. The family cannot usually undertake the cure alone: they are too closely involved.
■ The best starting point is the family doctor, especially if he or she has known the family for some time and has their trust. The doctor may wish to refer to a specialist (usually a psychiatrist or psychologist) if weight loss is extreme.
■ Parents often find it difficult to hand over control to the doctors: the psychiatrist, for example, has responsibilities to the patient and may not be prepared to discuss confidences with parents. Try to understand, and work with the doctors.
■ Parents often feel a need for more positive action than is first offered in terms of investigations and physical treatment. But the best result is for her to *want* to start eating again, not to be drugged and force-fed.

THE PATIENT'S PROBLEMS

■ She may have a distorted perception of her own size, and feel that she is large when she is thin. She may also be unable to assess what a normal plateful of food should be.
■ She may be deceitful about food and her weight. This is part of the illness.
■ There appears to be a deep-rooted fear that she will lose self-control if she gives in to the desire to eat.
■ She often feels insecure and incompetent.
■ She finds it difficult to ask for help because of her desire to retain control of her life.
■ Bulimia can be time-consuming: hours are devoted to secretly buying, eating and then vomiting up food.
■ Without treatment, the condition can progress to a point at which the patient is unable to help herself because of real malnutrition.

STRATEGY

Anorexia is a behavioral 'solution' to a state of internal conflict. The anorectic cannot be forced to give up anorexia before the process of recovery begins. Everyone needs defense mechanisms sometime.

■ Counselling and psychotherapy: Find someone the anorectic can trust, and talk with, as soon as possible. The therapist must be someone who allows her to re-

tain control of her treatment; if she does not, feelings of incompetence and insecurity will be compounded.
Drug therapy: The disadvantages usually outweigh the advantages. Because the drugs' action is essentially to lower resistance, they impair self-control, the very quality on which the therapist needs to work. Any decision to use drugs must be made with the anorectic's consent.

■ Hospital admission may be necessary if malnutrition is endangering the anorectic's life. A balanced diet of proteins, carbohydrates, fats, vitamins and minerals can be given by means of sedation, feeding via a tube into the stomach, or a drip into a vein.

Going into hospital can also be useful in removing the anorectic from a tense family situation. However, the emphasis in hospital tends to be on weight gain, rather than addressing the underlying problems. It is therefore essential for the anorectic and the family to consider what the hospital's approach will be before agreeing to admission. It ought to appreciate the importance of the patient retaining control where possible; treatment must not degenerate into a struggle of wills between her and the hospital staff.

One aspect of hospital treatment is behavior modification based on a reward system for co-operation. Privileges such as family visits, being allowed out of bed and participation in activities are made to depend on weight gain. This can involve loss of control by the patient: there may be a rapid weight gain, but after discharge there may well be an equally rapid weight loss, and possibly suicidal depression. Enforced bed rest until weight gain has been achieved can also be a torment for an already anxious, restless person. If there is to be a weight goal, it ought to be negotiated with, not dictated to, the patient.

Individual and group psychotherapy with family involvement ought to be the major part of any hospital treatment, but resources for psychotherapy are limited in some countries. Hospital treatment should, in addition, include occupational therapy.

Both in hospital and at home there must be total honesty over contents of food prepared for the anorectic. Secretly adding high calorie products will result in loss of trust and resistance to all food.

■ Chances of a happy outcome are significantly improved if the problem is presented to a doctor early, and if the onset is in the early teens, within three years of puberty. There is no correlation between disturbed behavior and the number of episodes.

SIGNS OF RECOVERY

A change in attitude towards eating; loss of obsession with food. Weight gain is not a reliable sign of recovery and menstrual periods take many months to return to normal. Recovery also involves a sense of the patient being in charge of her own life, with an ability to make her own decisions about what she wants, and an accurate sense of her worth.

Iron, folic acid, vitamin B12

NAMES YOU WILL HEAR
Iron
Generic name: ferrous sulphate; **trade names:** Eldec Kapseals, Feosol, Ferro-Folic, Ferrograd, Ferro-gradumet, Heptuna, Iberet, Irospan, Pramet, Slow Fe, Feospan, Ferrograd C, Feritard, Fespan, Fer-in-Sol, Fesofor, Ferrosan. **Generic name:** ferrous fumarate; **trade names:** Cevi Fer, Chromagen, Feostat, Ferancee, Ferrosequels, Ircon, Pramilet, Fersaday, Fersamal, Galfer, Bramiron, Fumiron, Feroton, Ferrofume. **Generic name:** ferrous gluconate; **trade names:** Albafort, Fergon, Ferralet, Fosfree, Iromin-G, Megadose, Ferro-G, Fersin, Glucohaem, Fertinic, Novoferrogluc. **Generic name:** ferrous glycine sulphate; **trade names:** Fe-cap, Ferrocontin Continus, Kelferon, Plesmet, Ferro-Chel. **Generic name:** ferrous succinate; **trade names:** Ferromyn, Cerevon, Kepler.

Injectable Iron Preparations
Generic names: iron dextran injection, iron sorbitol injection; **trade names:** Dextraron, Imferon, Jectofer.

Folic Acid
Generic name: folic acid; **trade names:** Biotin forte; Cefol, Cerifer, Eldec Kapseals, Eldercaps, Feosol, Pronemia, Vitafol, Niferex, Zincvit, Lexpec, Folettes, Folvite, Novofolacid.

Vitamin B12
Generic names: hydroxocobalamin, cyanocobalamin; **trade names:** B-C-Bid, Chromagen, Eldertonic, May-Vita Elixir, Redisol Injectable, Trinsicon, Vicon Forte, Cobalin-H, Neo-Cytamen, Cytacon, Cytamen, Hepacon-B12, Panalamine, Anacobin, Bedoz, Bio-12, Cyanabin, Neo-Rubex, Redisol, Rubion.

WHAT IS ANEMIA?

A lack of hemoglobin, the substance which gives blood its red color and which takes oxygen from the lungs to the tissues of the body.

Anemia may result in fatigue, breathlessness on exertion, palpitations, dizziness and headache. Sufferers may have an unusually pale skin, with loss of normal color in the lips, tongue and linings of the eyes. The pulse may be noticeably more rapid than usual, especially on exercising; people with heart disease or narrowing of the arteries may have worse symptoms if they become anemic.

The effects of anemia on the individual depend on its severity and on how quickly it has developed. Slowly-developing anemias allow time for the body to adapt and are thus better tolerated.

CAUSES Generally, anemias arise in main ways. In order to make blood properly, the bone marrow needs a supply of protein and essential vitamins and minerals such as folic acid, vitamin B12 and iron. Anemia can arise, therefore, from lack of these essential ingredients (see below); or from a disease of the bone marrow such as acute leukemia. Secondly, anemia can result from loss or breakdown of red cells at a rate which exceeds their production. This may occur in severe bleeding *(and see also page 226).*

CAUSES OF IRON DEFICIENCY Iron deficiency may arise from a poor diet, especially in the elderly, or from excessive blood loss, e.g. from a stomach ulcer or heavy menstrual periods.

FOLIC ACID DEFICIENCY A diet low in fresh fruit and vegetables can result in folic acid deficiency. The bowel may fail to absorb folic acid from the diet, for example in chronic diarrhea. Or there may be a high demand for extra folic acid, as in pregnancy, or in some bone marrow disorders; if folic acid supply does not keep up with the demand, anemia will follow.

CAUSES OF VITAMIN B12 DEFICIENCY Absorption of vitamin B12 from the stomach may be lowered if there has been surgery to the stomach, for example to treat ulcers. Another cause is pernicious anemia, which results from an immune response. Less commonly, vitamin B12 deficiency can result from disease or surgical removal or key parts of the small bowel. A tape worm acquired by eating raw meat or fish may compete (successfully) with the patient for the available vitamin B12 and so cause pernicious anemia.

PRESCRIPTION DRUGS

Iron deficiency will usually respond to taking iron by mouth. However, some people are truly unable to tolerate iron by mouth, or may have bowel problems preventing this remedy. These may require iron by injection. Treatment with iron corrects the anemia of iron deficiency in six to eight weeks. A further two to three months' treatment is often given to replace the body's iron stores.

Folic acid and vitamin B12 deficiencies are treated by pills; vitamin B12 deficiency is also treated by injection. Response to folic acid and vitamin B12 is rapid, with clear evidence of improvement within a few days. The anemia is usually completely corrected in four to six weeks. In folic acid deficiency, treatment is often continued for three to four months to replace body stores. Maintenance injections of vitamin B12 may be necessary and in this case are given every two or three months for life. It is dangerous to treat a vitamin B12 deficiency with folic acid. This may make the body use its dwindling reserves of vitamin B12 and cause severe neurological damage. Do not treat yourself with folic acid but seek medical help in determining what your problem is.

QUESTIONS TO ASK YOUR DOCTOR

- Am I anemic or is there some other cause for my symptoms?
- What sort of anemia do I have?
- Why have I become deficient in iron/folic acid/vitamin B12?
- Should I modify my eating habits?
- Is there an underlying cause for the anemia that needs investigation?
- How long will the treatment take to work?

OVER-THE-COUNTER TREATMENTS

Although the preparations containing iron and vitamin B12 are available at health food shops, don't attempt to treat yourself. This is a complex condition, and dosage has to be correct: many preparations contain too little iron or B12 to be effective.

SIDE EFFECTS

Iron: nausea, discomfort in the stomach, constipation and diarrhea. These effects are due to iron itself and an

PATIENT'S EXPERIENCE

"I am now 26 years old and I have suffered problems with sickle cell anemia since early childhood. My main problem at present is a tendency towards recurrent crises which produce severe pain particularly in my back and legs. I have found that over-exertion and rapid changes in temperature increase the likelihood of a crisis developing and I am careful to avoid them. If I feel a mild crisis starting, I keep warm, drink plenty of fluids and take simple painkillers. This is often all I need to do; however, sometimes the crisis worsens and I then need intensive treatment in the hospital. Fortunately this is infrequent."

NAMES YOU WILL HEAR

Generic name: oxymetholone; **trade names:** Anadrol-50, Anapolon 50, Adroyd. **Generic name:** antithymocyte immunoglobulin (ATG); anti lymphocyte globulin (ALG); **trade name:** Pressimmune (ALG). **Generic name:** methyl prednisolone hemi succinate; **trade names:** Solumedrol, Medrol·Depo-Medrol, Solu-Medrone, Solu-Medrol. **Generic name:** deferoxamine mesylate; **trade name:** Desferal Mesylate. **Generic name:** methyl prednisolone; **trade names:** Solumedrol, Deltasone, Prednicen M, Codelsol, Delta Phoricol, Deltacortril, Deltalone, Deltastab, Precortisyl, Prednesol, Sintisone, Nisolone, Delta-Cortef, Deltasolone, Prelone, Lenisolone, Meticortilone, Predeltilone.

alternative iron preparation may produce fewer side effects only because it contains less iron. All iron pills produce darkening of the feces. Iron given intramuscularly or intravenously may produce nausea, vomiting and flushing. Staining of the skin may also occur. Major reactions with collapse, low blood pressure and acute breathlessness are rare, but iron should not be given in this way to people with a history of allergy and asthma. **Folic acid and vitamin B12** are essentially free of significant side effects. Neither should be given, however, until a deficiency state has been properly diagnosed.

SELF-HELP

If you have iron, folic acid or vitamin B12 deficiency, eat a well balanced diet containing a full range of vitamins and minerals. Some diets do carry a risk of developing vitamin deficiencies, for example very strict vegetarian diets may contain insufficient vitamin B12. See page 228.

Look for and report immediately to your doctor any bleeding in the urine or feces, unusually heavy or abnormally-timed menstrual bleeding, and particularly bleeding from the vagina after menopause.

OTHER ANEMIAS

Aplastic anemia is a severe anemia caused by reduced production of normal blood cells in the bone marrow. This may be due to invasion of the bone marrow by abnormal cells, as in cancer; to a toxic effect of certain drugs such as phenylbutazone or chloromphenicol; or it may have no discernable cause.

Thalassemia occurs as a result of failure of the mechanism for producing normal hemoglobin. The red cells are broken down more easily than usual. It runs in families.

Sickle cell anemia is a similar hemolytic anemia occurring particularly in people of west African or West Indian extraction.

PRESCRIPTION DRUGS AND OTHER TREATMENTS

Aplastic anemia: Less severe cases may need no drugs; mildly or moderately affected people may benefit from attempts to boost bone marrow function. The agent most commonly used in this situation is **oxymethalone,** a drug similar to the male hormone testosterone. Severe (life-threatening) cases may be treated by bone marrow transplant. If this is not possible, drug treatment with the **anti-white cell agents** (immunosuppressive drugs) and the steroid **methyl prednisolone** may be tried.

Thalassemias: Most people with thalassemia need no treatment. However, a severe thalassemia (thalassemia major) causes a serious anemia in early childhood. This is not amenable to drug treatment but needs regular blood transfusions. This causes problems: transfused blood contains large amounts of iron which accumulate in the body and can damage vital organs such as the heart and liver. To rid the body of this excess iron, **desferoxamine** may be used – it binds the iron, enabling it to be excreted in the urine. Some children with severe thalassemia have been effectively treated by bone marrow *transplant,* although such treatment is not yet widely available.

Sickle cell anemia: People with sickle cell disease are unusually anemic but tolerate the condition well and often require no specific drug treatment other than regular folic acid. Children with sickle cell anemia should receive prompt treatment for bacterial infections – their resistance to infection may be diminished.

Sickle crises (severe pain in the legs, back or chest due to blockage of small blood vessels by the abnormal 'sickled' red cells) may respond to simple measures at home (see **SELF-HELP**).

SIDE EFFECTS

Oxymetholone can cause the following: acne, fluid retention leading to ankle swelling; in women development of facial hair, deepening of the voice and irregular periods. A serious side effect can be jaundice, a yellow discoloration of the skin and eyes indicating disturbance of liver function. See your doctor immediately.

The steroid methyl prednisolone can cause acute rise in blood pressure, fluid retention, muscle weakness, and, rarely, drug-induced diabetes *(see page 156)*; insomnia and depression; indigestion and heartburn and generally decreased resistance to infection. Long-term prednisolone's side effects are undeniably grave, but the drug's use is justified by the fact that it can be life-saving; that not all patients suffer the side effects; that careful monitoring can anticipate problems before they develop. Stopping the drug can itself be problematic, and must be done gradually under supervision.

Desferoxamine must be given by injection. It can, very occasionally, cause pain at the infusion site, and collapse with a sudden fall in blood pressure. This usually occurs at the start of the infusion; the first few doses must be carefully monitored.

Vitamin supplements

NAMES YOU WILL HEAR
Generic name: vitamin A; **trade names:** Aquasol-A, Eldercaps, Natalins, Tri-Vi-Flor, Ro-A-Vit, Afaxin, Arovit. **Generic name:** vitamin B1 (thiamine); **trade names:** Eldercaps, Mega-B, Therabid, Thiamine Hydrochloride Tablets. **Generic name:** vitamin B2 (riboflavine); **trade names:** Albafort, Eldertonic, Prenate, Riboflavine Tablets. **Generic name:** vitamin B6 (pyridoxine); **trade names:** Beelith, Prenate, Therabid, Benadon, Pydox, Hexa-Betalin, Lactosec. **Generic name:** folic acid; **trade names:** Biotin Forte, Fero-Folic 500, Zincvit, Lexpec, Folettes, Folvite, Novofolacid. **Generic name:** vitamin B12 (cyanocobalimin); **trade names:** Albafort, Cobolin M, Therabid, Redisol injectable, Cobalin-H, Neo-Cytamen, Cytacon, Cytamen, Hepacon B12, Panalamine, Anacobin, Bedoz, Hio-12, Cyanabin, Neo-Rubex, Radisol, Rubion. **Generic names:** vitamin C, ascorbic acid; **trade names:** Cevi Bid, Vicon C, Ferancee, Hy-C, Ascorbic Acid Tablets, Ascorb, Adenex, Cebion. **Generic name:** vitamin D; **trade names:** Cal-Bid, Prenate, Tri-Vi-Flor, Rocaltrol, Vi-De-3. **Generic name:** vitamin K; **trade names:** Konakion, Mephyton, Synkavit.

WHAT IS VITAMIN DEFICIENCY?

Vitamins are constituents of the diet necessary for the normal function of various organs in the body. Minimum requirements are recognized for each one.

CAUSES Restricted or deficient diet: typically a problem of vegans (those on ultra-restricted vegetarian diet); alcoholics who may not eat properly; old people living alone who find it too bothersome to cook; non-absorption of vitamins because of bowel disease; temporarily increased need for certain vitamins, for example in pregnancy or growth spurts. Certain drugs also interfere with vitamin absorption.

Vitamin A deficiency is rare in developed countries. It results in poor night vision, dry eyes, damage to the cornea and eventually blindness. The vitamin is found in animal fats, fruit and vegetables.

Vitamin B group – thiamine (B1), riboflavin (B2), pyridoxine (B6), cyanocobalamin (B12) and folic acid – are rarely deficient because they are found in a wide variety of foods. Deficiency occurs in disease of the gut, chronic alcoholism or as the result of an extremely restricted diet. Folic acid and B12 deficiencies result in anemia, *see page 224*.

Vitamin C deficiency causes scurvy. Mild symptoms are quite common, especially in the elderly, and include bleeding gums, bruising and delayed healing of wounds. The vitamin is found in citrus fruit, green vegetables and potatoes, but is destroyed by cooking.

Vitamin D deficiency causes rickets and is most commonly found in the elderly and in Asians who eat unleavened bread. It may also be seen in babies (especially those born prematurely) who are not given vitamin D supplements. The vitamin is necessary for hardening of bone and for normal strength in muscles. In young children the deficiency results in bending of the long bones; in the elderly the bones become soft. Vitamin D can be produced in the skin in the presence of sunlight; it is also found in fish oils and animal fat.

Vitamin K is important for chemicals necessary for blood clotting. Produced by bacteria in the bowel, and absorbed with fat, it may be deficient in the newborn because just after birth the bowel is sterile. It may also be lacking in people who cannot absorb fats from the bowel. Deficiency may also result from "crash diets" aimed at weight reduction. The vitamin occurs in milk and green plants. Deficiency causes prolonged bleeding.

REPLACEMENTS

Vitamin A can be given as a single daily dose, alone or in combination with Vitamin D or a multivitamin preparation. The recommended daily dose is 1,300 to 5,000 units. Higher doses can be given less frequently.

Vitamin B1-B6 taken by mouth, B12 by injection can be given by tablet or injection.

Vitamin C is given as a single daily dose of 200 mg to prevent or treat scurvy, particularly in the elderly or those on a poor diet.

Vitamin D can be given as drops for the very young, or as a tablet or injection. The usual daily dose is 400 units.

Vitamin K is given routinely by injection to newborn babies for reasons given above, and because a baby's liver tends to be immature at birth and, with reduced vitamin K, fails to produce enough clotting factors.

OVER-THE-COUNTER TREATMENTS

All the vitamins listed are available without prescription. Multivitamin preparations have no advantages over single preparations, and many are expensive.

QUESTIONS TO ASK THE DOCTOR

- If I am a vegetarian, do I need extra vitamins?
- Do old people need extra vitamins?
- Does my baby need vitamin supplements?
- Do I need to let you know if I am taking vitamins?
- Can I take extra vitamins during pregnancy?

SIDE EFFECTS

Vitamin A in excess can cause rough skin, dry, sparse hair and increased calcium in the blood. Very large doses can cause irritability and increased pressure within the brain. Large doses should be carefully avoided during pregnancy.

Vitamin B group and **vitamin C**:no significant side effects.

Vitamin D is potentially dangerous as high doses can increase the level of calcium in the blood. This can cause vomiting, dehydration, constipation and kidney stones. Do not use during pregnancy or while breast-feeding because of risk to the baby.

Vitamin K can cause excessive clotting in patients on anticoagulants, but has no other side effects.

SELF-MANAGEMENT

- A commonsense, balanced diet is all that is necessary to prevent vitamin deficiency.
- Restricted diets must be critically examined for vitamin content.

PATIENT'S EXPERIENCE

"I was feeling run-down in the middle of the winter and I went to see my doctor because I felt that I needed a vitamin tonic. She asked me questions about my diet, and said that although I was a vegetarian, my diet did contain sufficient vitamins. She took a blood test for anemia and when I returned for the results, it was normal. I was not convinced because I was still so tired and irritable. We spoke for a while about my job which hadn't been going very well. She said she felt that my job was affecting me and suggested that I take a vacation. This has helped a bit, and I am actively trying to cut down stress at work: maybe I do feel better."

VEGETARIANS

– Do not generally need extra vitamins if their diet is varied, but vitamin supplements may well be necessary.

VITAMIN PREPARATIONS

- The body's requirements for vitamins is generally much less than is contained in most of the vitamin preparations. There is no advantage to taking excessive doses of vitamins and in some cases, overdose can cause illness.
- Avoid multivitamin preparations: if there really is a deficiency of a vitamin, replace it with the correct dose.
- Vitamin D is usually added to baby formula feeds.

NAMES YOU WILL HEAR
Generic name: terfenadine; **trade name:** Seldane, Triludan. **Generic name:** astemizole; **trade name:** Hismanal. **Generic name:** cromolyn sodium; **trade names:** Intal, Nalcrom.

Other terms
Food intolerance; additivies; tartrazine; benzoates; sulfur dioxide; caffeine.

WHAT IS FOOD INTOLERANCE?

The expression ''One man's meat is another man's poison'' is of Roman origin: it has long been acknowledged that foods can produce adverse reactions in sensitive individuals. This phenomenon is now known by the general term of food intolerance and includes several recognized conditions:

Food aversion is a psychologically based inability to tolerate certain foods; an extreme, but typical example is **anorexia** – *see page 220.*

True food allergy is a sensitivity to a particular food mediated through the immune system. Fish allergy, associated with severe swelling of the lips, is a classic form. The allergy is readily demonstrated by a skin reaction when testing solution is applied. Many foods cause allergy, including nuts, eggs and mushrooms.

Chemical or pharmacological reactions produced in the body by some foods or drinks are normally minor, if noticeable at all, but if the subject is particularly sensitive or takes the food in large quantities, symptoms may appear. The commonest substance which acts in this way is the caffeine in coffee, tea and many carbonated beverages. Large quantities of coffee in sensitive subjects can produce headache, palpitations, anxiety and insomnia.

Enzyme deficiency: the body is unable to break down specific foods. Lactase, for example, is a bowel enzyme which breaks down milk sugar (lactose). Individuals lacking it develop chronic abdominal pain and diarrhea after eating dairy products.

Certain substances can, in addition, cause reactions in sensitive individuals by mechanisms which are not yet understood. These include substances which are added to food as preservatives, coloring agents, tasting agents and substances which affect texture and moisture. Monosodium glutamate, the flavour-enhancing agent in Chinese food, can cause pain and tingling in the chest which can be mistaken for a heart attack. Tartrazine, a yellow coloring used in many foods, can cause swelling of the lips, urticaria (large, itchy red lumps in the skin) and it can exacerbate asthma. Certain dyes, such as eosin, can produce hyperactivity in sensitive children.

PRESCRIPTION DRUGS

Drug therapy is of little value in food intolerance, as the main approach is to identify and then avoid any food which causes a major problem. However, an acute allergic reaction with swelling of the face and urticaria can be treated with an **antihistamine:** one of the newer types such as terfenadine (seldane) is best, since it does not cause drowsiness. **Cromolyn sodium,** a mast-cell stabilizer, will sometimes prevent an allergic reaction and is prescribed for food-allergic patients who are going out for a meal which may contain a food to which they are sensitive. It is not helpful on a regular basis.

OVER-THE-COUNTER TREATMENTS

None.

QUESTIONS TO ASK THE DOCTOR

- Do you think I have a true food allergy?
- Can you recommend a diet?
- Is it worth seeing a specialist dietician?

SIDE EFFECTS

The main problem with food intolerance is that it can produce a wide range of symptoms which can mimic many other diseases. It is, therefore, important that the patient should be assessed by a physician to exclude any serious disease prior to investigating food intolerance. The following symptoms can be caused by food intolerance: headache, catarrh, sneezing, depression, anxiety, sore throat; palpitations, asthma; chronic pain, bloating, diarrhea; rheumatism, eczema, urticaria.

For side effects of **antihistamines** *see* ***sinusitis,*** *page 262;* of **cromolyn sodium,** *see* ***asthma,*** *page 74.*

SELF-MANAGEMENT

1 Check with your doctor that your symptoms do not have another cause.
2 Avoid, for one week, any food which you suspect might be related to your problem.
3 If you do not suspect a particular food, try a general elimination diet for seven days. A simple one limits you to meat, fish, vegetables, salads, fruits and water. It excludes bread and all grains, dairy products, additives, tea and coffee. For the first few days you may feel unwell due to withdrawal symptoms, but an improvement should be evident within seven days.
4 If the symptoms resolve within seven days, foods should then be added back into the diet at 24-hour intervals to identify which was causing the problems.
5 If there is no improvement after seven days, food intolerance is unlikely; return to a normal diet. BUT:
6 If you still feel that food intolerance could be the cause of your problems, seek expert advice. It is dangerous to attempt more rigid elimination diets.

PATIENT'S EXPERIENCE

"I suffered severe migraine attacks every weekend. They occurred on a Saturday afternoon: agonizing – I was sick too, and I felt weak all over. My wife thought they were psychological: an excuse to avoid shopping with her on Saturday afternoons. Numerous drugs failed to help. Finally I went to see an allergist interested in food intolerance who noted that I regularly drank about ten cups of coffee each day when at work, but not at the weekend. He suggested that my weekend headache was similar to a drug withdrawal: the level of caffeine in my blood dropped at the weekend. I stopped drinking coffee at work during the week and, to my surprise, the headaches ceased."

Skeletal, joint and muscular disorders

The body has a complicated system of bones and joints which allow a great variety of movements. The joints are supported and strengthened by ligaments (fibrous strengthening around or inside the joints), muscles and tendons. Tendons connect the body of the muscle with fixed points on the bony skeleton. The joints are lubricated by synovial fluid produced by the membrane surrounding the joints. The upright posture of the human being has produced a range of adaptations from the basic four-legged animal skeleton, but our ''locomotor system'' is still prone to wear and tear and disease.

See also: *Fatigue, page 90.*

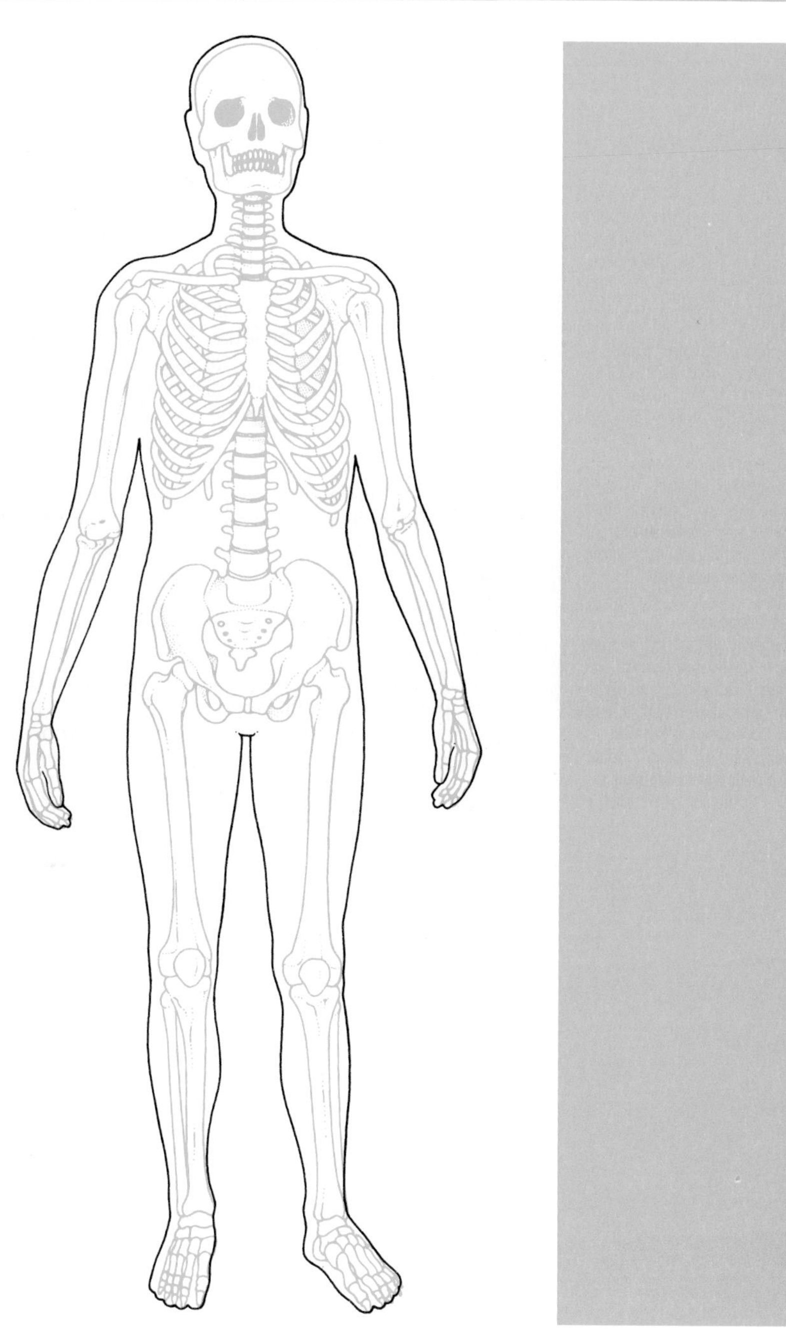

STRAINS AND SPRAINS

Simple analgesics, steroid injections, non-steroid anti-inflammatory drugs (NSAIDS), rubefacients

NAMES YOU WILL HEAR
Simple analgesics
Generic name: acetaminophen; **trade names:** Phenaphon, Panadol, Tempra, Tylenol, Pamol, Calpol, Tylenon, Paracin, Parmol, Panado, Ceetamol, Atosol, Exctol, Ennagesic, Ilvamol. **Generic name:** aspirin; **trade names:** Aspirin, Ascriptin, Ecotrin, Measurin, Astrin, Bi-Prin. *See also **pain,** page 106.*

NSAIDs
Generic name: ibuprofen; **trade names:** Motrin, Advil, Medipren, Nuprin, Rufen, Apsifen, Ebufac, Brufen, Fenbid, Ibumetin, Lidifen, Paxofen. **Generic name:** indomethacin; **trade names:** Indocin, Indocid, Artracin, Indoflex, Mobilan, Rheumacin, Arthrexin. **Generic name:** naproxen sodium; **trade names:** Naprosyn, Laraflex, Anaprox, Synflex. *See also **pain,** page 106.*

Steroid injections
Generic name: hydrocortisone; **trade names:** Hydrocortisone Injection, Solucortef, Efcortesol, Hydrocortistab. **Generic name:** dexamethasone; **trade names:** Dexamethasone Injection, Decadron, Oradexon. **Generic name:** methyl prednisolone; **trade names:** Prednisolone Injection, Hydeltrasol, Codelsol, Deltastab. **Generic name:** triamcinolone; **trade names:** Aristocort, Kenalog, Adcortyl.

SUDDEN OR REPETITIVE INJURIES

– Are covered in this section. They are responsible for a variety of problems in the muscles, tendons, ligaments and joints. Sudden injury is typically sustained in vigorous exercise; repetitive injury can result from as innocent an occupation as wringing out clothes.

Muscle injury results, typically, from a direct blow or by tearing the fibers; this can involve complete rupture, in which case the muscle loses its ability to contract; or it may be a partial tear – the painful ''pulled muscle'' typically sustained by athletes. If the muscle tear is situated near the skin, a large bruise can appear within a few days, sometimes some distance from the site of injury. Muscles are also affected by fibrositis, or soft tissue rheumatism. This usually appears in the neck, shoulder, or lower back and is often attributed to drafts, cold, anxiety or poor posture. The muscle fibers go into spasm in one specific area, and nodules, lumps or trigger points which or may not be painful can be felt.

Tendons connect the muscles to the bones. Although strong, they cannot stretch much; indeed with age they become even more inelastic, and thus more prone to injury. Tendons are usually surrounded by a sheath which produces a lubricating fluid with movement. Unaccustomed movement can cause pain known as tendonitis; it resolves within a few days without treatment. Tenosynovitis occurs when the tendon is overused or injured by repetitive movement such as a heel tab on a shoe constantly rubbing against the Achilles tendon. The tendon becomes painful and swollen, and movement is restricted. Tendons, like muscles, can be partially or completely ruptured: a painful experience which causes varying loss of function. Tennis elbow is an inflammation of the tendinous joint between the muscles of the forearm and the bone just above the elbow on the outside of the arm. Golfer's elbow is a similar condition affecting the inner aspect of the arm.

Ligaments and joints exist in various forms throughout the body. There are simple hinge joints (for example the fingers); and there are complicated ball-and-socket joints (for example the hip or shoulder). The stability of joints is maintained not only by the surrounding muscles and tendons, but by the **ligaments,** which are essentially bands of tissue. The more unstable a **joint,** the more ligaments are present. The knee is stabilized by a large number of ligaments not only around the joint but also within it.

PRESCRIPTION DRUGS

Simple analgesics or painkillers like acetaminophen or aspirin will relieve the pain and, to a lesser extent, reduce inflammation. The catch is that once the pain is relieved, there is a temptation to return to full activity at once, and thus to worsen the injury. Combinations with codeine increase the pain relief. *See **pain,** page 106.*

NSAIDS will reduce swelling, redness and tenderness around an injury, and quicken healing. As they also reduce pain, there is a similar temptation to return to full activity too soon. *See **osteoarthritis,** page 238.*

Steroid injections, given directly in the injured area, can have great effect in reducing local inflammation. They are particularly helpful in treating tennis elbow and joint swellings. *See **rheumatoid arthritis,** page 242.*

Rubefacients – agents which are rubbed in or sprayed on – act by counter-irritation of the skin: the feeling of warmth detracts from pain elsewhere. There is no evidence that they help with deep pain.

OVER-THE-COUNTER TREATMENTS

Apart from steroid injections, all the other treatments listed are available from pharmacists. The range of NSAIDS is limited; use them with caution.

QUESTIONS TO ASK THE DOCTOR

- How long should I rest after the injury?
- Would physiotherapy be helpful?
- What can I do to stop it happening again?

SIDE EFFECTS

Simple analgesics are relatively free of side effects: however, if combined with codeine, they are more likely to produce nausea, vomiting and constipation *(see **pain,** page 106* and ***common cold,** page 134).* Aspirin should not be used in children under 12 years of age. Allergic reactions can occur, often an itchy skin rash.

NSAIDs are related to aspirin and allergic reactions do occur. *See **pain,** page 106.*

Steroid injections, if repeated too frequently, can lead to joint and tendon damage.

Rubefacients should not be used on broken skin. Local allergic reactions are common.

NON-DRUG OPTIONS

Rest is usually necessary to allow the healing process to get under way. Strapping and resting an injured part are common measures. Physiotherapy, if available, is often helpful, especially ultrasonic sound therapy.

PATIENT'S EXPERIENCE

"It was around Christmas, on the ice, that I slipped while running and fell over on my left ankle. It was extremely painful, but I managed to walk the three miles home. Afterwards, my ankle was like a balloon: I was sure that it was broken, but the doctor said that it was just a bad sprain. I insisted on an X-ray, but he was right. It was taped up and I had daily ultrasonic treatment from a physiotherapist at the hospital. I needed crutches to get around. The swelling slowly went down, but even at Easter I could still feel the pain if I put it under pressure. If I hadn't had to walk home, I don't think it would have swelled up so much."

THE RICE PRINCIPLE

Apply the RICE principle for the first few days after the injury. R is for rest. This helps to stop bleeding, external and internal, and to minimize damage to the tissues. I is for ice, or application of cold water, applied for about 20 minutes every four hours. Take care: excessive cold can burn skin. C is for compression: firm bandaging will stop bleeding into the tissues. Don't apply too tightly. E is for elevation: raising the affected part allows fluid to drain away and reduces swelling.

A couple of days after most sudden or repetitive injuries, it is usually possible to start gentle exercise, massage, but if in any doubt consult a doctor or physiotherapist.

BACK PAIN

Simple analgesics, narcotic analgesics, non-steroid anti-inflammatory drugs (NSAIDS),

NAMES YOU WILL HEAR
Simple analgesics
Generic name: aspirin; **trade names:** Ascriptin, Ecotrin, Measurin, Aspirin, Astrin, Bi-Prin. **Generic name:** acetaminophen; **trade names:** Phenaphon, Panadol, Tempra, Tylenol, Pamol, Calpol, Tylenon, Paracin, Parmol, Panado, Ceetamol, Atosol, Exctol, Ennagesic, Ilvamol. *See also* ***pain,*** *page 106.*

Narcotic analgesics
Generic name: buprenorphine; **trade names:** Temgesic, Buprex. *See also* ***pain,*** *page 106.* **Generic name:** dihydrocodeine; **trade names:** DF 118, Onadex 118, Paramol 118, Rikodeine, Tuscodin, Paracodin, Fortuss.

NSAIDS
Generic name: ibuprofen; **trade name:** Motrin, Advil, Medipren, Nuprin, Rufen, Apsifen, Ebufac, Brufen, Fenbid, Ibumetin, Lidifen, Motrin, Paxofen. **Generic name:** indomethacin; **trade names:** Indocin, Indocid, Artracin, Indoflex, Mobilan, Rheumacin, Arthrexin. *See also* ***pain,*** *page 106.*

Muscle relaxants
Generic name: diazepam; **trade names:** Valium, Alupram, Atensine, Evacalm, Solis, Tensium, Valrelease. **Generic name:** orphenadrin citrate; **trade names:** Norflex, Norgesic, Disipal, Myotrol, Biorphen. **Generic name:** methocarbamol; **trade names:** Robaxin, Robaxisal. **Generic name:** chlormezanone; **trade names:** Trancoprin, Trancopal, Lobak.

THE BACK AND ITS PROBLEMS

The back bone, or spine, is divided into three main sections: neck (cervical spine), upper back (dorsal or thoracic spine), and lower back (lumbo-sacral spine).

The spine is actually a column of bones called vertebrae, separated from each other by discs, which are rings of tough fibrous tissue with an inner core made of a jelly-like substance. Their principal function is to absorb stress on impact, like a shock-absorber. With age they slowly stiffen, becoming brittle.

The vertebrae are secured by a system of ligaments and muscles which support the whole structure and allow a limited amount of movement. Each vertebra also has joints linking it with adjacent bones thus making a whole series of complex joints allowing co-ordinated movement. The spine also provides protection to the spinal cord, from which, between the vertebrae, fine pairs of nerves branch off and lead to the skin, muscles and joints of the body.

Similar causes give pain in any part of the back.

CAUSES OF BACK PAIN Movements which place abnormal stress or load on the spine will cause injury and pain. This can happen suddenly, as when lifting a heavy weight, or it can come on slowly, as when performing a repetitive task. The vertebrae can be compressed in a severe injury; indeed the arch bones at the back of the vertebrae can be broken in a severe twisting injury. Ligaments of the spine may be stretched, partially torn or may rupture completely. The small joints may be strained, or, even more serious, the discs may rupture and the jelly inside can protrude and compress nerves or the spinal cord itself.

"Referred pain" occurs when injury to the spine irritates a nerve supplying a specific part of the body. Perhaps the commonest example is sciatica, in which pain is felt in the legs, although the spine is the site of damage or inflammation. Fibrositis is a common back problem arising from muscle spasm, in turn caused by over-use of a muscle or muscles.

Arthritis in the spine is usually a "wear and tear" process; it may reflect previous injury, or be a gradual change associated with ageing. X-rays will reveal changes caused by early "wear and tear" arthritis in most people in their 20s or 30s.

PRESCRIPTION DRUGS

Simple analgesics – aspirin and acetaminophen – are often effective, relieving pain and reducing inflamma-

tion. *See* ***pain,*** *page 106,* as also for **narcotic analgesics.** **NSAIDS** reduce the swelling and inflammation around an injured area, thus giving pain relief.
How they work: *see* ***osteoarthritis,*** *page 238.*
Muscle relaxants are of some value, especially when most of the pain is due to muscle spasm. Diazepam, a sedative, can reduce associated tension and anxiety.

OVER-THE-COUNTER TREATMENTS

Aspirin and acetaminophen, available without prescription, should be tried before consulting a doctor. If you find that they are ineffective, this can be a useful basis on which to plan the next step in treatment.

Ibuprofen is available from pharmacists in many countries and can be tried if simple analgesics have failed.

Rubefacient creams are widely available. They are a way of applying local heat to the affected part.

QUESTIONS TO ASK THE DOCTOR

- What do you think has caused the pain?
- Would physiotherapy or spinal manipulation be helpful?
- Can I go to work/take exercise?
- Should I learn back-strengthening exercises?

SIDE EFFECTS

Simple analgesics, especially acetaminophen, are more or less free of side effects. However, aspirin should be used with caution and not at all in the under-12 age group. *See* ***pain,*** *page 106.*
Narcotic analgesics can produce drowsiness, unsteadiness and an inability to concentrate. Vomiting is sometimes a problem and most people become constipated if they take these drugs for an extended period. There is a danger of addiction. *See* ***pain,*** *page 106.*
NSAIDS are related to aspirin and have the same side effects but usually less so. Indigestion, a common side effect, can often be prevented by taking them with a meal, or with milk. *See* ***osteoarthritis,*** *page 238.*
Muscle relaxants are often sedative, but they can also cause dry mouth and blurring of vision, especially if taken in higher dosage. *See* ***anxiety,*** *page 84.*

SELF-HELP

- Take simple painkillers or NSAIDS as soon as the pain starts. Cold or ice treatment can be started immediately: apply cold pack or ice to the most painful area for twenty minutes, every four hours.

PATIENT'S EXPERIENCE

"I was working as a nurse on a geriatric ward when I got my first attack of low back pain. It was while we were lifting this old man: I had to twist and lift at the same time. The pain came on like a knife: I could hardly move. I had to go home, rest and take some painkillers. The pain went within ten days; I went back to work. However, the pain kept coming back, and I kept having to take time off.

This went on for more than a year: I was seriously thinking of changing my job when a physiotherapist at the hospital saw me in pain. She suggested some exercises, and advised me on how to lift patients the right way. It took some months for the benefit to come through; but now my back feels much stronger and I'm taking much less time off work."

REST

Once the pain has started, rest is the most important healing factor: anything that leads to further back strain should be avoided. Sitting will aggravate the pain unless the back is well supported with a cushion. A cervical collar or lumbar support may be of temporary benefit, but should not be used for too long.

PREVENTION

1 always lift weights with the knees bent and the back straight; **2** maintain strong back and stomach muscles by means of suitable exercises (ask a physiotherapist to show you the exercises); **3** sleep on a firm bed.

CAUTION

If there is much referred pain and numbness in the arms or legs, or if you are unable to pass urine, seek medical help immediately.

Simple analgesics, compound analgesics, non-steroid anti-inflammatory drugs (NSAIDs)

NAMES YOU WILL HEAR

Simple analgesics

Generic name: aspirin; **trade names:** Ascriptin, Ecotrin, Measurin, Aspirin, Astrin, Bi-Prin. **Generic name:** acetaminophen; **trade names:** Tylenol, Panadol, Pamol, Calpol, Tylenon, Paracin, Parmol, Panado, Ceetamol, Atosol, Exctol, Ennagesic, Ilvamol. **Generic name:** propoxyphene; **trade names:** Darvon, Dolene, Doloxene, Algaphan, Algodex, Depronal SA. *See also* ***pain,*** *page 106.*

Compound analgesics

Generic name: propoxyphene plus acetaminophen; **trade names:** Darvocet, Wygesic, Co-proxamol, Distalgesic; *see also* ***pain,*** *page 106.*

Non-steriod anti-inflammatory drugs

Generic name: aspirin; **trade names:** Ascriptin, Ecotrin, Measurin, Aspirin, Astrin, Bi-Prin. **Generic name:** indomethacin; **trade names:** Indocid, Artracin, Indoflex, Mobilan, Rheumacin, Arthrexin. **Generic name:** ibuprofen; **trade names:** Apsifen, Ebufac, Brufen, Fenbid, Ibumetin, Lidifen, Motrin, Paxofen. **Generic name:** ketoprofen; **trade name:** Orudis. **Generic name:** naproxen sodium; **trade names:** Laraflex, Naprosyn, Synflex. **Generic name:** phenylbutazone; **trade name:** Butazolidin. *See also* ***pain,*** *page 106.*

WHAT IS OSTEOARTHRITIS?

A degenerative disease of the joints. It may affect any joint, and it comes with age. It is particularly likely to develop in joints subjected to undue wear and tear. Thus in overweight people the joints in the lower back, hips and knees tend to be most severely affected. Minor degrees of arthritis are extremely common, but do not necessarily cause trouble.

Nature has designed most joints so that a smooth range of movement can occur. In a normal synovial joint (see diagram) the opposing bone ends are covered by areas of smooth and glistening hyaline cartilage. These are separated by a very thin layer of a lubricating substance called synovial fluid. In osteoarthritis (OA), there is thinning or complete loss of the normally smooth joint cartilage, as well as changes in the surrounding bone.

The severity of OA varies considerably: in mild forms there may be just slight loss of joint cartilage with no symptoms at all; in severe forms the cartilage may be completely worn away so that bone grates on bone and there may be considerable damage, disability and pain. Mild forms of OA are extremely common: in certain joints, such as the one at the base of the big toe, everyone develops some of these joint changes from as early as their 20s or 30s.

CAUSES The root causes of OA are not fully understood; certainly the ageing process, and general wear and tear, are implicated. A better understanding of the causes is perhaps gained by an awareness of the different types of OA:

Primary generalized OA affects many joints. It may begin in women in their 40s and 50s, but can affect men. You may notice bony swellings around the joints at the ends and middle of the fingers, and sometimes swelling at the wrist or the base of the thumb. Often these joints ache and may be a little stiff, particularly in the morning. These symptoms are usually much milder than the pain and stiffness of say, rheumatoid arthritis *(page 000).* Symptoms of pain and stiffness tend to vary. The joints commonly involved include the base of the big toe, the knees, the neck and the low back. Primary generalized OA tends to run in families.

Localized OA is confined to one or two weight-bearing joints such as the hip or the knee, and becomes increasingly common with age. Patients with primary generalized OA may also develop localized OA in weight-bearing joints.

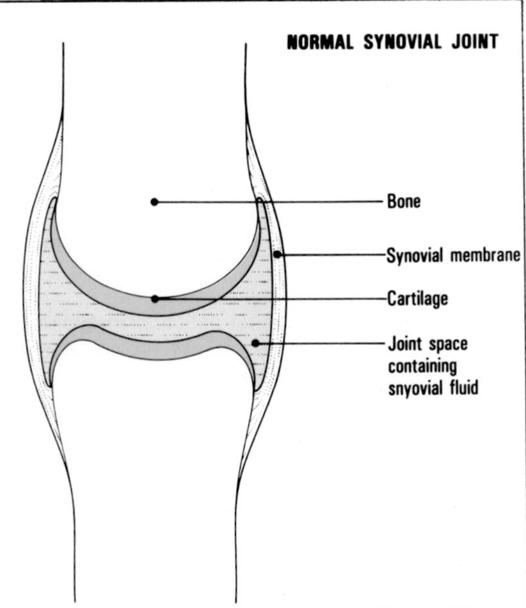

Above, *the appearance of a normal synovial joint, with cartilage intact and synovial fluid to lubricate movement; below, the effects of osteoarthritis on the same joint – cartilage lost, and bony swelling round the joint.*

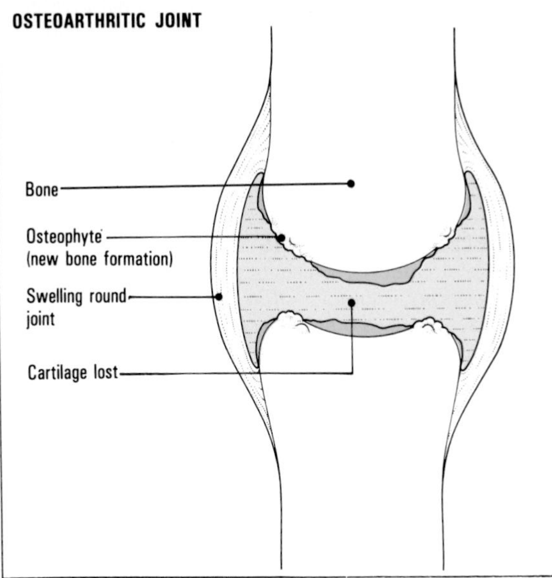

Simple analgesics, compound analgesics, non-steroidal anti-inflammatory drugs (NSAIDs)

Secondary OA may occur as the result of pre-existing joint disorders. These include rheumatoid arthritis and previous injury to the joint. Childhood joint problems may well be involved; the knees, typically of professional football players, are especially vulnerable.

TREATMENT

Drugs form a major element of treatment. For details on how analgesics and compound analgesics work, *see especially **pain**, page 106* and ***rheumatoid arthritis**, page 242.*

Primary generalized OA: In most patients, **analgesics** such as acetaminophen and aspirin will provide adequate pain relief. Where there is more severe stiffness, other more powerful non-steroidal anti-inflammatory drugs (NSAID) may be prescribed. But because this form of arthritis is typically very mild, a major part of the treatment will be reassurance from the doctor that no other, potentially more serious, form of arthritis is present. Your doctor may ask a physiotherapist to advise a simple hand exercise program, or exercises to strengthen muscles around other joints involved.

Associated problems such as neck stiffness may be helped by the use of a special foam collar, and low back pain by physiotherapy.

Localized OA in hip or knee: Again, analgesics as above tried first with other **NSAIDs** being reserved for more severe pain and stiffness. As with primary generalized OA, physiotherapy may be helpful. Weight reduction through dieting may also be advised in an attempt to reduce joint load. Splints and supports may be prescribed for unstable joints. Lastly, in severely affected joints, the patient may be referred to an orthopaedic surgeon for surgical joint replacement.

OVER-THE-COUNTER TREATMENTS

OA is best treated by prescription for the appropriate pain relief from a doctor; but in the event of a sudden painful flare-up, or a first bad spell, it is perfectly sensible to treat yourself with acetaminophen. Dose: a maximum of two 500 mg tablets four times daily.

No drug will restore an osteoarthritic joint to normal and the only function of medications in this condition is to relieve pain and stiffness.

QUESTIONS TO ASK THE DOCTOR

- Should I lose weight?
- How much exercise should I get?

■ What type of exercise is suitable?
■ Would a special diet help?
■ Do I need an operation?
■ What are the side effects of my pills?
■ Would relaxation exercises help?

SIDE EFFECTS

Acetaminophen in normal dosage is safer than, and does not have the gastric side effects of, **aspirin** and the other **NSAIDs.** However, in overdose, acetaminophen may cause fatal liver damage and **dextropropoxyphene** can cause respiratory depression and heart failure. *See **pain,** page 106.*

NSAIDs: the main side effects of these drugs include gastro-intestinal discomfort, nausea and sometimes bleeding. People with previous histories of chronic indigestion or gastric or duodenal ulcers are particularly suspectible. Other side effects include rashes, headaches, ankle swelling and a range of uncommon effects on other internal organs including the kidneys and liver.

SELF-MANAGEMENT

■ If you are overweight, lose weight by cutting down on sweets, sugar and alcohol. Ask your doctor for a diet sheet.

■ If you have OA in a weight-bearing joint, avoid overstressing it with excessive exercise. On the other hand, a certain amount of exercise helps to maintain muscle tone. Obtain advice from your doctor on the amount and type of exercise you need. Swimming is generally a useful form of exercise for OA as it allows muscular activity in an environment where the joints are relatively protected from gravity.

■ Local warmth is often helpful if the pain is restricted to one accessible joint. A heating pad, not hot enough to damage the skin, can produce short-term relief of pain and discomfort.

■ *See also **strains and sprains,** page 234, and **back pain,** page 236.*

FLARE-UPS

OA sufferers may have intermittent flare-ups which may be related to the release of crystals into the joint space. These attacks may be recognized by increasing pain, warmth and tenderness in the affected joint and they do require medical attention. This will often involve rest, sometimes local injections and prescription of regular analgesics or NSAIDs.

PATIENT'S EXPERIENCE

"I noticed that I was getting more and more pain in my hip. At first it was just uncomfortable but over two or three years it became worse; the joint began to get stiff and I had difficulty walking. I went to my doctor who told me to lose weight – I was rather heavy – and gave me some mild painkillers. I did manage to lose thirty pounds over a six-month period and my hip got better – but not for long. My doctor then sent me to see a surgeon, and he operated right away – my hip joint was replaced with a metal one. The pain relief was marvellous and I can now walk almost normally again."

NAMES YOU WILL HEAR

Non-steroid anti-inflammatory drugs

Generic name: aspirin; **trade names:** Ascriptin, Ecotrin, Measurin, Aspirin, Astrin, Bi-Prin. **Generic name:** indomethacin; **trade names:** Indocin, Indocid, Artracin, Imbrilon, Indoflex, Indolar SR, Indomod, Mobilan, Rheumanin, Arthpexin. **Generic name:** ibuprofen; **trade names:** Motrin, Advil, Medipen, Rufen, Brufen, Apsifen, Ebufac, Fenbid, Ibumetin, Lidifen, Amersol. **Generic name:** ketoprofen; **trade names:** Orudis, Alrheumat, Oruvail. **Generic name:** naproxen sodium; **trade names:** Naprosyn, Anaprox, Laraflex, Synflex. **Generic name:** acetaminophen; **trade names:** Anacin 3, Phenaphen, Panadol, Tempra, Tylanol. **Generic name:** phenylbutazone; **trade name:** Butazolidin. **Generic name:** fenoprofen; **trade name:** Nalfon. **Generic name:** piroxicam; **trade name:** Feldene. **Generic name:** tolmetin; **trade name:** Tolectin. *See also **pain,** page 106.*

Remission-inducing drugs

Gold salts

Generic name: sodium aurothiomalate; **trade name:** Myochrysine. **Generic name:** aurothioglucose; **trade name:** Solganal. **Generic name:** auranofin; **trade name:** Ridaura.

Antimalarial agents

Generic name: chloroquine phosphate; **trade name:** Aralen. **Generic name:** hydroxychloroquine sulfate; **trade name:** Plaquenil.

Others

Generic name: penicillamine; **trade names:** Cuprimine, Depen.

Steroids

Generic name: Prednisone; **trade names:** Deltasone, Meticorten, Orasone, SK-Prednisone. **Generic name:** methyl prednisolone; **trade names:** Solumedrol, Codelsol, Delta Phorical, Deltacortril, Deltalone, Deltastab, Precortisyl, Prednesol, Sintisone.

WHAT IS RHEUMATOID ARTHRITIS?

– A chronic inflammation of the joints, which results in deformity and disability. There is joint pain, swelling and stiffness, especially in the mornings. The hands and toes are often affected early in the course of the disease. Later the inflammation spreads to other joints; almost any joint may be involved. It is an episodic disease, with periods of severity and improvement. There is no cure, but the intervals between bad episodes can last for years.

Although the joints are often the worst problem, other organs can be affected too: fatigue, loss of appetite, weight loss, fever, skin nodules, muscle pain, dry eyes, anemia, and damage to nerves are all symptoms. Occasionally the lungs and heart are involved.

Rheumatoid arthritis can afflict children, in which case it is called juvenile rheumatoid arthritis (previously known as Still's disease). The condition usually disappears before adulthood, but damage to joints may occasionally be permanent.

CAUSES Unknown, but both inherited and environmental factors are involved.

PRESCRIPTION DRUGS

The aims of treatment are: to relieve the pain; to maintain function of joints; to prevent or minimize permanent deformity. The great variety of drugs available indicates that none is totally successful.

NSAIDS: Aspirin is still the first choice, but many suffer side effects (see below) from the high doses necessary. Aspirin needs to be taken every four hours if it is to work its best, and this is often inconvenient so slow release forms have been produced.

Indomethacin is also very effective, but again side effects can be problematic. Ibuprofen, ketoprofen, and naproxen are less likely to cause side effects than aspirin or indomethacin, BUT may be less effective.

There are numerous other preparations available, all with similar side effects. Their only advantage is that they have to be taken less frequently. It is often important to try various preparations: some respond better to one than another.

How they work: by inhibiting the body's production of prostaglandins, which play an important part in creating inflammation.

Slow-acting antirheumatic drugs: One of these may be included in the treatment as an extra if anti-inflammatory

drugs are not adequately controlling the pain and inflammation. About 80 per cent of patients will respond to one or other of these preparations, but it takes a few months for this type of drug to work properly.
How they work: unknown. Gold (sodium aurothiomalate) is thought to have some effect on the inflamed membranes of joints.
Steroids work well on joint inflammation but the benefit wears off as soon as they are stopped. Steroids have severe side effects if used continuously (see below) and should only be used when all other measures have failed to arrest severe progressive disease. They reduce the inflammation but do not restore the damaged joints. Steroids may also be given by injection directly into inflamed joints, satisfactory if only a few large joints, for example the knee or shoulder, are involved. The side effects of steroids by mouth are avoided in this way.
How they work: by blocking the chemical process which causes inflammation.

Surgery can improve the function of damaged joints, but the patient must be clear about the likely result.

OVER-THE-COUNTER TREATMENTS

Simple analgesics can of course be bought without a prescription, but this disease requires close cooperation between the patient and doctor. If the drugs your doctor has prescribed are failing to control the pain, it is best to discuss this and together plan a more effective form of treatment. Aspirin should not be used in combination with prescription drugs without the approval of a doctor: it can worsen the side effects of other drugs.

Acetaminophen, however, does not interfere with other drugs and can be used for severe pain until you can see a doctor.

QUESTIONS TO ASK THE DOCTOR

- Will joint deformity result?
- Will physiotherapy help? What about swimming?
- Should I rest painful joints?
- How long should I take the drugs?
- Will local heat treatment help?
- Am I anemic? Should I have a blood test?
- Is joint replacement likely to help me?

SIDE EFFECTS

NSAIDS: *see* ***osteoarthritis,*** *page 238.* **Aspirin:** *see pain, page 106.* **Slow-acting antirheumatic drugs** can cause skin rashes, mouth ulcers, nausea and vomiting. Occa-

PATIENT'S EXPERIENCE

"I developed rheumatoid arthritis when I was 35. My first symptom was tiredness; I found it difficult to get up in the morning. Soon I realized that this was because the muscles in my arms, legs and hands were stiff and painful. The stiffness improved during the morning, but after a week the symptoms were becoming so severe that I was unable to get up in time to take the children to school. I also had some swelling of my wrists, and my fingers were constantly painful. I went to see my doctor who did some blood tests and X-rays.

The results showed rheumatoid arthritis, and he referred me to a specialist. When I went to the specialist I was horrified to see other patients with severely deformed joints, many of them confined to wheel chairs. By the time that I saw the specialist I was in tears, as I imagined that this was what I would be like in a few years' time. The specialist explained that most patients were not severely affected and that with treatment, and some effort on my part, things wouldn't be too bad.

My GP had started me on large doses of aspirin, but I stopped taking it as it made me dizzy and gave me continuous ringing in the ears. The specialist prescribed Indocin suppositories at night to help the morning stiffness, and an Indocin capsule in the morning to help for the rest of the day. The Indocin had to be taken with food.

I also had to have physiotherapy three times a week. Here I learned the importance of exercising the muscles and not letting the joints become stiff and immobile. I also met another lady who had had several severe episodes of RA. She now had very little pain, but still continued her exercises regularly.

The pain has responded well to the treatment and I am feeling a lot more optimistic."

sionally abnormalities of the blood may occur. Chloroquine may cause eye damage and penicillamine and gold injections can affect the kidneys. Patients must have regular blood and urine checks to detect these complications, and patients on chloroquine need to have regular eye examinations. Serious side effects are rare if patients have these checks. Patients on gold injections should carry a card to this effect in case of sudden reactions.

Steroids cause few problems if given only over a week or so. The serious side effects come from more prolonged use and are dose-related: *see **anemia,** page 224.*

Steroids are, in addition, very difficult to stop. Not all of the side effects occur in every patient, but most occur in patients on steroids for more than a couple of months. The side effects are minimized if the lowest possible dose is given; taking steroids on alternate days only may decrease side effects. Against this list of grave drawbacks must be weighed the fact that steroids usually give marked relief to rheumatoid arthritis patients.

While on any of the prescription drugs described above: Let your doctor know immediately if you may be pregnant or are considering breast-feeding. Check with your doctor before taking any other drugs. This includes cold remedies, oral contraceptives, vaccines and many other prescription drugs. Avoid alcohol, while taking any of the drugs, until you have checked with your doctor.

All of the drugs used have significant side effects, but these must be balanced against the risk to the patient of letting the disease continue unchecked. Discuss the side effects of each new drug with your doctor.

SELF-MANAGEMENT

The disease has active and quiet periods. Joints become damaged at times of active inflammation.

- Prevention of or minimizing of permanent deformity depends to some extent on how much the patient can keep the joints mobile, even during an acute attack.
- Take drugs regularly and on time, with food, as instructed.
- Physiotherapy started during an acute attack should be continued to maintain mobility of the joints.
- Exercises should be done regularly at home – indefinitely.
- Aids and appliances are available to help patients who have problems in the home because of weakness or deformity of joints.

■ A firm mattress and one firm pillow prevent strain on the muscles and joints of the back.
■ Contact with rheumatoid arthritis groups are very useful in solving individual problems.
■ There are many useful publications about this disease in public libraries.
■ Obesity puts extra strain on joints and weight should be reduced to normal wherever possible.
■ Exercising in water is particularly beneficial.
■ Don't assume that the drugs can be stopped as soon as you feel better – check with your doctor.
■ Relaxation of body and mind help to control pain, anxiety and tension.
■ Remember, only a small proportion of patients with rheumatoid arthritis go on to develop severe disability.
■ 'Miracle cures' are usually the result of a spontaneous improvement – as far as doctors know. Climate and diet have no specific effect, but a healthy diet is always advisable.

Don't be fooled into paying money for 'cures'. Discuss them with your doctor.

SELF-HELP IN AN ATTACK

■ Find out from your doctor what extra medication you can take if the pain suddenly becomes more severe. If in doubt, take two acetaminophen tablets every four hours.
■ Make an appointment to see your doctor early in an attack, so that your treatment can be stepped up to meet the attack.
■ Warmth can ease the pain and a hot water bottle on an affected joint is helpful.
■ Take sufficient medication to reduce inflammation and relieve pain. This may mean regular pill-taking, even when you are not actually in pain.
■ Don't just retire to bed without consulting your doctor: stiff, deformed joints may result. A balance must be achieved between adequate rest of inflamed joints, and maintaining muscle power and preventing deformity. Physiotherapy plays an essential part in achieving this.
■ Splints can be useful, especially at night, to rest joints and prevent deformity. These may be ready-made, or made especially for you to rest the joint in the best possible position.
■ Remember, the more pain-free you are, the more you will be able to move your joints and keep them mobile. Don't delay seeing your doctor, and don't be afraid to take regular treatment to reduce inflammation.

Colchicine, steroid injections, allopurinol, probenicid

NAMES YOU WILL HEAR

NSAIDs

Generic name: indomethacin; **trade names:** Indocin, Indocid, Artracin, Indoflex, Mobilan, Rheumacin, Arthrexin. **Generic name:** ibuprofen; **trade names:** Motrin, Advil, Medipen, Rufen, Apsifen, Ebufac, Brufen, Fenbid, Ibumetin, Lidifen, Paxofen. **Generic name:** ketoprofen; **trade names:** Orudis, Alrheumat, Oruvail. **Generic name:** naproxen sodium; **trade names:** Naprosyn, Anaprox, Laraflex, Synflex. *See also* ***pain,*** *page 106.*

Others (acute gout)

Generic name: colchicine; **trade name:** prescribed by generic name in USA; elsewhere Colchicine Tablets. **Generic name:** hydrocortisone acetate; **trade name:** Hydrocortisone Acetate Injection, Cortef, Hydrocortone, SoluCortef.

Drugs which lower uric acid

Generic name: allopurinol; **trade names:** Zyloprim, Allopurinol Tablets, Zyloric. **Generic name:** probenicid; **trade name:** Benemid.

WHAT IS GOUT?

A metabolic disorder which results in an excess of uric acid in the blood (hyperuricaemia). This may be completely asymptomatic, or the uric acid may be deposited in joints causing acute or chronic arthritis, or occasionally, kidney stones. Uric acid may also be deposited in the skin, causing lumps (tophi).

The most common symptom is joint pain, often affecting the big toe, hands, knees and ankles. Almost any joint may be involved later in the course of the disease; early on, usually one joint is involved.

In acute arthritis, the onset is sudden, with the pain developing over a few hours. The joint is agonizing: even the pressure of a sheet is painful. In the chronic forms, the pain is usually milder, although acute attacks can occur. The frequency of these attacks varies from every few weeks to every few years. Without treatment, the joints gradually deteriorate, leading to deformity.

Gout is commonest in men, and in women after the menopause.

CAUSES The high uric acid levels in the blood may be due to an over-production of uric acid by the body, or a failure to excrete uric acid in adequate amounts. These abnormalities can be inherited.

PRESCRIPTION DRUGS

It is important to differentiate between the drugs used for the treatment of an acute attack and those used in the long-term control of the disease, which lower uric acid levels.

NSAIDS: Colchicine is most frequently used to treat an acute attack. Indomethacin is preferred by some physicians as the side effects are less severe. Given either as a tablet or a suppository, it usually gives relief within two to five days. Other anti-inflammatory drugs such as ibuprofen, ketoprofen and naproxen are also useful. They are slightly less effective than indomethacin, but tend to have a lower incidence of side effects. Aspirin should not be used in the treatment of gout, as it can raise the uric acid level and aggravates the symptoms.

How they work: *see* ***rheumatoid arthritis,*** *page 242.*

How it works: it is thought to act against the inflammatory process caused by uric acid.

Steroid injections into an acutely inflamed joint will relieve symptoms, but the treatment is only suitable for certain large joints.

How it works: *see* ***rheumatoid arthritis,*** *page 242.*

Long-term control: Drugs to lower the uric acid tend to be used only if the level is very high, or when there are recurrent attacks of acute arthritis. These drugs should never be started during an acute attack: they can make it worse; they are given with large amounts of fluid.

Allopurinol lowers the uric acid level. It can however precipitate an attack of gout, and to prevent this, anti-inflammatory drugs are usually given with it initially.

How it works: by preventing the formation of uric acid from other chemicals within the body.

Probenicid can be used instead of allopurinol or in conjunction with it.

How it works: by increasing uric acid excretion from the kidneys. It cannot be used if the patient has kidney stones or kidney disease.

OVER-THE-COUNTER TREATMENTS

There are no effective non-prescription treatments for gout. Acetaminophen can be used for the pain, but it is not strong enough to be effective.

QUESTIONS TO ASK THE DOCTOR

- For how long should I take the drugs?
- Will deformity result?
- Would a change of diet help?

SIDE EFFECTS

NSAIDS: *see **rheumatoid arthritis,** page 242.*

Colchicine commonly casuses nausea, vomiting, and abdominal pain. It can also cause severe diarrhea, rashes and kidney damage. Nerve damage and blood disorders are rare side effects.

Steroids: *see **rheumatoid arthritis,** page 242.*

Allopurinol is usually well tolerated, but it can cause rashes and mild gastro-intestinal disorders. Headache, hypertension, baldness and liver disorders are rare side effects.

Probenicid has few side effects, though occasionally nausea, vomiting or headache result. Very rarely, liver, kidney or blood disorders arise.

SELF-MANAGEMENT

- The disease has active and quiet periods; joint pain can become severe over a few hours, so always have an anti-inflammatory drug available.
- Resting the affected joint is essential.
- Drugs such as diuretics can make gout worse, so always remind your doctor that you have had gout if he wants to give you any new tablets.

PATIENTS' EXPERIENCES

"My first attack of gout started suddenly: I had no ides what it was. I had come home from work early, feeling exhausted. I had a slight feeling of discomfort in my right big toe, and over the next few hours the pain got so bad that by bed time I couldn't bear the weight of the bedclothes on my foot. I was in such pain that my wife called the doctor. He said that I had gout and gave me an indomethacin suppository to use immediately, plus one for the morning. When I saw him the following day, the pain had eased a bit, but I could not drive my car. He took a blood test for uric acid and said that I should continue on the indomethacin.

When I went to see him a few days later for the blood result, the pain had almost disappeared. My uric acid level was high, so he suggested that when the pain had completely cleared up, I should start on some tablets to lower the uric acid level in the blood. I told him I was worried about the outlook. My uncle suffered gout and by the age of 50, had severe joint problems. The doctor said that with appropriate treatment, and much-reduced alcohol consumption, I probably would not suffer too much. When I saw him again a month later he started me on allopurinol. I had to take a gradually increasing dose; he also put me back on the indomethacin for a few weeks to prevent further acute attacks.

That was three years ago. I'm still taking allopurinol. The single tablet a day is no problem to remember. It is certainly preferable to another attack of gout."

ALCOHOL AND GOUT

Alcohol (of any type) can increase the frequency of attacks and should be restricted. Drinking heavily can precipitate an attack.

ANKYLOSING SPONDYLITIS

Non-steroid anti-inflammatory drugs (NSAIDS), steroids, analgesics

NAMES YOU WILL HEAR

Non-steroid anti-inflammatory drugs (NSAIDS)

Generic name: aspirin; **trade names:** Ascriptin, Ecotrin, Measurin, Aspirin, Astrin, Bi-Prin. **Generic name:** indomethacin; **trade names:** Indocin, Indocid, Artracin, Indoflex, Mobilan, Rheumacin, Arthrexin. **Generic name:** ibuprofen; **trade names:** Motrin, Advil, Medipren, Nuprin, Rufen, Brufen, Apsifen, Ebufac, Fenbid, Ibumetin, Lidifen, Motrin, Paxofen. **Generic name:** ketoprofen; **trade names:** Orudis, Alrheumat, Oruvail. **Generic name:** naproxen sodium; **trade names:** Naprosyn, Laraflex, Anaprox, Synflex. For more comprehensive lists of trade names of the foregoing drugs, *see* ***pain****, page 106*. **Generic name:** phenylbutazone; **trade name:** Butazolidin. **Generic name:** piroxicam; **trade name:** Feldene. **Generic name:** diflunisal; **trade name:** Dolobid; **Generic name:** diclofenac; **trade name:** Voltarol.

Steroids

Generic name: methyl prednisolone; **trade names:** Solumedrol, Deltacortef, Sterane, Codelsol, Delta Phorical, Deltacortril, Deltalone, Deltastab, Precortisyl, Prednesol, Sintisone, Nisolone, Delta-Cortef, Deltasolone, Prelone, Lenisolone, Meticortilone, Predeltilone.

Analgesics

Generic name: acetaminophen; **trade names:** Anacin 3, Phenaphon, Datril, Panadol, Tempra, Tylenol, Pamol, Calpol, Tylenon, Paracin, Parmol, Panado, Ceetamol, Atosol, Exctol, Ennagesic, Ilvamol; *see also* ***pain****, page 106.*

WHAT IS ANKYLOSING SPONDYLITIS?

– A chronic inflammation of the joints of the back, occurring most commonly in young men.

The inflammation affects the joints between the vertebrae (the bones which make up the spine), and also the joint between the sacrum of the spine and the iliac bones of the pelvis (see diagram). This inflammation causes fusion of the vertebrae: the back loses its flexibility and becomes rigid. There may be arthritis of other joints in the body, for example the hips and shoulders.

Onset is gradual, with pain and stiffness in the lower back. Symptoms are worse in the morning and following inactivity. The pain occurs in bouts; at times there is no pain at all. As the disease progresses, the normal curvature of the lower (lumbar) spine is lost and the movements of the back are limited. This may lead to a characteristic posture: head and neck forward, upper back rounded, chest flattened. Limitation of movement can also affect deep breathing.

Ankylosing spondylitis can also produce inflammation of the eye, the main blood vessel from the heart (the aorta) and the aortic valve of the heart itself. The last is a rare cause of heart failure *(see page 52).*

CAUSES Unknown at present, but there is a strong familial pattern. The inherited antigen HLA B27 is linked with ankylosing spondylitis, and with some other inherited disorders.

PRESCRIPTION DRUGS

The principles of treatment are the same as for ***rheumatoid arthritis*** – *see page 242.* In ankylosing spondylitis the problem of rigidity is more severe, and every effort must be made to maintain the flexibility of the spine. This is done by using drugs to reduce pain and inflammation, by active physiotherapy and exercises to maintain mobility.

NSAIDS: *See* ***rheumatoid arthritis,*** *page 242.* The same range of drugs used in rheumatoid arthritis are appropriate.

Steroids: These are sometimes used to treat the eye inflammation as well as the joints: *see* ***rheumatoid arthritis,*** *page 242.* Local injections of steroids into the large joints may be helpful, just as in rheumatoid arthritis.

Surgery is necessary in a few cases to correct deformity of the spine. Hip replacement can be beneficial if the hip joints are badly affected. Treatment of heart failure as a result of the disease page 52.

OVER-THE-COUNTER TREATMENT

*See **rheumatoid arthritis**, page 242.*

QUESTIONS TO ASK THE DOCTOR

- Can I pass it on to my children?
- What can I do to prevent rigidity of the spine?
- Will physiotherapy help?
- What sports can I play?

SIDE EFFECTS

*See **rheumatoid arthritis**, page 242.* Phenylbutazone may (rarely) cause heart failure and stop normal production of white blood cells in the bone marrow.

SELF-MANAGEMENT

*See **rheumatoid arthritis**, page 242.* However, maintaining mobility is of such importance that patients and those concerned with them should realize that:

- More than 75 per cent of patients with ankylosing spondylitis can stay at work, moreover without taking a large amount of time off.
- This is a chronic disease, and the long-term outcome depends largely on how much effort is put into exercise. Get into the habit of exercising regularly at home and continue these exercises for the rest of your life.
- Physiotherapy is essential, both to prevent postural deformity, and to monitor progression of the disease.
- Take up non-contact sports such as swimming. Your doctor will advise.

SELF-HELP IN AN ATTACK

*See **rheumatoid arthritis**, page 242* – the remedial action to be taken is identical.

The Lower Spine and pelvic girdle

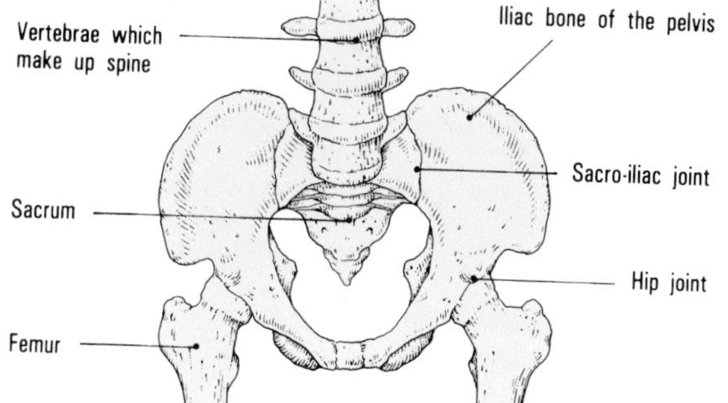

***The lower (lumbar) spine** and pelvis, showing the joints which become inflamed in ankylosing spondylitis, including those between the vertebrae, and between the sacrum and iliac bones of the pelvis (the sacro-iliac joints).*

PATIENT'S EXPERIENCE

"I started noticing pain in my lower back. It was bad in the morning and wore off during the day. Over the next month, it gradually got worse, and I found difficulty in getting out of bed. I saw my doctor, who examined my back. When he pressed in certain places, it hurt. He sent me for blood tests and X-rays. When I went for the results, he did a thorough examination, and told me that I had ankylosing spondylitis, which alarmed me as I had an uncle with the same problem. His back was so deformed that he was almost bent double. The doctor must have noticed my reaction, as he went on to assure me that with proper treatment and good co-operation on my part, it was unlikely that I would have any significant deformity. He started me on indomethacin suppositories at night, which relieved all the symptoms. He also referred me to the hospital, so that I could see a specialist and also start physiotherapy.

That was five years ago, and although I have had two episodes when the pain was severe, I still have only slight stiffness of the lower spine, and at present I am on no drugs at all. As soon as the back pain starts, I go on to indomethacin and see my doctor. The physiotherapist has given me exercises which I do every evening; I go sailing and wind-surfing in summer. In winter I play badminton every weekend. I see a specialist every six months, together with the physiotherapist, who monitors the mobility of my back.

Any chronic condition is unpleasant, but this has not been as bad as I anticipated."

CRAMP

Quinine bisulphate, cyclandelate, nicotinic acid, salt tablets

NAMES YOU WILL HEAR
Generic name: quninine bisulfate; **trade names:** Quinamm, Quindan, Biquin, Myoquin. **Generic name:** cyclandelate; **trade names:** Cyclospasmol, Cyclobral. **Generic name:** oxerutins; **trade name:** Paroven. **Generic name:** nicotinic acid; **trade names:** Nicobid, Hexopal, Linodil, Vasodil. **Generic name:** guaiphenesin + calcium gluconate + nicotinic acid + calciferol; **trade name:** Crampex.

WHAT IS CRAMP?

– Sudden painful spasm of muscles which control body movement. Mainly the calves, feet, thighs and less commonly the back, arms and hands are involved. Cramp occurs without warning and cannot be controlled. It lasts from a few seconds up to ten minutes, sometimes during sleep. The pain arises because the affected muscles ''lock up'' Though painful and unpleasant, cramp is not dangerous unless it occurs during activities such as swimming.

Writer's cramp affects those who use their hands for long periods performing delicate and intricate tasks. It is unlike the usual type of cramp and thought to be mainly the result of tension and other psychological conditions. It may last a long time.

CAUSES Not really understood: cramp can occur at any age, but is more common in the elderly. The problem may arise in some people because the body is deprived of fluids containing certain salts such as sodium or potassium. Other reasons may be injury to the muscle fibers and the nerves serving them, or medical conditions which prevent proper blood circulation. Certain drugs may also contribute. Some experts think arthritis of the spine with sciatica may precipitate attacks, especially in the elderly. Cramp is also common in pregnancy, but usually does not signify any serious underlying problem.

PRESCRIPTION DRUGS

For bedtime cramp the most commonly prescribed drug is **quinine bisulphate.** The dose may vary, but it is usually 300 mg taken before going to bed. Other drugs given are **cyclandelate** and **nicotinic acid.** For cramp after severe exercise in warm climates a doctor will suggest taking plenty of non-alcoholic fluid with added salt. Salt tablets may help in hot climates.
How they work: Not fully understood, but quinine is thought to decrease muscle membrane excitability and hence prevent the muscle from going into spasm. The others are thought to improve blood supply to muscles and prevent the onset of cramp.

Muscles become more irritable when deprived of surrounding body fluid and salts; extra fluid and salts replace those lost through sweating.

OVER-THE-COUNTER TREATMENTS

Quinine can easily be taken as a glass of tonic water, which contains the drug. Salt tablets are widely available; but consult your doctor before treating yourself: excessive salt can be dangerous.

QUESTIONS TO ASK THE DOCTOR

■ Am I on any pills which may cause cramp?
■ Do I need a treatment, or will my cramp just go?

SIDE EFFECTS

Quinine in the usually prescribed dose for night cramps has few side effects. Very occasionally nausea, vomiting, noises in the ear, abdominal pain, rashes, visual problems and allergy may occur: should you have any suspicion of these, stop taking it and report the symptoms to your doctor. It may cause fetal abnormalities so should NOT be taken during pregnancy. It may also interact with the heart drug digoxin. **Cyclandelate** and **nicotinic acid** may cause nausea, flashing and dizziness with very high doses. Care has to be taken when these drugs are given to patients with certain heart complaints.

SELF-MANAGEMENT

Prevention

■ Avoid loss of body fluids by prolonged sweating, vomiting or diarrhea. ■ Avoid risk of muscle stress by unaccustomed exercise when unfit. ■ Avoid extremes of temperature – cold can bring on an attack of cramp.

SELF-HELP IN AN ATTACK

■ Rub the muscle or apply a heating pad or ice pack. Or apply a firm bandage, but be sure not to cut off the circulation to the muscle. ■ Sudden cramp in a lower limb can often by cured by stretching the limb strongly or willing the opposite muscles to contract. For instance, if there is cramp in the calf, the foot should be pulled up and the leg straightened. ■ When cramp occurs in bed, try getting up and standing on the leg. ■ Analgesics such as acetaminophen are useful for treating the residual pain after an attack.

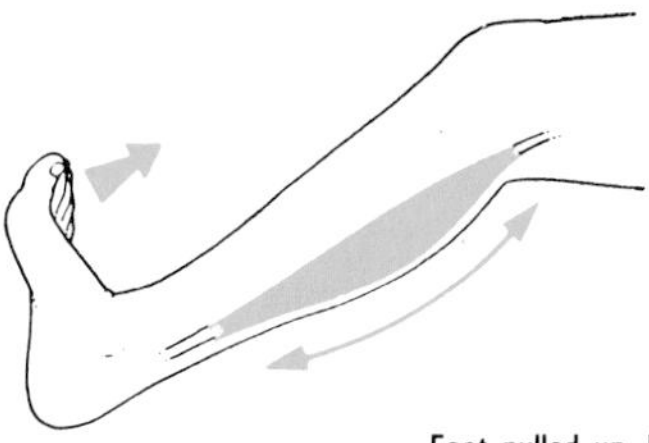

Foot pulled up, leg straightened

PATIENT'S EXPERIENCE

"I am in my middle forties and work as vice president of a bank. Some months ago I noticed I was getting fat and unfit. I decided to start playing tennis again and joined a local club. I am an average player, but I like to play hard, so I sweat a lot. I play if possible once a week for about two hours. I found a few weeks after starting to play that I was experiencing night cramns. These began to worry me so I went to my doctor. He suggested that when I got home after playing I elevate my legs, supporting them from the ankle to the buttocks with cushions, and that I drink about a pint-and-a-half of fluid over two to three hours before I go to bed. He also suggested I take a container of non-alcoholic fluid with me to drink between games. I followed the advice and some weeks later, the night cramps had gone."

Ear, nose and throat and eye

Ear, nose and throat problems are traditionally looked after by "E.N.T." surgeons – here we have also included problems with the eyes. Infection plays a large part in the common disorders mentioned here, many of which can become a great nuisance.

See also: *Influenza, page 138; common cold, page 134.*

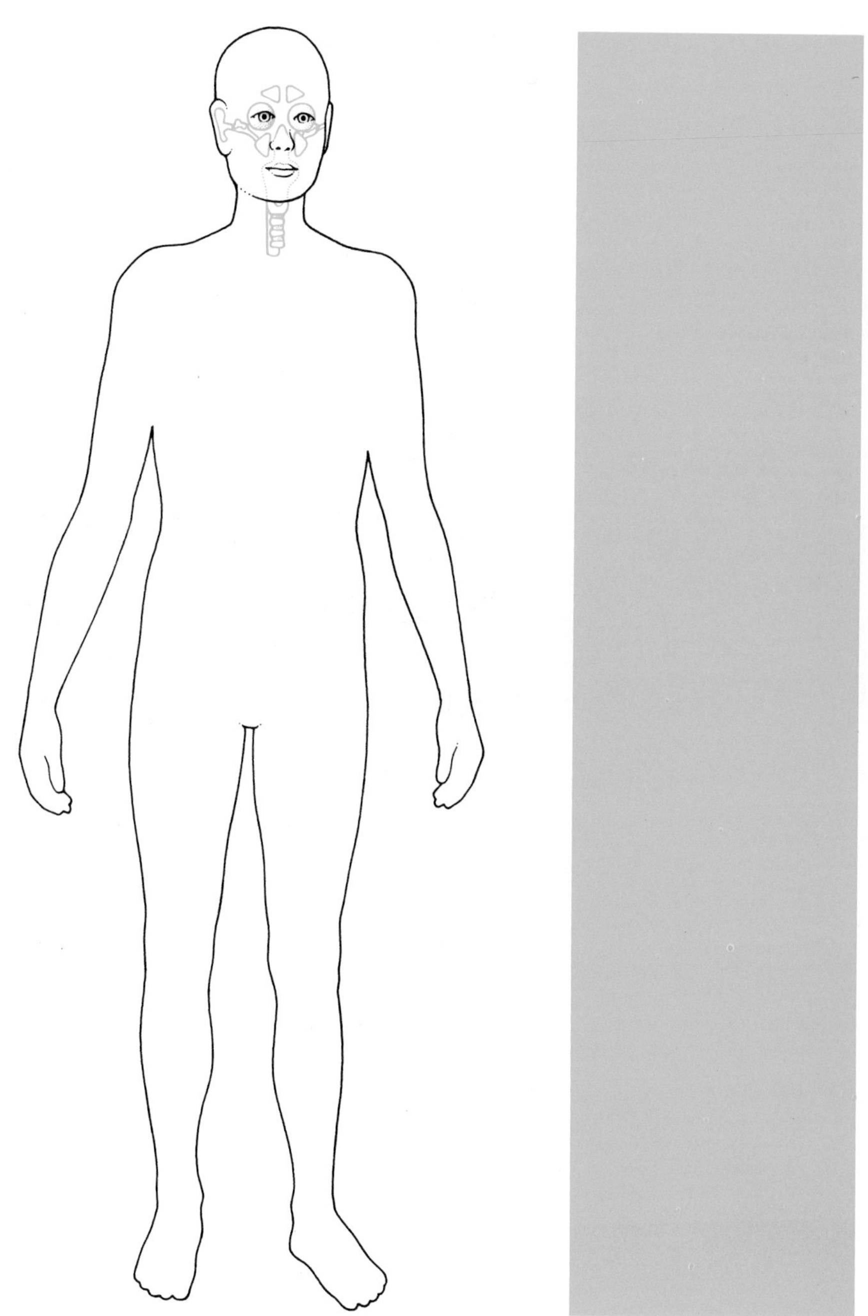

NAMES YOU WILL HEAR

Anti-emetics

Generic name: prochlorperazine; **trade names:** Compazine, Stemetil, Anti-Naus, Mitil, Vertigon. **Generic name:** cyclizine; **trade names:** Marzine, Valoid. **Generic name:** cinnarizine; **trade name:** Stugeron. **Generic name:** promethazine theoclate; **trade name:** Avomine. **Generic name:** meclozine; **trade names:** Ancoloxin, Ancolan, Bonamine, Navicalm.

Drops for removal of wax from ear

Generic name: turpentine oil mixture; **trade name:** Cerumol. **Generic name:** docusate sodium; **trade names:** Waxsol, Soliwax, Molcer, Dioctyl. **Generic name:** carbamide peroxide; **trade name:** Debrox.

WHAT IS DEAFNESS?

Partial or complete loss of hearing; in older patients especially, it may be associated with tinnitus (noises in the ears) and vertigo. **Vertigo** (''dizziness''), *see page 96,* is a feeling of movement, either of one's own body or of objects around one, and it is often more troublesome than the deafness itself.

CAUSES Obstruction in the canal leading into the ear; interference with the hearing apparatus within the ear; damage to the nerve from the ear to the brain (see diagram). The first can be a result of wax, or occasionally a foreign body, in the external ear canal. The second arises from damage to the ear drum, or disease such as ear infection in which fluid within the middle ear prevents the hearing mechanism from working properly. The last can be present from birth (as in children whose mothers have rubella during pregnancy); can develop suddenly due to damage to the nerve caused by meningitis or head injury; can develop gradually as part of the process of ageing.

PRESCRIPTION DRUGS

Antiemetic drugs may help with the nausea associated with vertigo.

How they work: by acting on the brain, suppressing the stimulus to vomit.

The treatment of deafness depends, of course, on the cause. Wax in the ear can be removed by drops which liquify the wax. If this is inadequate, syringing may be necessary. **Middle ear infections** are treated in varying ways – *see page 256.* Damage to the ear drum or other parts of the hearing apparatus may be corrected by surgery. Lastly, hearing aids can restore a degree of hearing by increasing the sounds in the ear. Different types suit different forms of hearing loss; selecting the right one for the individual requires specialist help.

OVER-THE-COUNTER TREATMENTS

Ear drops such as Debrox, can be bought without a prescription; provided manufacturer's instructions are followed, self-treatment is appropriate.

QUESTIONS TO ASK THE DOCTOR

- Will my hearing recover, stay the same, or get worse?
- What can be done for the vertigo and tinnitus?
- What help is available to deaf people?

■ Will a hearing aid help me?

SIDE EFFECTS

Antiemetics cause drowsiness in many people and should not be taken when driving or working in a potentially dangerous environment. *See also* ***lung cancer,*** *page 202.*

Ear drops for removing wax can cause an allergic skin reaction: stop immediately if this occurs.

SELF-MANAGEMENT

One of the major causes of deafness in children can be prevented by immunization against rubella (German measles) before becoming pregnant. Hearing problems in young children are detected by early screening tests at the doctor's office. Even milder cases need specialist help if schooling is not to suffer.

Severely or totally deaf people have to face up to communication problems without delay. Totally deaf people should learn lip-reading and finger-spelling as early as possible while hearing aids can help the partially hearing child or adult. Many partially hearing or deaf people underestimate their capabilities; self-help groups can help a patient acquire or regain confidence. Tinnitus may be less noticeable when the patient is mentally occupied.

Mechanical aids for the home are worth investigating: a flashing door bell light is available, for example.

If deafness is associated with impaired balance, walking in the dark and working at heights should be avoided.

Hearing aids take some getting used to, but it is well worth persevering and having the aid regularly serviced.

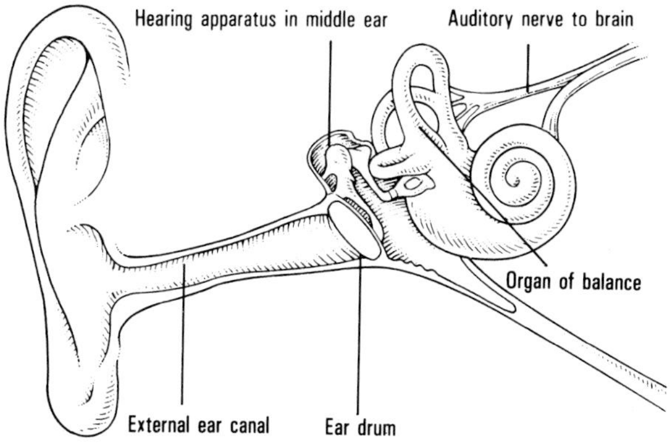

PATIENTS' EXPERIENCE

"My deafness had been increasing gradually for a few years, but over the last year, since I retired, it has become much worse. I can no longer follow a conversation or watch television.

I had a hearing aid fitted a few years ago, but I found it very difficult to use. I went to see my doctor because of the noise in my ears, and problems with balance. Sometimes I would feel dizzy and sick. The consultation was difficult because he was busy and I couldn't understand what he was saying. He gave me some pills to help with the nausea, but they made me sleepy, so I stopped taking them. They did not do much good, anyway. I got a different hearing aid later, and that helped for a few years.

I live alone and the deafness makes me more and more depressed. The constant noise in my ears is very disturbing; but at least if I make the effort to get out and do things, it takes my mind off the noise."

"My little boy aged three seemed to have become very naughty. He paid no attention when I told him to behave. Also, he had become rather clumsy: he seemed to fall about more than usual. He had had a slight cold the week before.

I took him to the doctor who looked in his ears and diagnosed an ear infection. He gave him antibiotics and within a few days he was much better and his balance had improved.

The doctor asked me to take him back after a week to make sure that the fluid in his ears had cleared. It had, and it is obvious to me now that he was just not hearing properly when he had the ear infection."

Sound waves enter the external ear canal and hit the ear drum. This vibrates, causing the tiny bones of the hearing apparatus to vibrate too. This activates the auditory nerve, which conducts the sound message to the brain.

MIDDLE EAR INFECTIONS

Antibiotics, decongestants, antihistamines

NAMES YOU WILL HEAR

Antibiotics

Generic name: phenoxymethylpenicillin, penicillin-V; **trade names:** Betapen, Penicillin V, V Cillin K, Veetids, Crystapen V, Distaquaine V-K, Stabillin V-K, V-Cil-K, Abbocillin-VK, Bramcillin, Cilicaine VK, Falcopen VK, LPV, Pfipen V, Propen VK, PVK, PVO, Rocilin, Viraxacillin-V, Ledercillin VK, Nadopen-V, Novopen-VK, PVF V, V-Cillin K, VC-K, Copen, Darocillin, Deltacillin, Fenoxypen, Incil-VK, Jatacillin, Novo-VK, Nutracillin. **Generic name:** ampicillin; **trade names:** Omnipen, Polycillin-N, Principen, Ampifen, Penbritin, Pentrexyl, Vidopen, Austrapen. **Generic name:** cephalexin; **trade names:** Keflex, Ceporex.

Decongestants (oral)

Generic name: pseudoephedrine hydrochloride; **trade names:** Atrohist, Co-Tylenol Cold Medication, Fedahist, Novahistine, Robitussin, Sine-Aid, Tylenol Maximum Strength Sinus Medication, Actifed, Sudafed, Sudelix, Drixora Repetabs, Eltor.

Decongestants (nasal)

Generic name: xylometazoline; **trade names:** Otrivin, Otrivine Nasal Drops or Nasal Spray, Otrivine Paediatric Nasal Drops, Otrivine-Antistin, Otrix, Sinutab.

Antihistamines

Generic name: astemizole; **trade name:** Hismanal. **Generic name:** brompheniramine; **trade names:** Dimotane, Dimetane. **Generic name:** chlorpheniramine; **trade names:** Dallergy, Chlortrimeton, Haymine, Piriton, Chlor-Tripolon, Histalon. **Generic name:** clemastine; **trade names:** Tavegil, Tavest, Trabest. **Generic name:** mebhydrolin; **trade name:** Fabahistin. **Generic name:** terfenadine; **trade name:** Triludan. **Generic name:** trimeprazine tartrate; **trade names:** Vallergan, Panectyl. **Generic name:** triprolidine; **trade names:** Actidil, Pro-Actidil. **Generic name:** promethazine; **trade names:** Phenergan, Avomine, Progan, Prothazine, Histantil, Lenazine, Prohist.

WHAT ARE EAR INFECTIONS?

When "germs" from an infection of the nose and throat spread up the Eustachian tube to the middle ear it gets inflamed, causing severe ear ache, sometimes with dizziness, vomiting and a high temperature. It can cause impaired hearing. In babies, who cannot complain of ear ache, the symptoms are vague: loss of appetite, vomiting, diarrhea, fever, irritability. Sometimes the ear drum perforates under pressure, discharging green or yellow pus. The pain often goes away when this happens. The perforation nearly always heals, and hearing is unimpaired; but in view of the small risk of lasting deafness, doctors – and patients – need to monitor the condition carefully. The problem is commonest in children under ten: they are generally more susceptible to respiratory infections.

CAUSES Middle ear infections usually start a few days after a cold. Other causes include pressure changes (such as experienced when flying), enlarged adenoids (in young children), and diving into water (especially in children with colds). Some children are especially vulnerable: those with allergies, such as hay fever, and those born with a cleft palate.

PRESCRIPTION DRUGS

Antibiotics are often prescribed for all except the mildest degree of ear infection, although research has shown that most ear infections will clear up without them. Their use is sometimes justified by the need to prevent the serious complications: mastoiditis (rare) and chronic (persistent) discharging ear. The antibiotics most commonly used for this condition are listed.

How they work: by destroying the bacteria responsible for the more serious ear infections. However, they have no effect on the viruses which cause most of the milder forms of middle ear trouble.

Decongestants help to relieve blockage of the Eustachian tube; taken either as drops or spray applied up the nose, or as medicine or tablets taken by mouth.

How they work: by shrinking the swollen linings of the nose and Eustachian tube.

Antihistamines are often found in combination with decongestants, and are used whenever allergy is thought to be playing a part in the illness.

How they work: by reversing the effects of allergies.

OVER-THE-COUNTER TREATMENTS

Decongestants and antihistamines, usually in combination, are widely available, as of course are simple analgesics such as acetaminophen. But if ear ache does not clear up with acetominophen and a decongestant, consult a doctor within a few days.

QUESTIONS TO ASK THE DOCTOR

- Do I really need an antibiotic?
- For how long should the antibiotic be taken?
- Could the infection cause deafness?
- What about swimming?
- How can I get the most from these drops?

SIDE EFFECTS

Antibiotics are usually prescribed for seven days. Some people become allergic to certain antibiotics; this is shown by a rash, or itchy swelling of the face. More common side effects include diarrhea, nausea, or feeling generally ill. *See also page 79.*

Decongestants taken by mouth, such as pseudoephedrine, can interfere with sleep, and children can also develop hallucinations and behavior disturbance. Mild symptoms of this nature are probably quite common; they clear when the medicine is discontinued, and should not cause anxiety. Decongestant sprays or drops will irritate the nose if used for more than about one week, leading to further blockage and running (called vasomotor rhinitis). Patients with a history of high blood pressure should not take these drugs.

Most **antihistamines** (except newer types such as terfenadine) cause drowsiness, which can be an advantage in helping children to sleep at night. *See also* ***cough,*** *page 68* and ***hay fever,*** *page 260.*

SELF-MANAGEMENT

For mild ear ache in older children who have a cold, acetaminophen and decongestant nose drops or medicine will often relieve the pain and fever and prevent a full-blown ear infection from developing. DO NOT PUT DROPS INTO THE EAR, as they will not help, and if the ear drum has perforated, will cause damage. *See the diagram below on using nose drops.*

If ear ache persists for more than 24 hours, or becomes severe, consult your doctor.

Ideal position for instilling nose drops.

PATIENT'S EXPERIENCE

"My sisters are both deaf with perforated ear drums, so when my son got ear ache I took him straight to the doctor, who gave antibiotics and advised me to bring him back for more if it occurred again. Now he is ten, and he hasn't had any trouble for a whole year. We keep him off swimming whenever he has a cold. They checked his hearing at the clinic, but it was quite normal."

EXTERNAL EAR INFECTION

Astringent drops, antibiotics, anti-fungal drugs, steroids, wax-softeners

NAMES YOU WILL HEAR

Astringent drops
Generic name: aluminum acetate; **trade name:** Aluminum Acetate Ear Drops, Otic Domeboro Solution.

Antibiotic drops/ointment
(indicates steroid also present)*
Generic name: chloramphenicol; **trade name:** Chloromycetin Otic, Chloromycetin. **Generic name:** neomycin; **trade names:** Audicort*, Betnesol-N*, Neo-Cortef*, Otosporin*, Predsol-N*, Tri-adcortyl Otic*. **Generic name:** framycetin; **trade names:** Framycort*, Framygen, Sofradex*, Soframycin. **Generic name:** gentamicin; **trade names:** Garamycin, Cidomycin, Genticin, Gentisone HC*. **Generic name:** tetracycline; **trade names:** Achromycin, Sumycin. **Generic name:** oxytetracycline; **trade name:** Oxymycin, Terramycin, Terra-Cortril*. **Generic name:** clioquinol; **trade names:** Vioform, Vioform-hydrocortisone, Locorten-Vioform*.

Anti-fungal drops
Generic name: clotrimazole; **trade name:** Lotrimin, Canesten. **Generic name:** nystatin; **trade names:** Micostatin, Nilstat, Tri-Adcortyl Otic*.

Antibiotic tablets/medicine
Generic name: dicloxacillin; **trade names:** Panthocil, Dynapen, Veracillin. **Generic name:** flucloxacillin; **trade names:** Floxapen, Flopen. **Generic name:** erythromycin; **trade names:** Erythrocin, Ilotycin, E-mycin, Staticin, Erythromid, EpMycin, Erostin, Emu-V, Ethryn, Eromel, Ilocap, Ilosone.

Steroid drops
Generic name: betamethasone; **trade names:** Diprolene, Betnesol, Vista-Methasone. **Generic name:** methyl prednisolone; **trade name:** Solumedrol, Deltacortef, Hydeltrasol, Predsol.

Wax-softening drops
Generic name: carbamide peroxide; **trade name:** Debrox. **Generic name:** dioctyl sodium sulfosuccinate; **trade names:** Dioctyl, Molcer, Soliwax.

WHAT IS EXTERNAL EAR INFECTION?

The external ear is simply a tube of skin lining the passage from the outside to the middle ear, which is separated from it by the ear drum. The outer part carries hairs and produces wax. Bacteria can enter the skin if it is broken, causing pain, swelling, and an offensive discharge. A boil can develop at the base of a hair, causing severe pain because the skin is closely attached to the bone, leaving little room for swelling.

CAUSES Irritation of the skin by accumulated wax, shampoo, water or a foreign body (such as an insect); or any pre-existing itchy skin condition, which causes scratching. Hot weather seems to encourage this condition, probably due to increased sweating and humidity.

PRESCRIPTION DRUGS

Astringent drops – aluminum acetate – are the simplest and often the only treatment necessary. They may be applied as drops, or by soaking a strip of gauze which is inserted into the ear by a doctor or nurse.
How they work: by drying up inflamed tissues, so helping the natural healing process.
Antibiotics are usually applied as drops or ointment, but in severe cases will be given by mouth.
How they work: provided the bacteria responsible for the infection are sensitive to the particular antibiotic being used, and provided the drops can reach the infected skin, then the antibiotic should destroy those bacteria. Removal of dead skin and other matter from the ear canal, by syringing or mopping (a job for the doctor), is essential for the effective use of topical antibiotic drugs.
Anti-fungal drugs: Because some ear infections are caused by yeasts (Candida or thrush) often developing after treatment with antibiotics, anti-fungal drops may be prescribed.
How they work: in the same way as antibiotics, but only if the cause is this particular fungus or yeast.
Steroids: Antibiotic drops marked with a * in the NAMES YOU WILL HEAR list also contain one of these cortisone-like drugs, which reduce the irritation and swelling that often accompanies external ear infections.
How they work: steroids suppress the body's response to infection, injury and allergy. They are particularly effective in reducing the symptoms of eczema or dermatitis, which can occur in the ear.

Wax-softening drops will be prescribed to prepare the wax for syringing. Wax is a normal occurrence in the ear, and is only treated if it is completely blocking the ear canal, causing either deafness or pain and inflammation.

OVER-THE-COUNTER TREATMENTS

Drops for softening and removing wax are widely available. The simplest are the safest: olive oil, almond oil, glycerine or mineral oil are cheap, safe and effective. The softened wax will often flow out without the need for syringing. Proprietary ear drops, apart from those listed, can irritate the ear, and are best avoided.

QUESTIONS TO ASK THE DOCTOR

■ What is the best way to insert the ear drops or ointment?
■ For how long should I use the drops/ointment?
■ Is the infection contagious?
■ What happens if I develop an allergy to the drops?

SIDE EFFECTS

Astringent drops cause mild, transient stinging, which is normal and to be expected. **Antibiotics** applied to the skin anywhere, including the ear canal, can cause an allergy. The irritation will get worse rather than better, and you might notice redness spreading out from the ear. If this happens, stop the treatment and report to your doctor. Some antibiotics, such as neomycin, gentamycin, and polymyxin, cause damage to the inner ear if applied to a perforated ear drum. If you know you have a perforation, always remind your doctor. **Steroid drops** can mask the effects of infection, and can lead to new infections developing. They should be used only for short periods, up to one week, and only under medical supervision.

SELF-MANAGEMENT

■ Take care to keep your ears dry, using disposable ear plugs or cotton smeared in vaseline to prevent water getting in while washing your hair or swimming.
■ DO NOT use Q-tips or anything else to try to remove wax. This usually pushes it further in; it can only be removed by syringing.
■ If you suffer from a pre-existing skin disease, seek your doctor's advice on the best preparation to use in your ears.
■ Avoid scratching your ears. It may cause an infection.

PATIENT'S EXPERIENCE

"My ears were producing a lot of wax, which I tried to remove with Q-tips. One day, after I had washed my hair, I went completely deaf. I bought some wax-removing drops, but they made my ears itchy. The next day, the whole side of my face was swollen, red and itching, so I had to go to the doctor. He said I had an infection of the outer ear, and also an allergy to the ear drops. The nurse syringed my ears when the infection had settled down – a lot of wax and some white stuff came out. The doctor prescribed some antihistamine tablets for the allergy. My doctor suggested I use a little warm olive oil in each ear if I felt them getting blocked, and that I should keep the water out when washing my hair."

Decongestants, steroids, sodium cromoglycate, antihistamines

NAMES YOU WILL HEAR

Decongestants

Generic name: xylometazoline hydrochloride; **trade names:** Otrivin, Otrivine Nasal Drops or Nasal Spray, Otrivine Paediatric Nasal Drops, Otrivine-Antistin, Otrix, Sinutab. **Generic name:** antazoline; **trade names:** Antistin, Vasocona. **Generic name:** oxymetazoline; **trade names:** Afrin, Dristan, Oxymetazoline Nasal Solution, Afrazine Nasal Drops or Nasal Spray, Afrazine Paediatric Nasal Drops, Drixine, Nafrine. **Generic name:** ephedrine hydrochloride; **trade name:** Ephedrine Nose Drops.

Topical steroids

Generic name: beclomethasone dipropionate; **trade names:** Beconase, Vancenase. **Generic name:** betamethasone sodium phosphate; **trade name:** Betnesol. **Generic name:** budesonide; **trade names:** Preferid, Rhinocont. **Generic name:** flunisolide; **trade names:** Syntaris, Rhinalar.

Cromolyn sodium

Generic name: cromolyn sodium; **trade names:** Nasalcrom, Rynacrom.

Oral antihistamines

Generic name: brompheniramine; **trade names:** Dimotane, Dimetane, Dimotapp. **Generic name:** chlorpheniramine; **trade names:** Expulin, Expurhin, Teldrin, Chlor-Trimeton, Haymine, Piriton, Chlor-Tripolon, Histalon, Novopheniram, Allertex, Chlortrimeton, Histamed, Allergex, Bramahist Chloramine, Histaids, Teledrim. **Generic name:** clemastine; **trade names:** Tavegil, Tavist, Trabest. **Generic name:** mebhydrolin; **trade name:** Fabahistin. **Generic name:** terfenadine; **trade names:** Seldane, Triludan. **Generic name:** trimeprazine; **trade names:** Temaril, Vallergan, Panectyl. **Generic name:** triprolidine; **trade names:** Actidil, Pro-Actidil. **Generic name:** astemizole; **trade name:** Hismanal.

Allergent extract vaccine

Generic name: alum precipitated extracts from aqueous pyridine.

WHAT IS HAY FEVER?

– An allergic reaction causing sneezing, watering and irritation of the eyes and nose, and obstruction of the nose. It is common in adults aged 15-45 years; the symptoms tend to recur seasonally, as the responsible agent appears.

CAUSES Inhaled allergens, usually grass or tree pollens and molds. The reaction is mediated by chemicals such as histamine which are produced in "mast cells" in the conjunctiva, and the lining of the nose, soon after exposure to pollen.

PRESCRIPTION DRUGS

Local applications

Decongestant eye drops give only temporary relief; likewise nose drops, indeed they can make symptoms worse if used for long periods. See SIDE EFFECTS. Neither are therefore the first choice of treatment.

How they work: *see **sinusitis**, page 262.*

Steroids and **cromolyn sodium** are available as nasal sprays and eye drops. Start cromolyn preferably before the hay fever season begins, to prevent attacks. Steroid nasal sprays are effective in preventing an attack. These drugs are usually taken two to four times a day, and as their effect is cumulative, they need to be continued for several weeks, or even months.

How they work: by stabilizing mast cells, thus stopping the allergic reaction. Cromoglycate only works to prevent future attacks, not to help during an acute episode.

Oral drugs

Antihistamine tablets help both eye and nose symptoms. They are usually used to stop attacks in courses lasting a few days, but they may also be used continuously.

How they work: by preventing released histamine from gaining access to its receptor. Antihistamines occupy the same receptor as histamine, thus preventing histamine having its effects.

Steroids are a powerful expedient for very severe attacks. Relief of symptoms can be quite dramatic, but they are normally used for short periods only.

How they work: by blocking both allergic and inflammatory reactions.

Desensitization injections can be given in courses before the hay fever season starts. They work by slowly acclimatizing the body to the various allergens and thus reducing the reaction when next exposed.

OVER-THE-COUNTER TREATMENTS

Many of the nasal decongestants and antihistamine preparations can be bought over the counter. Steroids and steroid preparations are only available on prescription. In all but the most severe attacks, self-treatment is appropriate. See IN AN ATTACK.

QUESTIONS TO ASK THE DOCTOR

■ Can treatment prevent attacks, or only treat them?
■ Can I treat myself in future attacks?
■ Can I have the type of antihistamine that causes the least drowsiness?

SIDE EFFECTS

Decongestants: prolonged use – typically more than two weeks continuously – can damage the lining of the nose. Also, stopping them can cause a rebound effect: the symptoms not only recur, but are actually worse than if the drops had not been used at all.
Topical cromolyn and **steroid preparations** have no significant side effects.
Antihistamines: The main side effect is drowsiness which can make driving or operating machinery dangerous (the effect is additive with alcohol). Some of the newer antihistamines, for example terfenadine, cause less drowsiness. Chlorpheniramine, by contrast, can make some people very drowsy. Other effects include dry mouth and blurred vision.

Desensitization injections have the risk of a rare but grave side effect called anaphylactic (allergic) reaction.

SELF-MANAGEMENT

■ Avoid exposure to pollen: stay indoors, particularly on hot days, and when the pollen count is high. ■ Sufferers should particularly avoid freshly mown grass and hay fields, or other known source of allergen.

IN AN ATTACK

Go indoors if possible. Avoid bright sunlight: it puts extra strain on already irritated and watering eyes. Dark glasses can help. During a mild attack, try topical steroids or cromolyn drops or sprays. If the symptoms are more severe, or you want more effective relief, start yourself on antihistamine pills straight away and continue for several days. Both these preparations can be used simultaneously if necessary. With very severe attacks, or when attacks are so frequent that they warrant continuous treatment, consult a doctor.

solutions; **trade name:** prescribed by generic name.

Oral steroid
Generic name: methyl prednisolone; **trade names:** Solumedrol, Codelsol, Delta Phoricol, Deltacortril, Deltalone, Precortisyl, Prednesol, Sintisone, Nisolone, Delta-Cortef, Deltasolone, Prelone, Lenisolone, Meticortilone, Predeltilone.

PATIENT'S EXPERIENCE

"My hay fever used to make me feel desperate – gasping for air, swollen eyes and face, blocked nose, throat and chest. I often wondered whether to call a doctor. I used a decongestant spray bought from the pharmacist. It gave real relief – but only for about five minutes.

Then, this spring, I went to the allergy clinic I had heard about at the local hospital. The specialist advised me to stop using the spray immediately: he told me it could be making the symptoms worse. I did what he said. So far this summer the symptoms have been much less aggravating than usual: maybe it's partly because there is less pollen around, but the improvement is so dramatic that I suspect dropping the spray has helped. The specialist said that my doctor could prescribe the cromolyn spray just before the pollen count rises next spring."

Decongestants, antihistamines, antibiotics

NAMES YOU WILL HEAR

Decongestants (oral)
Generic name: pseudoephedrine hydrochloride; **trade names:** Actifed, Atrohist, Co-tylenol Cold Medication, Dimetane-DX Cough Syrup, Fedahist, Novahistine, Robitussin, Sine-Aid, Tylenol Maximum Strenth Sinus Medication, Sudafed, Sudelix, Drixora, Repetabs, Eltor.

Decongestants (nasal)
Generic name: xylometazoline; **trade names:** Otrivin, Otrivine Nasal Drops or Nasal Spray, Otrivine Paediatric Nasal Drops, Otrivine-Antistin, Otrix, Sinutab. **Generic name:** oxymetazoline; **trade names:** Oxymetazoline Hydrochloride Nasal Solution, Afrazine Nasal Drops or Nasal Spray, Afrazine Paediatric Nasal Drops, Drixine, Nafrine. **Generic name:** ephedrine hydrochloride; **trade name:** Ephedrine Nose Drops. **Generic name:** phenylephrine hydrochloride; **trade names:** Biomydrin, Neophryn, Phenophrin, Mydfrin, Nasalmed.

Oral antihistamines
(Prescription-only types)
Generic name: astemizole; **trade name:** Hismanal. **Generic name:** brompheniramine; **trade names:** Dimotane, Dimetane, Dimotapp. **Generic name:** chlorpheniramine; **trade names:** Haymine, Piriton, Chlor-Tripolon, Histalon, Novopheniram, Allertex, Chlortrimeton, Histamed, Allergex, Bramahist Chloramin, Histaids, Teledrim, Expulin, Expurhin. **Generic name:** clemastine; **trade names:** Tavegil, Tavest, Trabest. **Generic name:** mebhydrolin; **trade name:** Fabahistin. **Generic name:** terfenadine; **trade name:** Triludan. **Generic name:** trimeprazine tartrate; **trade names:** Vallergan, Panectyl. **Generic name:** triprolidine; **trade names:** Actidil, Pro-Actidil.

Antibiotics
*See **cystitis,** page 142 and **pneumonia and pleurisy,** page 78.*

WHAT IS SINUSITIS?

The sinuses are spaces in the bones of the face and forehead, lined by a form of skin similar to that on the inside of the nose, and connected to the nose by small openings or passages. True sinusitis is an infection of one or more of these spaces, which occurs when the opening becomes blocked due to swelling of the lining, as happens frequently during a cold. Bacteria invade the lining of the sinus and the bone itself. The spaces fill with yellow or green pus, causing severe pain and a high temperature; you feel very ill indeed. Serious complications such as cerebral alsun may ensue if the condition is not diagnosed and treated.

The condition commonly called "sinusitis", is in fact a less severe form of true sinusitis: one or more sinuses become blocked with mucus, causing discomfort.

CAUSES anything which leads to blockage of the sinus openings, including allergies and hay fever, but the common cold is the most usual.

PRESCRIPTION DRUGS

Decongestants: the first line of treatment; the drops or sprays should not be used for more than five days, since they eventually worsen the congestion.
How they work: by shrinking the swelling inside the nose, allowing mucus or pus to drain. See SIDE EFFECTS.
Antihistamines: often found in combination with decongestants in medicines such as Actifed or Dimetapp.
How they work: by reversing the effects of allergies. Thus they may be helpful in sinus blockage caused by hay fever, or allergy to dust or animals.
Antibiotics: commonly prescribed, but probably unnecessary for the milder sinus pain described above. Many varieties: those most commonly used are listed.
How they work: by destroying certain bacteria, but not the viruses that cause colds and flu. In true sinusitis they stop the infection, relieving pain and fever.

OVER-THE-COUNTER TREATMENTS

Decongestants, both nasal and oral, are widely available, and often advertized on TV. Combination medicines with antihistamines are ever more common. Provided the side effects are noted, self-treatment with these preparations is entirely appropriate in mild cases.

QUESTIONS TO ASK THE DOCTOR

■ How long should I take the medicine(s)?

■ Can I take simple painkillers as well?
■ Can I drive my car, or drink alcohol?

SIDE EFFECTS

Decongestants taken by mouth, such as pseudoephedrine, can interfere with sleep, and in children can also cause hallucinations and behavior disturbance. Mild symptoms of this nature are probably quite common; they clear when the medicine is discontinued, and should not cause anxiety. Decongestant sprays or drops will irritate the nose if used for more than about one week, leading to further blockage and running (called vasomotor rhinitis). Patients with a history of high blood pressure should not be given these drugs.

Most **antihistamines** cause drowsiness, and impair coordination. The depressant effect of alcohol will be increased. Don't drive, or operate machinery when on these drugs: concentration is significantly impaired. One or two of the newer antihistamines are relatively free of this effect (eg Terfanedine or Triludan).

Antibiotics are usually prescribed for five to ten days. Some people become allergic to certain antibiotics and develop a rash or itchy swelling of the face. These should be reported at once to your doctor. More commonly side effects include diarrhea, nausea, or feeling generally ill. *See also **pneumonia** and **pleurisy,** page 000.*

Women taking ampicillin, or other broad spectrum antibiotics, may develop thrush.

SELF-MANAGEMENT

Because the initial cause of an attack of true sinusitis is obstruction of the openings into the nose, treating a blocked nose by simple steam inhalation (see margin), or carefully sniffing cold water (with a little salt dissolved in it), or using a decongestant spray for not more than three or four days may prevent sinusitis.

SELF-HELP IN AN ATTACK

■ Whenever your nose feels blocked, try to identify the cause – a cold (virus infection), an allergy such as hay fever, or an irritant.
■ Use decongestant drops or nasal spray three or four times a day for three or four days only; or, if you prefer, a decongestant pill or medicine. (Avoid pills or medicine if you are pregnant – see SIDE EFFECTS.)
■ Fresh air often helps. Avoid hot, dry atmospheres, central heating and air conditioning.
■ Simple analgesics, aspirin or acetaminophen, may be taken to give pain relief three or four times a day.

PATIENT'S EXPERIENCE

'I used to suffer from sinusitis every time I got a cold, and often had to get antibiotics from the doctor. Then I gave up smoking to save money, and also changed my job from a smokey office to a supermarket; since then I have hardly had any trouble. I'm sure the smoking was causing catarrh. And I don't get breathless now, either.'

Cut away diagram of the face to show the two main sinuses, and their connections with the nose.

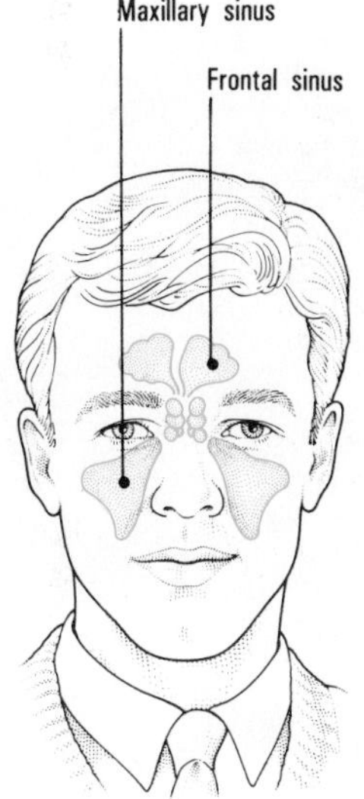

STEAM INHALATION

Sit at a table with a pitcher of water that has only just boiled (take due care). Place a towel over your head and the pitcher, and breathe in the steam for five to ten minutes. Try to breathe through your nose. Repeat as often as you feel the exercise is useful. Preparations to add to the water for inhalation are widely available, but of unproven worth – apart from their pleasant smell. The real value is in the steam, which liquifies the excess mucus in the passage.

Disorders of THE MOUTH

Antiseptic mouthwashes, low-potency steroids, iron, antibiotics, anti-fungals.

NAMES YOU WILL HEAR

Antibiotics and antifungals
Generic name: chlortetracycline; **trade name:** Aureomycin. **Generic name:** nystatin; **trade names:** Mycostatin, Nilstat, Nystex, Nystan. **Generic name:** amphotericin B; **trade name:** Fungizone, Mysteclin F, Fungilin. **Generic name:** miconazole; **trade names:** Monistat, Daktarin.

Antiseptic mouthwashes
Generic name: chlorhexidine; **trade names:** Peridex, Corsodyl, Hibitane, Eludril. **Generic name:** benzydamine; **trade name:** Difflam.

Steroids
Generic name: triamcinolone; **trade names:** Aristocort, Kenalog, Adcortil. **Generic name:** hydrocortisone pellets; **trade name:** Corlan.

WHAT ARE MOUTH DISORDERS?

– Three distinct types of problem occur:

Mouth ulcers, from which most people suffer from time to time, are areas of soreness and swelling on the inside of the mouth, often associated with infection. Though fairly painful, they are not sufficiently so to prevent eating. There are, however, many kinds of mouth ulcer, and even the simplest may occasionally be associated with minor degrees of anemia and similar conditions. It is therefore essential to mention any persistent mouth ulcer to a dentist or doctor. If you are told that it is simple ulceration, then self-treatment is appropriate. Any ulcer which lasts for more than two weeks without showing signs of healing should have expert attention.

A sore mouth has many causes, some obvious – such as the fitting of new dentures – and some less so. If you have a sore mouth or tongue which lasts for more than a week or two for no obvious reason, consult a dentist or doctor. If there is no clear reason for the problem, an investigation such as a blood test may be advised. Many diseases which affect the skin also appear in the mouth, sometimes before the skin is seen to be involved. You may need a biopsy – the removal of a small section of the mouth lining (a local anesthetic eliminates any pain) for microscopic examination. This does not necessarily mean that some sinister disease is suspected. In a few patients, usually women at or around the time of the menopause, no cause is ever found for the complaint.

Thrush is an infection of the mouth by a fungus. The organism is usually present in healthy mouths, but only becomes active when an individual is weakened by illness. It appears as white flecks on the lining of the mouth; it is usually moderately sore. Thrush may occur also in young or old patients with no other significant illness, and in patients taking certain drugs – particularly steroids and, sometimes, antibiotics.

PRESCRIPTION DRUGS

Antiseptic mouthwashes will be suggested for mild ulceration.

Bear in mind that whatever the treatment, there is no cure for mouth ulcers; the best you can hope for is improvement until they clear of their own accord.

Iron and/or vitamin tablets may be given if a sore mouth is associated with anemia *(see page 224)*. Since a sore mouth can be caused by a number of conditions, treatments vary widely. **Antifungal preparations** are prescribed for thrush; they are usually given as lozenges, gels, creams, or suspensions for use in and around the mouth. Only occasionally will they be in a form designed to be swallowed.

OVER-THE-COUNTER TREATMENTS

There is an enormous range of mouthwashes, pastilles and lozenges which can effectively relieve the symptoms associated with mouth ulcers. However, it is essential to have any persistent ulceration or soreness checked out by a doctor/dentist rather than persist with self-treatment.

QUESTIONS TO ASK A DOCTOR OR DENTIST

■ How often should I use the mouthwash/lozenges?
■ How long should I use the mouthwash/lozenges?
■ Should I keep on using them when my mouth is better?
■ What should I do if the treatment seems to be making my mouth worse?
■ Is the treatment a permanent cure?

SIDE EFFECTS

Mouthwashes and iron tablets have no significant side effects. For ***antibiotics*** and ***antifungals,*** *see pages 79 and 285.*

SELF MANAGEMENT

■ Oral hygene is enhanced by regular brushing of the teeth in the correct fashion, with a toothbrush of the size advised for you individually. Ask your dentist.
■ Additional oral hygene, again on the advice of a dentist, may be necessary for people with disorders of the structure – gums, bone and other tissue – supporting the teeth. Measures include use of dental floss and wooden picks for removing plaque.

PATIENT'S EXPERIENCE

"I've had mouth ulcers ever since I was seven years old. Once, they got so bad I had to go to hospital for tests. They told me they couldn't find anything wrong to account for the; all I can do is use the mouthwashes they prescribed. It's a help, but the problem still keeps on coming back."

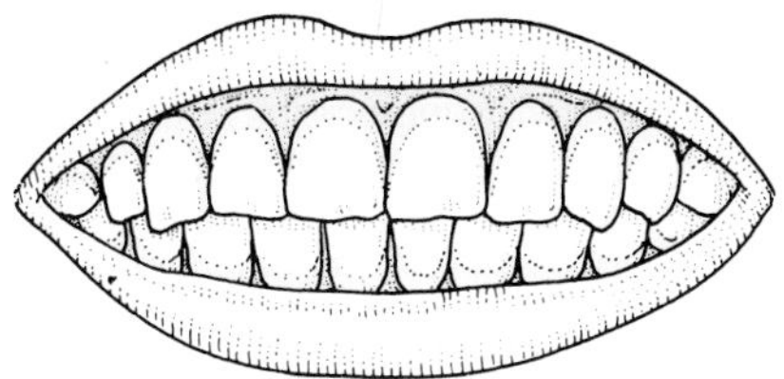

Plaque – bacterial deposits – *is revealed by chewing a disclosing tablet. This procedure can be an invaluable aid to maintaining a clean mouth and avoiding mouth disorders.*

LARYNGITIS AND CROUP

Local anesthetic lozenges, analgesics, cough suppressants, antibiotics

NAMES YOU WILL HEAR

Antibiotics

Generic name: amoxicillin sodium; **trade names:** Amoxil, Augmentin, Triniox, Wymox, Moxacin, Moxilean, Novamoxin, Penamox, Polymox. **Generic name:** co-trimoxazole; **trade names:** Septra, Septra DS, Bactrim, Fectrim, Nodilon, Septrim. **Generic name:** erythromycin; **trade names:** Benzamycin, Erymax, Ilotycin, Pediamycin, Pediazole, Arpimycin, Erycen, Erythroped, Retcin, Erythrocin, Erythromid, EpMycin, Erostin, Emu-V, Ethryn, Eromel, Ilocap, Ilosone, Rythrocaps.

Local analgesics

Generic name: benzocaine; **trade names:** AAA Spray, Tyrozets, Benzocaine. **Generic name:** benzocaine and dequalinium chloride; **trade name:** Dequacaine.

Analgesics

Generic name: acetaminophen; **trade names:** Anacin 3, Phenaphon, Panadol, Tempra, Tylenol, Pamol, Calpol, Tylenon, Paracin, Parmol, Panado, Ceetamol, Atosol, Exctol, Ennagesic, Ilvamol. **Generic name:** aspirin; **trade names:** Alka-Seltzer, Ascriptin, Bayer, Ecotrin, Measurin, Aspirin, Astrin, Bi-Prin. *See also **pain,** page 106.*

Cough suppressants

Generic name: codeine phosphate; **trade names:** Ambinyl Cough Syrup, Dimetane DC Cough Syrup, Robitussin DC Cough Syrup, Traimine Expectorant with codeine, Codeine Linctus, Codeine Syrup, Dimotane Co, Galcodine, Phensedyl, Tercoda, Terpoin, Uniflu. **Generic name:** pholcodine tartrate; **trade names:** Dia-Tuss, Duro-Tuss, Pholtex, Copholco, Copholcoids, Davenol, Expulin, Galenphol, Pavacol D, Pholcomed, Rinurel.

WHAT IS LARYNGITIS?

- An inflammation of the voice box (larynx) resulting in hoarseness or total loss of voice. Acute laryngitis comes on suddenly and lasts a few days. It is usually associated with a sore throat and sometimes there is a dry cough.

Acute laryngitis can cause croup in young children. Swelling of the air passage results in obstruction to breathing – the airways are relatively narrower in young children. The child has a hoarse cry and makes a noisy sound (stridor) when breathing in. If the obstruction is severe, the child will start to breathe rapidly, with straining of the breathing muscles.

Chronic laryngitis comes on more gradually and lasts a longer time. It is usually not painful.

CAUSES Acute laryngitis is usually caused by a viral infection such as the common cold, influenza or measles. Chronic laryngitis may be caused by faulty voice production and shouting, habitual over-indulgence in alcohol or tobacco, or chronic sinus infection. Hoarseness may also be caused by nodules or tumors on the vocal cords.

PRESCRIPTION DRUGS

Antibiotics are usually unnecessary in the treatment of acute laryngitis, as the cause is most often a virus, but they may be used in the treatment of associated bacterial infection such as sinusitis or ear infection. For details of these antibiotics, *see **pneumonia and pleurisy,** page 78.*

OVER-THE-COUNTER TREATMENTS

A **local anesthetic** in the form of a lozenge will ease the sore throat by decreasing the conduction of nerve impulses near the site of application, so making the throat less sensitive.

Analgesics such as aspirin and acetaminophen will also help the sore throat and the general symptoms associated with acute laryngitis. *See **common cold,** page 134.*

Cough suppressants will suppress the cough. Laryngitis is one of the few good reasons for the use of cough suppressants. The cough is usually irritating and nonproductive, and persistent coughing may further inflame the larynx. *See **cough,** page 68.*

QUESTIONS TO ASK THE DOCTOR

- How long will it last?

■ Will stopping smoking help?
■ Will resting my voice help?
■ Will antibiotics help?
■ (If a baby has croup) How can I stop the hoarse cough? What danger signs should I look for?

See SELF-MANAGEMENT.

SIDE EFFECTS

Antibiotics: *see **pneumonia and pleurisy,** page 78.*
Local anesthetics are generally very safe. Occasionally they cause an allergic reaction which results in mild irritation of the mouth.
Analgesics: *see **common cold,** page 134.*
Cough suppressants: *see **cough,** page 68.*

SELF-MANAGEMENT

■ The usual cause of laryngitis and croup is the common cold; *see the advice on page 136.*
■ If you have laryngitis, rest your voice: this really is important – talking will aggravate the condition.
■ Treat your sore throat regularly with analgesics, either in the form of anesthetic lozenges or tablets (for example aspirin or acetaminophen). If you are not sure which is best, *see **common cold,** page 134.*
■ If there is any difficulty in breathing associated with hoarseness, especially in a child, consult your doctor at once.
■ Hoarseness which persists for more than three weeks should be investigated by your doctor to rule out cancer.

TREATING CROUP

Croup can usually be treated at home if it is mild.
1 It is important to control the temperature *(see **common cold,** page 134):* the condition worsens if the child is hot, irritable and crying.
2 Increase the humidity in the child's room, both to minimize the problem, and to treat the acute attack. Simply boil a kettle, with the windows and doors closed, or sit the child in a steamy bathroom.
3 Encourage the child to drink clear fluids: dehydration can occur as a result of rapid breathing and sweating due to high temperature.
4 Keep the child calm: croup becomes much worse as soon as the child starts to cry.
5 If a child is breathing fast (chest heaving more than 50 times a minute), or having difficulty breathing, call a doctor.

PATIENT'S EXPERIENCE

"I had a sore throat and lost my voice. The problem was, I had an important presentation to make at a business meeting the following day. I asked my doctor to give me something for it, but he explained that laryngitis is usually due to a virus and that antibiotics cannot cure viral infections. He gave me some lozenges which helped the sore throat and my voice gradually returned over the next few days. However, I had to postpone my presentation."

PARENT'S EXPERIENCE

"My one-year-old developed croup a few days before Christmas. At first she seemed quite well, apart from a croaky voice and a slight cold. That night she woke at about midnight. Her temperature was high and when she breathed in, she made an awful hoarse noise. I gave her a teaspoon of acetaminophen and put her in a cool bath. She was miserable, so I got into the bath with her and played with her until she felt quite cool. She still had a hoarse voice, but she was no longer breathing fast and the noisy breathing had almost completely disappeared – the steamy atmosphere of the bathroom must have helped. I lay down on the bed with her in my arms and she fell asleep. Over the next few days she improved, but I noticed that the croup was always worse at night. Within a week she was completely better."

NAMES YOU WILL HEAR
Generic name: chloramphenicol; **trade names:** Chloromycetin, Sno Phenicol, Chlomin, Chloroptic, Chloramol, Chlorsig, Opclor, Fenicol, Isopto Fenicol, Chloramex, Chlorcol, Lennacol, Troymycetin. **Generic name:** gentamicin; **trade names:** Garamycin, Genticin, Alcomicin, Refobacin, Cidomycin, Lugacin. **Generic name:** neomycin; **trade names:** Cortisporin, Lazersporin, Graneodin, Neosporin, Neopt, Neomate, Neosulf, Quintress-N, Siguent Neomycin, Myciguent, Herisan Antibiotic, Neocin, Emelmycin, Neo-Gelicil, Neopan. **Generic name:** framycetin; **trade names:** Framygen, Soframycin. **Generic name:** tobramycin; **trade names:** Tobralex, Nebcin.

PATIENTS' EXPERIENCES

"When I was gardening last weekend a branch sprang back and poked me in the eye. It was painful, and it felt as if there was something in my eye. My doctor douldn't find anything, but said I had a corneal abrasion and gave me an antibiotic ointment to use four times a day. I found it hard to understand why my eye still felt as if there was something in it and I had to take two days off work. Anyway, by the third day it was better, and I have had no trouble since."

"My first attack of blepharitis was 15 years ago when my eyes suddenly became red and sore. I had several courses of different antibiotic ointments, drops and pills, but apart from slight improvements each time, they weren't much use. After a few weeks or months, back would come the redness and soreness. Eventually I was told to clean my eyelids regularly and I then realized that there had always been lots of crusty matter in my lashes. Once I started cleaning, my attacks happened much less often and weren't as bad either. Now I can live with it, at least."

WHAT IS RED EYE?

– A general term for several distinct eye conditions:

CONJUNCTIVITIS

– Gritty, irritable eyes with discharge during the day and stickiness in the morning.

CAUSE Usually a bacterial infection, but sometimes a virus. Viral conjunctivitis often occurs in epidemics.

PRESCRIPTION DRUGS

Antibiotics: many are available; the commonest is chloramphenicol. All may be given as drops or ointment – drops should be used two-hourly, ointment four times a day. Seven day's of treatment should clear a bacterial infection. Pull down the lower lid and apply one to two drops or a $\frac{1}{2}$-inch (1.5 cm) squeeze of ointment to the inside of the lid.
How they work: by killing bacteria. There is no treatment for viral conjunctivitis, but it clears in 14–21 days.

BLEPHARITIS

– Red, sore, itchy eyelids. The condition is usually longstanding (chronic). Two types occur: bacterial, with pus and ulceration along the lid margins; and squamous, with flakes of skin among the eyelashes.
CAUSES Bacterial blepharitis is due to the bacterium *staphylococcus* and tends to wax and wane. Squamous blepharitis is a manifestation of a skin disease known as seborrheic dermatitis – the eyebrows and scalp are usually involved as well. Secondary bacterial infection can occur in squamous blepharitis.

PRESCRIPTION DRUGS

Antibiotics: Ointment applied to the lid margins four times a day should clear a flare-up of bacterial blepharitis, but will not prevent a recurrence. Drops are of no value. Occasionally, antibiotics may be given.

OVER-THE-COUNTER TREATMENTS

Medicated shampoos: treating the scalp and eyebrows with one of these will improve squamous blepharitis when combined with lid hygiene.

CORNEAL ABRASION AND FOREIGN BODIES

Any injury or foreign body can scratch the cornea, the front of the eye. Your doctor will remove the foreign body and give antibiotics against secondary infection.

A corneal abrasion heals over two to three days in

much the same way as a scratch or graze on the skin, and only rarely causes long-term damage. During the healing process, however, it feels as if there is still something in the eye and it hurts to look at bright lights. Wear dark glasses and rest; stop the antibiotic when the sensation clears.

QUESTIONS TO ASK THE DOCTOR

- Should I cover the infected eye?
- Is my eye contagious? Can I protect the rest of the family from catching it? Should I stay away from work?

SIDE EFFECTS

Antibiotic ointment blurrs the vision for about 30 minutes, so don't drive until this has cleared. All eye treatments can occasionally cause allergy, ointment more commonly than drops. The allergy is to the preservatives or base rather than the active ingredient and appears as swollen red lids and conjunctiva. It can be dramatic, but clears once treatment is stopped.

SELF-MANAGEMENT

Do not use over-the-counter eye treatments unless first advised by a doctor. At best, they have no effect on the underlying condition and frequently cause an allergic reaction. In blepharitis, lid hygiene is the mainstay of control. Every morning, clean the eyelids with cotton wool and warm water ensuring that all crusts and flakes are removed from the margins. If necessary, use a Q-tip – rub it along the lash bases. Repeat as often as necessary through the day. In a flare-up, increase cleaning to four times a day and apply ointment.

OTHER CAUSES OF A RED EYE

These include acute glaucoma *(see page 270)*, acute iritis, corneal ulcer and corneal abscess. They are all uncommon and very painful with marked blurring of vision. As these can seriously affect your sight, every painful red eye should be seen by an ophthalmologist.

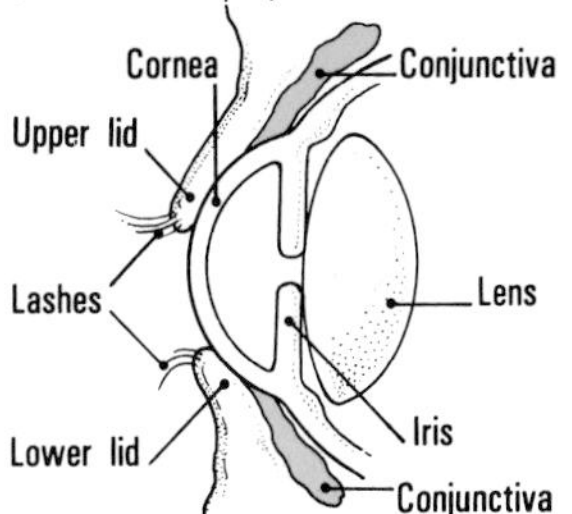

The lids *are in contact with the cornea and spread tears over its surface by blinking. The under surface of each lid is covered with conjunctiva which loosely spreads out above and below the eye to form potential spaces. Ointment or drops can be applied into the lower of these spaces by gently pulling down the lower lid.*

DRY EYE

This common problem occurs usually with age and causes a number of troublesome symptoms including itching, burning, discomfort, heaviness of the lids, frontal headaches and transient blurring of vision. It is not painful and the eye does not go red except in severe cases. It is worse in smoky or dry atmospheres and in the evening.

CAUSE Tear production falls below a level at which the lids can adequately wet the cornea.

Treatment Artificial tears usually contain water soluble polymers such as cellulose esters or polyvinyl alcohol. Clearz, Isopto Tears, Tearisol are examples of tear substitutes with cellulose derivatives. Liquifilm Tears, Tears Plus and Total are examples based on polyvinyl alcohol.

Self-help Understanding the condition: if tears are insufficient, dry spots occur. These cause the symptoms, which come on over four to six hours and last for about 24 hours. Instil the artificial tears regularly and frequently enough to ensure wetting at all times: **1** Put the drops in every two hours to start with. **2** If the symptoms are going to clear, this will take at least a day, so don't give up. **3** If, after a few days, there is no improvement, increase the drops to hourly or even half-hourly: there are no side effects. **4** When there has been an improvement, gradually reduce the frequency every other day to a level which keeps the eyes comfortable: use trial and error.

CHRONIC GLAUCOMA

Beta-blociers, sympathomimetics, pilocarpine, acetazolamide

NAMES YOU WILL HEAR

Beta-blockers

Generic name: timolol; **trade names:** Timoptic, Timoptol. **Generic name:** carteolol; **trade name:** Teoptic. **Generic name:** metipranolol; **trade name:** Glauline. **Generic name:** betaxolol; **trade name:** Betoptic. **Generic name:** nadolol; **trade name:** Optgard.

Sympathomimetics

Generic names: adrenaline, epinephrine; **trade names:** Adrenalin, EpiPen, Susphrine, Eppy, Epifrin, Isopto Epinal, Simplene, Epinal, Eppy/N, Glaucon, Micronefrin, Epitrate, Sus-Phrine. **Generic name:** dipivefrin; **trade name:** Propine. **Generic name:** Adrenoline plus guanethidine; **trade name:** Ganda.

Pilocarpine

Generic name: pilocarpine; **trade names:** Isopto Carpine, Pilopine, Sno pilo, Pilopt, Neutracarpine, Adsorbocarpine, Isopto Carpine, Pilocar.

WHAT IS CHRONIC GLAUCOMA?

– Gradual, painless rise of pressure in the eyeball causing loss of vision over several years. It starts as islands of reduced vision away from the central field. These islands slowly enlarge, but are not usually noticed until the late stages when only a small area of central vision is left (tunnel vision) before blindness takes over.

Acute glaucoma is by contrast usually sudden in onset, very painful, with altered vision and a red eye.

CAUSE Inability of the fluid within the eye to escape from the eye quickly enough. The intraocular pressure rises gradually until it is high enough to cause damage to the optic nerve. The optic nerve carries the nervous messages of sight from the eye to the brain and when it is completely destroyed, blindness results.

PRESCRIPTION DRUGS

Antiglaucoma drugs are usually given as drops, occasionally as ointment. They are often used in combination to achieve better control, and are taken for life.

Beta-blockers: Timolol is the commonest, given as drops twice a day.

Sympathomimetics are also used twice a day mainly in people with chest disease, who may suffer potentially serious side effects if given beta-blockers.

Pilocarpine drops are used three or four times a day and often added to timolol or adrenaline.

Acetazolamide is taken as pills two or four times a day; not often used due to side effects.

If these drugs do not control the pressure, a minor operation may be necessary to create a new drainage channel: this is known as a trabeculectomy.

How they work: They all lower the intraocular pressure by reducing the production of aqueous, except pilocarpine, which allows it to escape more easily.

OVER-THE-COUNTER TREATMENTS

None.

QUESTIONS TO ASK THE DOCTOR

- How often should I take the drops?
- What happens if I miss the drops once or twice?
- What strength should I use?
- What happens if the drops don't work?
- What are the side effects?

SIDE EFFECTS

Beta-blockers usually have no side effects; however if

they make you short of breath; stop them immediately and report it to your doctor.

Sympathomimetics: adrenaline causes eye redness in many people; dipivefrin does not and is thus more widely used.

Pilocarpine may cause headache for 30 minutes after use, but this problem usually fades in a week. It makes the pupil constrict, and can dim the vision particularly where there is also a cataract. It also paralyzes the eye's ability to focus and may make life very difficult for younger people.

Acetazolamide has many side effects: numbness and tingling in the fingers and toes, lethargy, loss of appetite, nausea, weight loss and confusion. Occasional but serious side effects are diabetes and kidney stones. Use is rarely justified, except in people who happen not to be prone to these effects.

SELF-MANAGEMENT

■ Take the drops and pills regularly to keep the pressure normal throughout the day. This way you will slow down or halt progress of the disease.

■ Take the treatment as usual on the day you go to the clinic so the specialist can get an idea of what the pressure is between visits.

■ If you are taking more than one type of drop, leave five to ten minutes between each: this prevents the first being washed away before it can work.

■ Glaucoma runs in families, so if you are told you have it, inform all close blood relatives. Parents, brothers and sisters over 40 should visit an optician for a check.

PATIENT'S EXPERIENCE

"I went to the optician for reading glasses but he found that my eyeball tension was high and referred me to a specialist. I was surprised because all I had wanted was reading glasses and I hadn't noticed any pain or blurring of vision. I had needed several changes of reading glasses, though, during the last few years. The specialist told me I had glaucoma, gave me drops and said that I would go blind if I didn't use them. I told my elder sister, who went to her optician and found that she also had glaucoma. Hers was worse than mine: she could hardly see out of one eye and the other wasn't much better. She went blind after a few years. I have been using the drops regularly; I am thankful my eyesight has stayed good over these last 12 years."

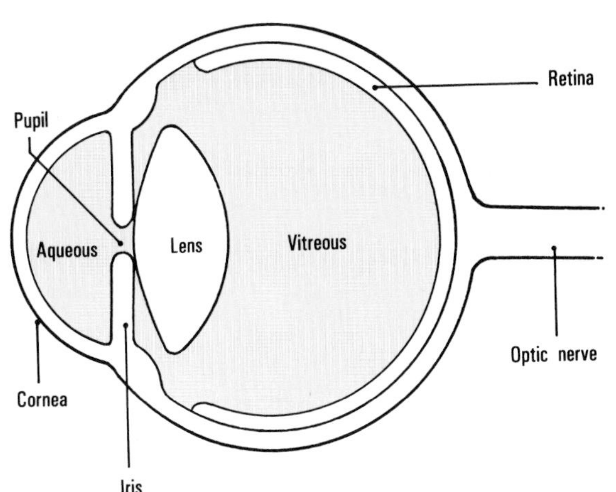

Light passes through the cornea, *pupil and lens and focuses on the retina. The retina converts the image into nervous impulses which travel down the optic nerve to the brain. A degree of intraocular pressure is essential to give the ocular structures their support. But the eye's interior is essentially a non-expandable space, and if pressure in the aqueous builds up, as in glaucoma, this is transmitted all over the eye, which then becomes tight and hard. This in turn damages the optic nerve, which leads off to the brain at the back of the eye, but has numerous endings in the retina.*

Skin and hair

The skin is the largest organ in the body and has a number of functions. To keep working well, it is constantly replaced – in fact everyone's skin is totally replaced every two to three weeks. The old skin falls off as flakes of dry skin which are rarely seen but which account for much of the dust in houses. Hair is a specialized form of skin.

See also: *Shingles, page 140; middle and external ear infections, page 256.*

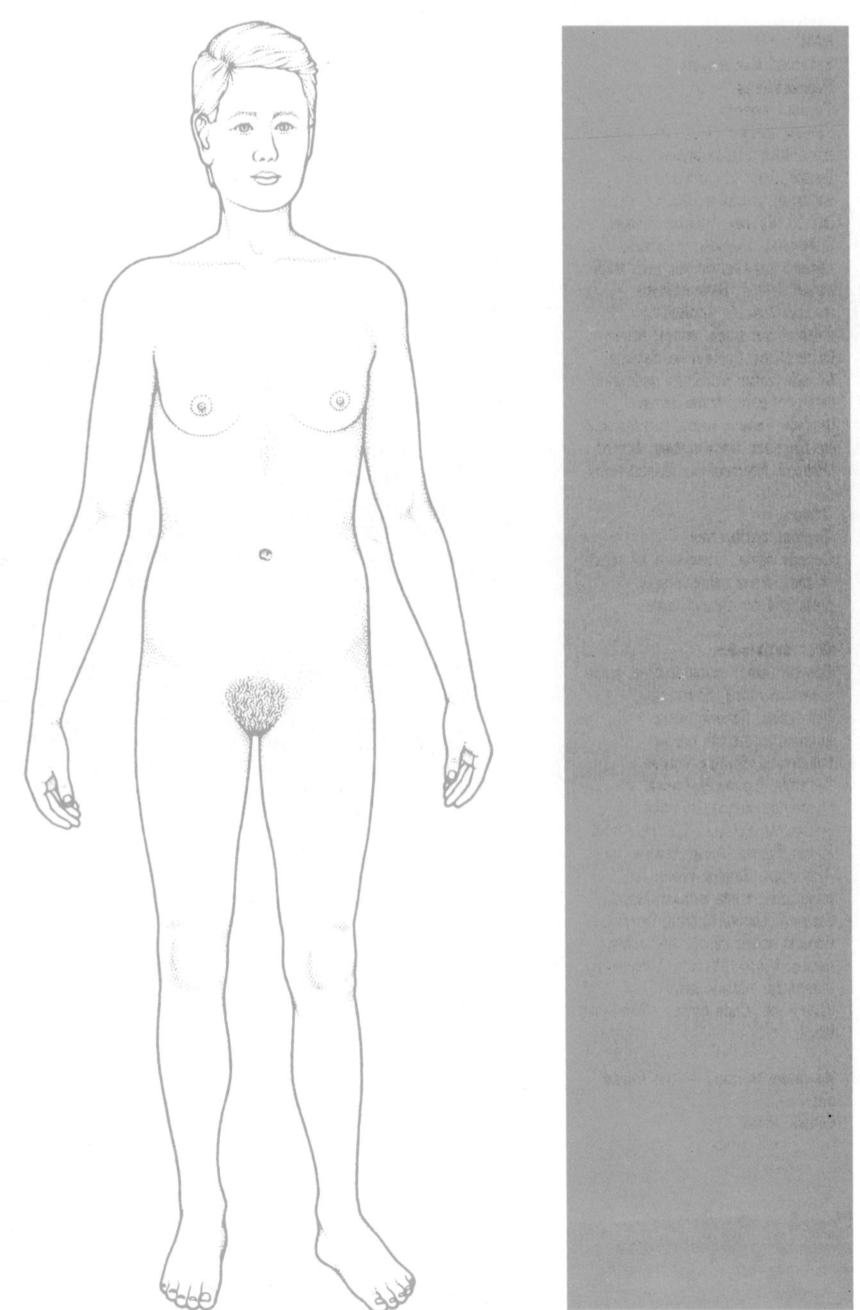

Benzoyl peroxide, abrasives, antibiotics, isotretinoin, the Diane pill, acne soaps and face washes

NAMES YOU WILL HEAR
Selected Commercial Preparations
Topical agents
Generic name: benzoyl peroxide preparations; **trade names:** Clearasil, Benzac, Acetoxyl, Acnegel, Benoxyl, Benzagel, Debroxide, Nericur, Oxy-5, Oxy-10, Stri-dex, Panoxyl Aquagel, Quinoderm, Theraderm. **Generic names:** tretinoin, retinoic acid; **trade name:** Retin-A. **Generic name:** resorcinol/salicylic acid/sulphur preparations; **trade names:** Acnomel, Castel-Minus, Dome-Acne, Eskamel. **Generic name:** aluminum oxide in detergent paste; **trade name:** Brasivol. **Generic name:** corticosteroid combinations; **trade names:** Actinac, Medrone, Neomedrone, Quinoderm HC.

Others
Topical antibiotics
Generic name: tetracycline for topical solution; **trade name:** usually prescribed by generic name.

Oral antibiotics
Generic name: oxytetracycline; **trade names:** Bactocill, Bramcycline, Betacycline. **Generic name:** erythromycin; **trade names:** Benzamycin, Erymax, Ilotycin, Pediazole, Arpimycin, Erycen, Erythroped, Retcin, Erythrocin, Erythromid, EpMycin, Erostin, Emu-V, Ethryn, Eromel, Ilocap, Ilosone, Rythrocaps. **Generic name:** co-trimoxazole; **trade names:** Septra, Bactrim, Fectrim, Nodilon, Septrim. **Generic name:** minocycline; **trade names:** Minocin, Vectrin, Minomycin, Ultramycin. **Generic name:** doxycycline; **trade names:** Vibramycin, Dioxin.

Hormone therapy – 'the Diane' pill
Generic name: isotretinon or 13-cis retinoic acid; **trade name:** Roaccutane.

Acne soaps and face cleansers
Clearasil, Fostex, pHisoDerm, Acne Aid, Biactol, Dome-Acne Cleanser, Hibiscrub, Phiso-Med, Ionax Scrub.

WHAT IS ACNE?

– Inflammation of the skin involving the sebaceous or oil glands. It occurs in areas of skin rich in those glands: the face, back and upper chest.

Nearly all teenagers have acne, though the severity varies enormously. Surprisingly, some people do not develop it until their early 20s; though mild, it may unfortunately persist until the mid to late 30s.

CAUSES The chain of events which leads to acne is understood, but not the root cause(s). At puberty, the skin becomes especially oily (sebhorrhea); the increased flow of grease (sebum) irritates the lining of the grease duct (see diagram) so that debris is produced. This builds up, blocking the duct opening. The debris may be pushed out by the sebum (blackhead); or the opening may remain blocked (whitehead) so that the sebum accumulates in the channel, ruptures its lining and escapes into the skin, causing the inflammation. The stagnation of the sebum leads to a change in the bacteria living in the sebaceous duct which produce substances which aggravate the inflammation produced by the duct rupture.

It is not infectious, and strictly speaking, it is not inherited: just because a father had severe acne, it does not mean his son will. However, there are unusually severe variants which do tend to run in families.

Ten per cent of teenagers have no acne at all, and 30 per cent have pimples now and again – "physiological" (almost normal) acne and require no treatment. About 40 per cent have mild acne with mostly blocked pores (blackheads and whiteheads) and a few red- (papules) and yellow-headed (pustules) spots. About 20 per cent have moderate or severe acne with many papules and pustules which require prescription treatment with both topical agents and oral antibiotics.

Dermatologists see most patients at 12-14 years when the acne is just starting and then they are not sure what it is; at 16 (females) or 18 (males) when the acne is at its peak and most stubborn; and in early 20s when it should have cleared up, but has not.

TREATMENT

Topical agents (ie applied to the skin) are largely based on **benzoyl peroxide.** They can be successful in treating mild to moderate acne, clearing both blackheads and whiteheads and papules and pustules. The preparation needs to be applied to the whole acne-prone area, not just the individual spots. In some preparations, benzoyl

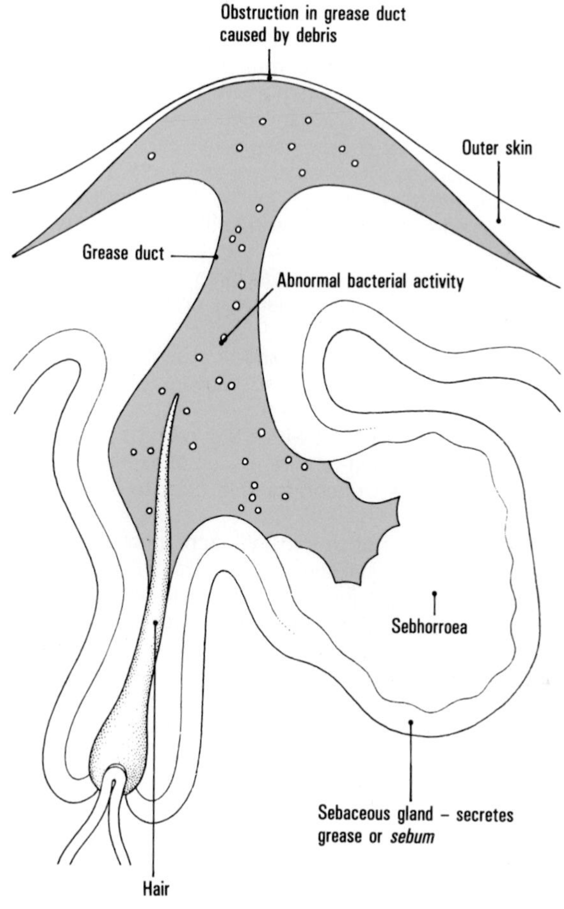

PATIENT'S EXPERIENCE

"I've had acne for two years, but over the last six months, I've been getting more and more spots. I'd tried different creams from the pharmacist but they hadn't helped. My doctor suggested treatment with antibiotics; they helped initially, but made me sick. When I complained he tried another antibiotic. It didn't have such bad side effects, and the spots did clear over four months or so. I haven't had any trouble since."

peroxide is combined with a topical steroid to settle the inflammation, and an antibiotic.

How they work: by relieving the blockage of the sebaceous ducts and destroying the bacteria which live in the ducts. Other topical agents are abrasives, based on resorcinol, sulfur, salicylic acid and aluminum oxide.

Acne soaps and antiseptic face washes are also useful. See OVER-THE-COUNTER TREATMENTS.

How they work: by relieving the obstruction in the sebaceous ducts.

Oral antibiotics are the mainstay for moderate or severe acne. They take time to work, and need to be taken for three to six months to produce maximum improvement. Unfortunately, acne frequently recurs on discontinuing the antibiotics. Often a low dose has to be continued on a long-term basis. A change from one type of antibiotic to another may give further improvement.
How they work: by killing bacteria in the ducts, so preventing inflammatory damage to the acne. They do not help get rid of blackheads and whiteheads – in which there is no inflammation.

In recent years, research has been directed at finding drugs to deal with the underlying problem of acne – greasiness of the skin.
Isotretinoin or **13-cis retinoic acid** is a synthetic form of vitamin A, reserved for the most severe forms of acne. It can reduce seborrhea by 90 per cent and improves the acne by 70 per cent within four months. There is a 1:2 chance of a long-term remission of over two years. However, it is an uncomfortable drug to take – see SIDE EFFECTS.

Most patients notice that their acne improves in the summer and artificial sunlight (ultraviolet light) therapy is sometimes prescribed. There are long-term problems with this therapy *(see **skin cancers,** page 292)* so it is only given for a short time.

As a general rule, diet has no part to play in the treatment of acne, though certain individuals may have exacerbations after eating specific foods such as chocolate.

Another remedy is the **Diane Pill** (not however prescribed in the USA). It is a hormone preparation which can reduce sebborhea by 30 per cent. It takes six to 12 months to produce best results and does not provide a long-term cure. Its side effects include weight gain, breast tenderness and headaches.

OVER-THE-COUNTER TREATMENTS

Many of these contain benzoyl peroxide, sulfur, resorcinal or acetyl salicylic acid (examine the package) and are genuinly useful for mild to moderate acne. Self-treatment with acne soaps and face washes (often containing abrasives) is also appropriate for mild to moderate acne. Don't be misled by the advertisements: no treatment can perform miracles, and all need to be used with persistence, and according to the directions.

QUESTIONS TO ASK THE DOCTOR

■ How long should I use this treatment for?

■ Should I be on any particular diet?

SIDE EFFECTS

Benzoyl peroxide causes redness and dryness, better tolerated if application is gradually increased from two hours each evening during the first week to (subsequently) morning and evening applications.
Antibiotics may cause gastro-intestinal upset (nausea or diarrhea) and vaginal yeast infections. Topical antibiotics, especially clindamycin erythromycin, meclocycline and tetracycline may be as effective as oral antibiotics in mild to moderate cases. Systemic side effects are rare unless the patient has a predisposing condition such as ulcerative colitis.
Isotretinoin causes dry, cracked lips, dry eyes, a dry nose and nose bleeds, dry rashes on the hands, headaches and joint pains. It can also damage the fetus, and is thus prescribed with extreme caution to females and is contra indicated in pregnancy.

SELF-MANAGEMENT

■ Acne can cause scars. The commonest are tiny pits in the surface of the cheeks known as icepick scars. Not so well recognized are flat white blemishes over the back. Occasionally thick, raised, overgrown scars called keloids occur on the chest and shoulders. Plastic surgery can help repair the damage but the only satisfactory answer to scarring is lasting and purposeful treatment of the acne.
■ Career prospects: acne becomes worse in hot humid environments, especially the Far East. The armed forces used to be very reluctant to take teenagers with moderately severe acne, though the use of isotretinoin is changing this attitude. A hot humid kitchen is similarly not to be recommended. Prejudice against skin disease, unjust as it may be, is prevalent and acne sufferers are probably best advised not to court disappointment by applying for jobs with a high public profile while their acne problem lasts.
■ Accept – realistically, but optimistically – that acne is part of being a teenager. Don't be cynical of the value of skin cleansing, diet and UV treatment as recommended by a doctor: in moderate or severe cases, these are an essential back-up to the mainstay drug treatments.
■ Don't use heavy oil-based cosmetics. Water-based and light powdered cosmetics are however harmless and indeed have an essential role in hiding the more unsightly acne.

DOCTOR'S EXPERIENCE
"Phillip, a 14-year-old who had had acne since he was nine, was teased continuously at school and often stayed at home locked in his bedroom. His family doctor tried various antibiotics, and sun-lamp treatment, for three years with no success. At that stage he was referred to the skin specialist who prescribed isotretinoin. His lips cracked, and his face and hands became dry and scaly. He was inclined to give up – but then the acne began to improve, and so he persisted with the treatment. The drug was stopped after four months, but the acne continued to clear. Three years later he is still free of spots."

NAMES YOU WILL HEAR
Steroid creams
Generic name: hydrocortisone/hydrocortisone-acetate; **trade names:** Cetacort, Cort-Dome Cream, Hytone, Dioderm, Dome-Cort Cream, Efcortelan, Hydrocortisyl, Hydrocortistab, Emo-Cort, Hydro-Cortilean, Unicort, Carimol, Hydro-Cortemel, Egocort, Cortef, Derma-Cort 'O', Hydrocortisyl, Hydrosone, Squibb-HC.

Antihistamines
Generic name: chlorpheniramine; **trade names:** Chlor-Trimeton, Teldrin, Haymine, Piriton, Chlor-Tripolon, Histalon, Novopheniram, Allertex, Chlortrimeton, Histamed, Allergex, Bramahist Chloramin, Histaids, Teledrim. **Generic name:** promethazine; **trade names:** Phenergan, Histantil, Lenazine, Prohist, Progan. **Generic name:** trimeprazine; **trade names:** Temaril, Vallergan, Panectyl.

*See also **pain,** page 106, for **analgesics.***

WHAT IS SUNBURN?

– Inflammation of the skin caused by exposure to sun rays of a certain wavelength technically known as middle wave ultraviolet light or UVB. UVA is by contrast the tanning element in sunlight. Sunlight has four effects on skin:

1 Initial redness (erythema) which occurs while in the sun but soon disappears. This is followed two to four hours later by a second phase of erythema which lasts for about 48 hours. These is associated with a variable degree of inflammation, pain, heat and blistering.

2 Tanning, which follows the second phase of erythema, is a protective response by the skin, mainly the result of increased production of the brown pigment melanin. Dark skin is rich in melanin, and so can cope more easily than pale skin with strong sunlight.

3 Skin aging, causing major facial wrinkles before the age of 30.

4 Skin cancer – *see page 292.*

Some drugs, such as tetracyclines, sulphonamides, chlorothiazides and phenothiazines increase sensitivity to sunlight. If you are on regular medication, ask your doctor before sunbathing.

CAUSES There are three important factors which determine how sunburnt you become: the degree of pigmentation prior to exposure; duration of exposure; the strength of the sun. The more vertical the sun's rays, the more damage to the skin. Exposure at midday, when the sun is at its highest, is the most damaging.

TREATMENT

Self-management (see below) is of course the answer to most sunburn. If a doctor sees a really serious case, the options are:

Analgesics: aspirin and acetaminophen, *see **pain,** page 106,* are the first choice for moderate or mild cases; acetaminophen plus codeine preparations are effective in more severe cases.

How they work: *see **pain,** page 106.*

Antihistamines: If the problem is itching more than pain, these may be useful.

How they work: in this context, mainly a sedative effect.

OVER-THE-COUNTER TREATMENTS

For protection: **Sunscreens** contain aminobenzoic acid or amyl dimethyl aminobenzoate, essentially their only active ingredient. It ''filters out'' a proportion of the harmful rays; burning can still occur. The sun protection factor (SPF) gives an indication of the degree of protection offered. The higher the SPF, the greater the protection. *For treatment:* **Calamine lotion** is an effective anti-itch and cooling preparation. It has several active ingredients including calamine, zinc oxide and glycerol. There are no side effects and it can be used as often as desired.

Low-strength **steroid creams** ($\frac{1}{2}$ per cent hydrocortisone) are now available over-the-counter. See SIDE EFFECTS.

Simple analgesics and also antihistamines are widely available from pharmacists.

Some natural oils (for example coconut oil) and some commercial preparations are claimed to promote tanning, and indeed may appear to do so; but there is no scientific basis for the claim.

QUESTIONS TO ASK THE DOCTOR

■ Will the pills I take regularly make me more likely to get sunburn?
■ What do I do if blisters develop?
■ How long will it take to subside?
■ Can I drink alcohol with pills containing antihistamine or codeine?

SIDE EFFECTS

Analgesics: *See **pain,** page 106.*
Steroid creams, which might be used for severe sunburn, are low-strength, and sunburn is a short-lived condition. The serious long-term side effects of their use *(see **eczema,** page 280)* are not an issue here.
Antihistamines increase the sedative effects of alcohol, so vacation drinking needs to be moderated; avoid driving or using machinery.

COMMONSENSE PRECAUTIONS

■ Don't sunbathe, or expose your bare skin, for long periods at the start of a vacation. Build up exposure gradually over a period of days, starting with half an hour to an hour, and increase exposure by no more than 45 minutes daily. Avoid sun between 10 am and 4 pm. You can become badly burned without realizing it while sitting in a cool breeze.
■ Use a sunscreen.
■ If swimming or snorkelling, your back may get badly burned, despite its feeling cool in the water. You can also get sunburned through clothing.
■ A sun-bed can cause sunburn (even though most of its light is UVA, the tanning part of ultraviolet light).

PATIENT'S EXPERIENCE

"When I was a teenager I had a super complexion. I used to spend the whole summer on the beach with the guys, swimming and sunbathing and getting a real deep tan. Now my face is all lined and wrinkled, like an old woman – and I'm not even 30."

ONCE YOU ARE SUNBURNED . . .

■ Avoid further exposure.
■ Towels soaked in cold water applied gently over the affected areas may help reduce the inflammation.
■ Calamine lotion has a soothing effect.
■ Take simple painkillers.
■ Local steroid cream may help short-term.
■ Get plenty of rest.
■ Moisturizers used daily will help to prevent the skin becoming excessively dry and also help to minimize peeling.

ECZEMA

Topical steroids, antihistamines, moisturizers, shampoo

NAMES YOU WILL HEAR
Topical steroids
Very strong
Generic name: clobetasol propionate 0.05%; **trade names:** Temovate, Dermovate. **Generic name:** diflorasone diacetate; **trade name:** Florone. **Generic name:** diflucortolone valerate 0.3%; **trade name:** Nerisone Forte. **Generic name:** halcinonide 01.%; **trade names:** Halog, Halciderm.

Strong
Generic name: fluocinolone acetonide 0.025%; **trade names:** Synalar, Cortoderm, Fluoderm, Dermalar, Synamol. **Generic name:** betamethasone dipropionate 0.01%; **trade names:** Betatrex, Beta-Val, Diprosalic, Diprosone, Diproderm. **Generic name:** betamethasone valerate 0.1%; **trade names:** Betnovate, Betaderm, Celestone-M, Celestone-V, Valisone, Betacort, Betaderm, Calestoderm-V. **Generic name:** diflucortolone valerate 0.1%; **trade names:** Nerisone, Temetex. **Generic name:** fluocinonide 0.05%; **trade names:** Lidex, Metosyn, Topsyn, Lidemol. **Generic name:** hydrocortisone butyrate 0.1%; **trade name:** Locoid. **Generic name:** triamcinolone acetonide 0.025%; **trade names:** Aristocort, Kenalog, Adcortyl, Ledercort. **Generic name:** fluclorolone acetonide 0.025%; **trade name:** Topilar.

Moderate to mild
Generic name: clobetasol dipropionate 0.05%; **trade name:** Temovate. **Generic name:** clobetasone butyrate 0.05%; **trade names:** Eumovate, Trimovate. **Generic name:** flurandrenolone 0.0125%-0.05%; **trade names:** Haelan, Drenison. **Generic name:** desoxymetasone 0.05-0.25%; **trade names:** Topicort, Stiedex.

Weak
Generic name: hydrocortisone 0.1%-2.5%; **trade names:** Dioderm, Dome-Cort Cream, Cort-Dome Cream, Efcortelan, Hydrocortistab, Hydrocortisyl, Emo-Cort,

WHAT IS ECZEMA?

– An itchy rash in which the skin is typically red and may develop small blisters which are then scratched, leaving raw areas. In long-standing eczema, the skin becomes thickened and the normal skin markings may be accentuated. There are five main types:
1 Atopic eczema usually starts in childhood and in some cases is associated with asthma and hay fever. There is often a family history of one or more of these conditions. In children it typically affects the face, the elbow creases, and behind the knees. In adults the common areas are the face, neck and elbow creases. In about 85 per cent of children with infantile eczema, the rash clears spontaneously during childhood. In a small number of individuals atopic eczema may be provoked by allergy to foods or to the house dust mite. **2 Seborrhoeic eczema** causes flaking and itchiness of the scalp, face, eyebrows and eyelids, sometimes with a rash on the chest, under the arms, and in the groin. **3 Discoid eczema** usually occurs after middle-age and causes circular itchy patches, often scattered on the limbs. **4 Varicose eczema** occurs on the lower legs in association with varicose veins and leg ulcers. **5 Contact eczema** is caused by sensitivity to substances which touch the skin. This may be due to allergy, for instance to metals such as nickel which is found in costume jewellery; or to chronic irritation, for example detergents causing "housewive's hand". This rash may spread.

PRESCRIPTION DRUGS

Steroid ointments and **creams** reduce the amount of inflammation in the skin and heal the eczema. The weakest possible preparation should be used for maintenance treatment, but in acute exacerbations, strong steroids may be required for a short time. When the skin is dry, the steroid drugs in ointment form, which are greasy, are much better absorbed than creams. Sometimes preparations which combine a steroid with an antibiotic are used if the eczema has become infected.
How they work: by blocking the inflammatory reaction.
Tar preparations *(see **psoriasis,** page 290)* are sometimes used in the treatment of long-standing eczema: they can reduce the itching and inflammation.
Antihistamines reduce itching and have a sedative effect. They can help you get a good night's sleep.

OVER-THE-COUNTER TREATMENTS

Moisturizers and bath oils are commonly available and

essential in the treatment of atopic eczema in which the skin is usually very dry. They should be used freely and frequently. In seborrheic eczema, antidandruff shampoos benefit an itchy, flaking scalp. Low potency steroid creams are available in most drug stores.

QUESTIONS TO ASK THE DOCTOR

■ For how long should the treatment be continued?
■ Which preparation is the moisturizer, and which the topical steroid?
■ Will the treatment cause staining?

SIDE EFFECTS

Strong topical steroids, used for long periods, cause thinning of the skin and easy bruising. This thinning occurs particularly under the arms and in the groin, where stretch marks may develop. Strong steroids can also eventually cause redness and a rash on the face. Stunting of growth may occur if potent steroids are used in childhood for extended periods. However, most of these side effects are caused by abuse and/or overuse: strong steroids are extremely valuable when used strictly as prescribed. Steroid creams and ointments should always be applied sparingly and rubbed in well. **Antihistamines** cause drowsiness; patients taking them should not drive or operate machinery. They have an additive effect with alcohol, and can also cause a dry mouth, blurred vision, and difficulty urinating.

SELF-MANAGEMENT

■ Atopic eczema usually causes a very dry skin; regular use of moisturizers is essential. See advice in margin on avoiding allergens.
■ Soaps and detergents such as bubble baths can irritate eczema, and should be avoided.
■ Children with eczema are more comfortable in cotton clothing. Wool next to the skin increases itchiness.
■ Clothing, especially bedclothes, should be cool and loose; itchiness tends to be worse if the body is hot.
■ Adults with a history of eczema should always protect their hands by wearing gloves when washing dishes and other chores.
■ Parents of children with eczema should warn them against occupations which can damage the skin, and particularly the hands. These include hairdressing and garage repair work.
■ Varicose veins and varicose eczema are helped by the use of support tights or bandages which also help to prevent ulcers forming on the leg.

Antihistamines
Generic name: promethazine: **trade names:** Phenergan, Mepergan, Avomine, Progan, Prothazine, Histantil, Lenazine, Prohist, Profan. **Generic name:** trimeprazine tartrate; **trade names:** Temaril, Vallergan, Panectyl. *See also* ***hay fever, page 260.***

Moisturizers
Acid Mantle Cream; Cetaphil Lotion; Kepi Lotion; Lacticare Lotion; Lubriderm Cream; Moisturel; Nivea Cream; Nutraderm Cream; Shepards Skin Cream; Sofenol-5; Aqueous Cream; Emulsifying Ointment; Alpha Keri Bath Oil; Balneam Bath Oil; Oilatum Emollient; Boots E45 Cream; Unguentum Merck; Ultrabase Cream; Aquadrate: Aveeno Bath Emollient.

PATIENT'S EXPERIENCE

"I had eczema behind my knees as a child, but grew out of it when I was about seven years old. I had almost forgotten I had had it – until just after my first baby was born. My hands became extremely red and sore, and the skin started splitting and peeling off. I had been doing a lot of laundry with all the diapers and the baby's clothes, but have never worn rubber gloves – I don't like their clammy feel. My doctor told me I should stop using soap on my hands and always wear rubber or plastic gloves when doing wet work, particularly rinsing out the diapers after they had been soaking in soap powder. I started to use a moisturizer regularly on my hands, and followed the advice about gloves. It was worth the effort: my hands soon started to heal."

AVOIDING ALLERGENS

Atopic eczema sufferers, particularly those who have asthma as well, should keep their bedrooms as dust-free as possible in order to minimize allergic reaction to the house-dust mite. *See* ***asthma,*** *page 72.* Avoid contact with any substance which causes a reaction.

NAMES YOU WILL HEAR
Generic name: formaldehyde 3% solution; **trade name:** usually prescribed by generic name. **Generic name:** 1.5% formaldehyde in gel; **trade name:** Veracur. **Generic name:** salicylic acid (sometimes combined with lactic acid), salicylic acid plasters (20-40%) and salicylic acid collodion (12%), a sticky preparation applied to warts on hands of feet; **trade names:** Duofilm, Verrugon, Salactol, Cuplex (latter also contains copper acetate). **Generic name:** glutaraldehyde 10%; **trade names:** Glutarol, Diswart, Verucasep. **Generic name:** benzalkonium chloride-bromine; **trade name:** Callusolve. **Generic name:** podophyllin; **trade name:** usually prescribed by generic name; used in variety of strengths and applications prepared by the pharmacist. **Generic name:** 20% podophyllin, 25% salicylic acid; **trade name:** Posalfilin. **Generic name:** inosine pranobex; **trade name:** Immunovir.

WHAT DO VIRAL WARTS LOOK LIKE?

Appearances differ, but they usually occur as raised, skin-colored, thickenings of skin. They may take the form of small nodules, as on the hand, otherwise known as common warts, or small flat lesions, known as planar warts. On the soles of the feet, warts appear as hard nodules, similar to calluses, or as multi-faceted, flatter lesions, known as mosaic warts. These are also known as plantar warts, or verrucae. Because they are weight-bearing, they tend to grow in, rather than out.

Genital warts (and occasionally other types), project out from the skin, with a feathery or cauliflower-like, pedunculated appearance. Ano-genital warts tend to be small and multiple, and may occur in massive crops. Elsewhere on the body projecting warts are often described as filiform.

Some people are anxious that warts may be linked with skin cancer, but see below.

WHO GETS VIRAL WARTS?

Virtually everyone, but some are more prone than others. Common warts and plantar warts are most frequent in children. As immunity develops, the warts resolve. The vast majority of people with warts do not have a defect of immunity, but those with altered immunity, for example, atopic eczema sufferers, may be more severely affected. People receiving immune-suppressing drugs, and AIDS patients, run the more serious risk of developing florid wart infections. The sexually promiscuous are more likely to get ano-genital warts. Whether warts are contagious depends on the site and type of wart: common hand and planar warts are not particularly so and as the virus is prevalent it is likely that those without resistance will eventually get warts and those with immunity will not. There is no reason for children to avoid contact with other children who have hand or plantar warts: banning children with plantar warts from swimming is unnecessary.

In general, there is no known link between common warts or plantar warts and cancer. In females with genital warts involving the cervix there is an increased risk of cancer of the cervix. Large warty lesions, particularly in the elderly, may be skin tumors, not viral warts: seek medical advice.

CAUSES Papilloma-viruses: over 40 different forms have been identified and many are specific to certain types of infection. The virus locally takes over division of skin cells, reproducing itself.

Most people recognize viral warts without much difficulty. However, there may occasionally be doubt about diagnosis, in which case consult the family doctor.

TREATMENT

Common and plantar warts in children are best left untreated unless they are causing problems; they often resolve spontaneously in a few years. If required, **topical salicylic acid, cantharidin** or **podophyllin preparations** can be used, but are best avoided on the face and in the ano-genital region.

In older patients, freezing with liquid nitrogen is often appropriate, but this is painful and can cause blistering. Warts on the soles, which have become thickened, should either be pared down with a sterile blade or rubbed down with an abrasive emery board before treatment. Then one of the above mentioned preparations can be applied; salicylic acid plasters are particularly useful at this site; alternatively, a **podophyllin compound** can be used. If these are unsuccessful, freezing and other destructive methods may be tried.

Genital and peri-anal warts are infectious: patients and their sexual partners should be examined in a specialist department. Females may require an internal examination for warts. Podophyllin 5-25% is commonly used externally: it is washed off after four to six hours and is normally started at low concentration, then built up. Some stinging and discomfort can occur, and if severe it should be stopped. Podophyllin should not be used during pregnancy. Freezing and/or surgery are further options.

Laser therapy has proved useful in treating certain cases of ano-genital and cervical warts.

OVER-THE-COUNTER TREATMENTS

These can be helpful, but avoid use on the face or ano-genital regions.

QUESTIONS TO ASK THE DOCTOR

- Is it a viral wart, and does it need to be treated?
- Is it infectious? Do I need to see a specialist?

SELF-MANAGEMENT

- Common and plantar warts do not require treatment unless they cause discomfort. Don't share razors.
- Don't place undue faith in old wives' tales for curing warts, even if they do seem to work: many viral warts have a tendency to resolve of their own accord.

PATIENT'S EXPERIENCE

"I first developed warts on my fingers when I was eleven years old. My mother used all sorts of things on them from the pharmacist, but they didn't make much difference. I was taken to my family doctor, who suggested that they be left alone; my mother was not very happy with this. The doctor gave me some liquid to apply from a bottle: it worked on a few of the warts, but I was still getting new ones. My parents were getting impatient, and asked the doctor if I could see a specialist. When I saw him, he explained that the warts would go in due course, but that he could not say when. As I had been teased at school, my mother insisted that something was done. The doctor, who was a dermatologist, said that we could have some liquid to apply to them, but this was the same as our doctor had given me. Alternatively, he said they could be frozen, but he was not very keen on this: he said it would sting and often required many freezings. In the end, my mother got her way and the warts were frozen with a spray of cold gas. It hurt; when I got home my finger was throbbing with blisters where the warts had been frozen. Several of the warts dropped off, but when I went back to the doctor they had started to grow back again. I told the doctor I didn't want any more freezing and he agreed. New warts stopped coming after six months; the old warts started to go after a year and they had all gone in two years.

Two years later I got warts on my feet. The doctor told me to soak my feet in warm water; after drying, we had to rub the hard, thickened areas with an emery board. Salicylic acid plasters were then put on and this was repeated every evening. The warts went after about six months and I haven't had any trouble since."

Imidazoles, hystatin preparations

NAMES YOU WILL HEAR
Generic name: econazole; **trade names:** Ecostatin, Gyno-Pevaryl. **Generic name:** miconazole; **trade names:** Monistat, Dermonistat, Daktacort, Daktarin. **Generic name:** clotrimazole; **trade names:** Mycelex, Canesten. **Generic name:** nystatin; **trade names:** Mycostatin, Nilstat, Nystex, Multilind, Nystaform, Nystan, Nystatin-Dome, Timodine, Diastatin, Nadostine, Candex, Korostatin. **Generic name:** griseofulvin; **trade names:** Fulvicin, Grigulvin, Fulcin (125), Grisovin, Griseostatin, Grisactin, Gris Peg. **Generic name:** ketoconazole; **trade name:** Nizoral. **Generic name:** amphotericin B; **trade names:** Fungizone, Mysteclin, Fungilin. **Generic name:** tolnaftate; **trade names:** Zeasorb AF, Timoped, Tinaderm, Aftate, Tinactin, Tinacidin. **Generic name:** chlorphenesin; **trade names:** Maolate, Mycil. **Generic name:** undecylenic acid; **trade names:** Desinex, Ceanel, Monophytol, Mycota, Caldesene Curex, Tineafax. **Generic name:** selenium sulphide; **trade names:** Exsel, Selsun, Lenium, Sebarex.

Preparations combining several ingredients
Whitfield's Ointment and Castellani's Paint.

WHAT IS A FUNGAL INFECTION?

– A tiny living organism which grows in long strands. It can live as mold on cheese, or mold in a damp house; and some varieties prefer to live on human skin. In doing so they cause infections such as athletes' foot, ringworm, ''jock itch'' and thrush. Usually they affect the top layers of skin only, making it dry, scaly and likely to flake off. The skin may be slightly itchy. The fungi thrive on warm, moist skin, so are common under the arms, beneath the breasts, in the groin and in the mouth. But different fungi have different patterns of growth and prefer particular sites, including hair, skin, nails, mouth and vagina. Fungal infections are rarely serious or life-threatening, but they do sometimes take a long time to clear up.

CAUSES *Candida* (thrush) normally lives in small numbers in the gut. Sometimes for no reason at all, and sometimes if an individual is run down, it multiplies and causes infection. Taking antibiotics for other bacterial infections also makes one more vulnerable to thrush: *see **pneumonia and pleurisy**, page 78.*

People who have diseases which decrease the body's defenses (for example, leukemia and AIDS) are also vulnerable to thrush. Babies may also develop thrush in the form of a diaper rash.

Athletes' foot and ringworm are usually caught from other people. Occasionally humans catch fungal infections from animals, for example cats and cattle, and these can also cause extensive rashes which take time to clear up.

If you or your doctor are uncertain whether the rash is fungal, it may be necessary to scrape off a sample of cells from the skin and examine them under a microscope.

PRESCRIPTION TREATMENTS

Lotions, creams, sprays or ointments are given according to the individual's needs and the type of infection. Creams wash off most easily and are easier to put on. Ointments are greasy and keep air off the affected area. Lotions are liquid and are particularly helpful when a large area of skin is affected or when the skin needs cooling because it is hot and inflamed. Dusting powders help to dry up wet rashes like athletes' foot, but will not cure the infection because they cannot penetrate the layers of affected skin.

Imidazole creams are the commonest treatments, for example miconazole and clotrimazole. Depending on the severity of the infection, all of these may have to be used for several weeks and often much longer to penetrate all the layers of skin and kill off all the fungi. **Whitfield's Ointment** and **Castellani Paint** are long-established and quite effective treatments, but increasingly superceded by the creams mentioned above which are easier to apply and more widely available.

Infections of the nails can be a particularly severe problem because replacement of infected tissue is slow. Long-term treatments such as **griseofulvia** and **ketoconazole** tablets may be necessary for up to a year.

QUESTIONS TO ASK THE DOCTOR

■ How do I know that I have a fungal infection and not eczema or psoriasis?

■ What will happen if I stop treatment too soon?

SIDE EFFECTS

Sometimes the skin will develop a secondary infection – another organism will take advantage while the skin's defenses are poor. If the skin becomes bright red and tight around the rash, a bacterial infection may be developing and a course of antibiotics may be required: see a doctor.

Some people develop an allergy to the cream they are using: a different rash develops. Stop applying it immediately and see a doctor. **Ketoconazole** will only be prescribed by a specialist because it sometimes impairs liver function.

SELF-MANAGEMENT

Try to prevent warm, moist skin conditions by:

■ Washing regularly – particularly groin, armpits, feet and hair.

■ Drying the skin carefully – especially between the toes.

■ Avoiding shoes which make the feet sweat or which have no ventilation. Similarly avoid tight jeans.

■ If you do have naturally sweaty feet, use antifungal dusting powder.

■ Avoid walking in wet areas in bare feet.

Also:

■ Eat well to keep up the body's defenses.

■ If you suffer from a condition which weakens your resistance to infection, for example diabetes, look after skin and feet and stick to any recommended diet.

■ Avoid close contact with animals or with people who have fungal infections.

PATIENT'S EXPERIENCE

"My nine-month-old had been having a slight diaper rash on and off for a few months. Then suddenly it started spreading in little patches on to the rest of his body. The doctor said it was thrush; the cream cleared it up, but it took much longer than I expected."

Benzyl benzoate, lindane

NAMES YOU WILL HEAR
Scabies treatments
Generic name: benzyl benzoate; **trade name:** prescribed by generic name in USA; elswehere Ascabiol. **Generic name:** monosulfiram; **trade name:** Tetmosol. **Generic name:** lindane or gamma benzene hexachloride; **trade names:** Kwell, Scabene, Esoderm, Lorexane, Derbac Soap, Quellada, Scabex. **Generic name:** crotamiton; **trade name:** Eurax.

Nits and lice treatment
Generic name: malathion; **trade names:** Prioderm, Suleo-M, Derbac with Malathion. **Generic name:** carbaryl; **trade names:** Carylderm, Clinicide, Derbac with Carbaryl, Suleo C.

WHAT ARE PARASITES?

– In the medical context, they are a number of different mites which live on human skin or hair, many of which do no harm. **Scabies** burrow their way under the skin and lay their eggs. These hatch out after two to three weeks and make the skin around them itchy and red. Areas affected are the hands (between the fingers), insides of the wrists, the elbows, the genital area, the arms and the feet. **Nits** prefer the hair, laying little white eggs which stick to the hairs and make the scalp itchy; do not confuse with dandruff, which can be shaken off. **Crabs** live on pubic hair – tiny whitish specks, accompanied by their white eggs as well. **Body lice** are a less common sort of parasite which cause itching all over the body and can be found in seams of clothes.

All parasites are transmitted by close contact with someone else who is infected: indeed one can catch head lice by using another person's comb or hat. People who live in poor housing or who have poor washing facilities are more vulnerable because of overcrowding. People who catch scabies are not necessarily dirty: it is easy for anyone to contract them.

Pubic lice are usually transmitted by sexual or very close bodily contact. If you have pubic lice, you may have some other sexually transmitted disease too, so have a check-up. Your doctor or a sexually transmitted disease clinic can arrange the tests.

PRESCRIPTION TREATMENTS

The lotions listed under NAMES YOU WILL HEAR for scabies, crabs and lice are applied all over the body except on head and neck. The lotion is put on after a bath and then washed off after the time stated in the instructions. The itching may continue for a while after the treatment.

Crotamiton cream – Eurax – can help relieve the itching before the treatment has had its effect.

For nits a lotion or a shampoo is applied all over the hair: keep it away from eyes and mouth. A nit comb may also be useful.

How the treatments work: by killing both mites and eggs.

OVER-THE-COUNTER TREATMENTS

Most of the treatments listed under NAMES YOU WILL HEAR are available from pharmacists without prescription, including nit combs. Self-treatment is fine – just follow the directions carefully. And remember that scabies can persist even after the treatment; if this happens, see a doctor.

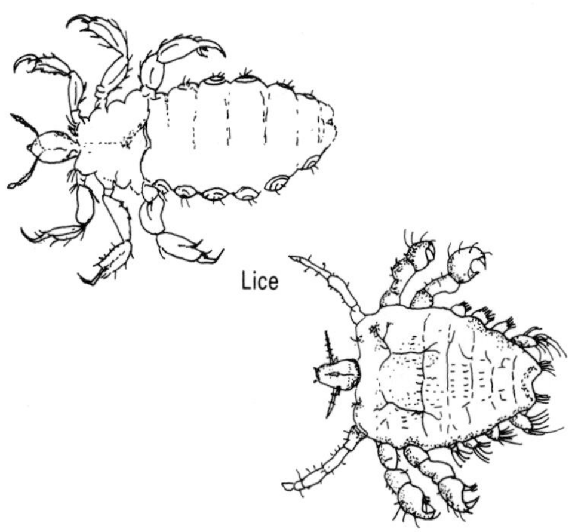

PATIENT'S EXPERIENCE

"My daughter Alice noticed some itchy red spots on her legs – sometimes the itching woke her up at night. When the doctor told her that she had scabies, she remembered she had noticed her husband scratching too. She, her husband and their baby all had to treat themselves with Kwell."

QUESTIONS TO ASK THE DOCTOR

- For how long will I be infectious?
- Can I get it again?

SIDE EFFECTS

Some people's skin can be irritated by these lotions; and sometimes infected yellow spots develop on top of the rash: a doctor may then need to prescribe antibiotics. **Malathion** and **carbaryl,** (not available in USA) contain alcohol, and are inflammable. Having applied either of them to the hair, after washing it, NEVER DRY THE HAIR BY A FIRE OR WITH AN ELECTRIC HAIR DRYER. There is a small, but real risk of the hair catching fire.

SELF-MANAGEMENT

- Immediately after using the treatment, wash all clothes and sheets which have been in use. Wash combs and brushes if the problem has been hair lice.
- Anyone who has been in close bodily contact with an infested person should also have treatment – children, parents and sexual partners. It is not necessary to shave the head if there have been nits, but cutting hair shorter is helpful.

SELF-HELP

To prevent infection:

- Take a bath as often as possible.
- Change clothes every day, and bedclothes regularly.
- Do not use other people's combs/brushes.

NAMES YOU WILL HEAR
Generic name: tetanus toxoid; **trade name:** prescribed by generic name in USA, elsewhere Adsorbed Tetanus Vaccine. **Generic name:** anti tetanus serum; **trade name** prescribed by generic name. **Generic name:** rabies vaccine; **trade names:** Imovax, Merieux Rabies Vaccine. **Generic name:** rabies immune globulin; **trade names** Hyperab, Imogam. **Generic name:** anti rabiesserum; **trade name** prescribed by generic name. **Generic name:** antivenin (caotalidae) polyvalent antivenin (pit viper antidote); **trade name** prescribed by generic name. **Generic name:** North American coral snake antivenin; **trade name:** prescribed by generic name. **Generic name:** Black widow spider antivenin; **trade name:** prescribed by generic name. **Generic name:** snake venom antiserum; **trade name:** Zagreb Antivenom. Outside the USA, different countries have their own specific and polyvalent antiserum against local venomous snakes, spiders and scorpions. **Generic name:** adrenaline; **trade name:** Adrenaline Injection.

Antibiotics
Generic name: benzylpenicillin; **trade name:** Crystapen. **Generic name:** amoxycillin sodium; **trade names:** Amoxil, Moxacin, Moxilean, Novamoxin, Penamox, Polmox. **Generic name:** erythromycin; **trade names:** Benzamycin, Erymax, Ilotycic, Pediazole, Arpimycin, Erycen, Erymax, Erythroped, Retcin, Erythrocin, Erythromid, Illotycin, EpMycin, Erostin, Emu-V, Ethryn, Eromel, Ilocap, Ilosone, Rythrocaps.

Local antihistamine
Generic name: mepyramine maleate; **trade name:** Anthisan.

DIFFERENT TYPES, DIFFERENT PROBLEMS

■ **Animal bites** – typically by dogs, monkeys and humans – can be serious: a human bite is especially liable to cause infection. Rabies is another hazard of animal bites (or of getting infected saliva in an open wound. ■ **Insect bites:** reaction to all of these is similar and varies only in degree. The insect injects a substance into the skin which causes irritation and slight redness and swelling. Complications occur if the bite is scratched, breaking the skin so that bacteria enter and cause infection. ■ **Insect stings** by bees, wasps or hornets can be painful and unpleasant. The symptoms gradually improve over a few hours. Allergy to a specific sting produces a severe reaction, sometimes life-threatening. ■ **Snake bites** inject a poison into the body. Poisonous snakes in the USA include the coral snake and various pit vipers (rattlesnake, copper head and water moccasin). Though death is rare, the seriousness of a snake bite is increased by (a) extremes of age, (b) ill health, (c) bites on the head and trunk, (d) exertion after the bite, (e) infection of the bite.

PRESCRIPTION DRUGS

Animal bites: The chief danger is contracting tetanus, a potentially fatal condition affecting the nerves and inducing muscle spasm. **Tetanus toxoid** will prevent it if given by injection within a few days of a bite, and it should be given for any animal bites if the patient has not received the immunization within the last 5-10 years. Most young people are routinely immunized during their school years. **Antibiotics** are not given routinely for dog bites, but they are always given for monkey and human bites, which almost always become infected. **Rabies vaccine** may be given to people at high risk, eg those working in quarantine stations.

Insect bites and stings: Calamine lotion is a useful agent for soothing the irritation of insect bites. **Antihistamines** can be taken as pills or given by injection. They will promptly alleviate irritation and allergic reactions to stings. **Adrenaline** and **steroids,** also given by injection, are used to treat severe allergic reactions which may complicate stings by bees, wasps, hornets and fire aub. Antihistamine creams are available, but may cause allergic reactions and are not recommended.
Spider bites Strong analgesics may be needed. There is a specific anti-venom for black widow bites.
Scorpion An anti-venom is available.

Snake bites: Analgesics are usually necessary. There are specific **anti-venoms** for pit viper and coral snake bites.

QUESTIONS TO ASK THE DOCTOR

- Is tetanus toxoid necessary?
- Can I be sure this squirrel bite won't cause rabies?

SIDE EFFECTS

Tetanus toxoid injection can cause pain and redness at the injection site, but this is not usually very severe and subsides within a few days. A lump may remain at the site for a few weeks. Allergy is rare. **Antibiotics:** *see **pneumonia and pleurisy**, page 78.* **Rabies vaccine** can cause allergic reactions. **Calamine lotion** has no side effects.

Antihistamine creams and **ointments** commonly cause allergic rashes: calamine lotion, or antihistamine pills are generally preferred. Antihistamines by mouth do have side effects: *see **hay fever**, page 260* Antihistamines should not be taken during pregnancy: *see page 184.* Adrenaline can cause tremor, dry mouth, rapid heart rate and irregular heart rhythm. These effects are related to the dose and are quickly reversible; even so, the drug should not be used in the elderly or those with heart disease, except if life is threatened. **Steroids** do not have significant side effects when used for short periods, as in the case of allergic reactions. **Analgesics:** *see **pain**, page 106.*
Snake anti-venom may itself cause a severe allergic reaction, leading to wheezing, swelling of the throat and shock. Thus anti-venom is usually given in hospital.

SELF-MANAGEMENT

Animal bites:

■ Clean the wound and cover with clean dressing. ■ See a doctor if the wound requires stitching, or if the patient has not had a tetanus toxoid injection within the last five years. ■ Consider whether there is a rabies risk. If so, see a doctor as soon as possible.

Insect bites and stings:

■ Prevent bites by wearing long pants and a long-sleeved shirt. Use insect repellant, and a mosquito net, particularly in areas where malaria is common. ■ If bitten, try to identify the spider or insect responsible. ■ Remove a bee's needle-like sting by scraping across the skin with a blade. Forceps will squeeze more venom into the wound. ■ Patients allergic to bee stings should carry a card or wear a Medic-alert bracelet. They should also carry a bee sting kit with them at all times.

Oral antihistamines
Generic name: promethazine; **trade names:** Phenergan, Avomine, Progan, Prothazine, Histantil, Lenazine, Prohist, Profan. **Generic name:** chlorpheniramine; **trade names:** Dallergy, Chlor-Trimeton, Teldrin, Haymine, Piriton, Chlor-Tripolon, Histalon, Novopheniram, Allertex, Chlortrimeton, Histamed, Allergex, Bramahist Chloramin, Histaids, Teledrim.

Calamine
Generic names: calamine, zinc oxide glycerol; **trade name:** Calamine Lotion.

PATIENT'S EXPERIENCE

"On a camping trip I was stung on the leg by a spider. It soon began to hurt and then the pain spread in waves all over my body. It was awful. I was taken to hospital. Fortunately I'd been able to kill the spider, and I showed it to the doctor, so he knew the pain was due to that and not to some other disease. He identified it as a black widow. He gave me morphine for the pain and the specific anti-venom, and I got better. I don't ever want to go through that again."

SNAKE BITES

■ If at all possible, identify the snake. ■ Reassure the victim and keep him calm and still. ■ Apply tourniquet if bitten on a limb (it should not be very tight). ■ Unless help is available within 15 minutes incise wound (straight cuts) and suck poison out. ■ Do NOT apply ice packs. ■ Hospitalize as soon a possible.

PSORIASIS

Tar preparations, dithranol, topical steroids, retinoids, cytotoxics

NAMES YOU WILL HEAR
Generic names: coal tar, as paste or paint, coal tar and salicylic acid ointment, liquor picis carbonis; **trade names:** Denorex, Fototar, Pentrax, Zetar, Alphosyl, Carbo-Dome, Clinitar, Gelcotar, Ionil T, Polytar Emollient & Liquid, Psoriderm, Psorigel, Pragamatar, Polytar, Gelcotar, Tarbonis. Note: these products are not necessarily exact counterparts – different combinations are used in different countries. Goeckerman regime is a term encountered in English worldwide for a combination of UVB light and tar treatment.
Generic name: dithranol or anthralin – often made up in stiff paste called Lassar's Paste; **trade names:** Anthraderm, Drithocreme, Drithoscalp, Lasan ointment and cream, Anthranol, Dithrocream, Psorodrate. Ingram regime is a term encountered in English worldwide for a combination of UVB and dithranol treatment. Short contact therapy is the term for dithranol treatment left on for only a short period.

Topical steroids
Generic names: hydrocortisone (often called HC), betamethasonesters, fluocinolone acetonide and many more; **trade names:** numerous and confusing – slight modifications of chemical name and concentration make significant differences in potency.

Retinoids
Generic name: etretinate; **trade names:** either Tigason or Tegison.

Cytotoxics
Generic names: methotrexate and hydroxyurea; **trade names:** the chemical names tend to be used instead.

WHAT IS PSORIASIS?

A skin condition which usually appears as raised red patches, often covered by silvery white scales. These plaques vary in size and can occur at almost any site, but commonly involve elbows, knees, hands and scalp. The nails may also be affected.

Different terms are used for psoriasis in its different appearances and distributions. Guttate psoriasis is common in children and may follow a sore throat. Pustular (blistering) forms of psoriasis are more stubborn and serious.

Psoriasis cannot be caught from someone else. There is no way of predicting how the disease will progress. Diet does not usually influence it. It can start at any age, and has phases of exacerbation, improvement and remission, which may be related to stress.

CAUSES The root cause is unknown. There is an excess local turnover of skin cells; it may be inherited. In some patients it is made worse by beta-blockers.

PRESCRIPTION DRUGS

There is no cure: treatment is aimed at reducing the number of plaques. It is not always possible to achieve complete clearance. In mild to moderate psoriasis, topical therapies (applied to the skin) are the mainstay.
Tar, though messy in its crude form, is now available in more useful preparations. They are applied directly to the skin, used in the bath, or as a shampoo. In extensive cases, tar can be combined with ultraviolet light.
Dithranol, another topical therapy, is effective in clearing even severe psoriasis. It is best avoided in delicate skin areas, especially the face. Dithranol is also combined with ultraviolet light for severe cases.
Topical steroids vary in potency. Mild to moderate potency topical steroids require long-term use to maintain an improvement; but this can cause side effects. They are often used to treat delicate skin areas. Potent steroids may be used on small areas of stubborn psoriasis.
Salicyclic acid, a descaling agent, may be mixed with other preparations to enhance efficacy.

Ultraviolet light helps psoriasis.

Retinoids: Etretinate, a drug derived from vitamin A, is particularly useful in severe forms, and may be combined with ultraviolet light therapy.
Cytotoxics: Methotrexate and hydroxyurea have a role in problem cases.
How they work: Most of the drugs mentioned act by limiting the rate at which skin cells are produced. Some

of the additional treatments, or components of the treatments, are moisturizing or de-scaling agents.

OVER-THE-COUNTER TREATMENTS

See **SELF-MANAGEMENT.**

QUESTIONS TO ASK THE DOCTOR

- How often and how long should I use it?
- What should I do if the treatment burns or irritates?

SIDE EFFECTS

Tar and **dithranol** may stain the skin transiently and the clothing permanently. Dithranol may burn the skin. **Topical steroids** can cause skin thinning, and other important side effects such as fluid retention *(see page 280).* If used excessively, they cause rebound of psoriasis on stopping the steroid treatment. **Ultraviolet light** therapy may increase the risk of skin tumours if prolonged. Take care to avoid burning. **Etretinate:** Dryness and cracking of the lips are common, as is also a small increase in hair loss. Etretinate also causes fetal abnormalities if pregnancy occurs during therapy or for up to a year after stopping so these drugs should NOT be given to women with child-bearing potential (all psoriasis drugs taken by mouth are avoided in pregnancy). Elevation of blood fats and liver and bone problems can also occur. **Methotrexate** and **hydroxyrea** can cause bone marrow and liver problems.

Side effects of the last three drug types are potentially grave; so drug administration is carefully managed under a dermatologist's supervision. The risks are carefully weighed with the patient's needs.

SELF-MANAGEMENT

Extremes of environment are best avoided; stressful situations may exacerbate the condition. Moisturizing creams and lotions are useful in reducing dryness and cracking. A dispersable bath oil and a moisturizing soap substitute are also helpful. Sunlight, with moderation, is often beneficial. Topical steroids are now available for anyone to buy over-the-counter, but do not use these for psoriasis without consulting your doctor.

SELF-HELP IN AN ATTACK

If psoriasis is red and angry all over and associated with shivering, you may be developing erythrodermic psoriasis. Keep warm, drink plenty of fluids and only use gentle moisturizers. See your doctor quickly.

PATIENT'S EXPERIENCE

"I first developed psoriasis when I was eight, following a severe sore throat. It was a spotty, all-over, red rash, which went away in six weeks, with little treatment; my doctor actually gave me penicillin for future sore throats. I didn't have any further trouble until I had another sore throat, which I didn't treat. This time the rash was treated with a coal tar cream and although it helped, it was difficult to use because there were so many small spots everywhere.

I had no further trouble with psoriasis until I was 17, when I had an accident; the rash developed in the healing scar. Soon after, the rash appeared on my scalp and on my knees. The knees were treated with a dithranol cream, which worked quite well – the brown marks soon cleared, but my bed linen was ruined with the stains. For my head, I was given a rather messy coal tar and salicyclic acid preparation, which was rubbed in at night and washed out in the morning with a coal tar shampoo. Once I had got used to the smell, it wasn't too bad.

On one occasion I got some psoriasis around my genitals. Unfortunately the dithranol was too strong, so the doctor gave me a mild topical steroid cream; occasional use of this kept the rash in the groin at bay.

This combination kept my psoriasis reasonably clear, but when I moved away from home I found it embarassing to continue the treatment when sharing a house with friends. So my new doctor suggested I use a much stronger dithranol cream applied for only 15 minutes, then washed off. I can do this in the bathroom at night and it is much more convenient. My psoriasis tends to be quite variable; if I have a bad time at work it is worse, but on vacation it nearly clears up."

NAMES YOU WILL HEAR
Topical cytotoxic drug
Generic name: 5-fluorouracil cream; **trade names:** Efudex, Fluoroplex, Efudix.

Sun screens
Generic name: para-aminobenzoic acid compounds; **trade names:** Presun, Solar Cream SPF, Spectraban 4 and 15. **Generic name:** benzophenones; **trade names:** Coppertone Supershade 15 (also contains aminobenzoic acid), Elizabeth Arden Sundown Extra. **Generic name:** cinnamates; **trade name:** RV Paque, Piz Buin, available with various SPFs (also contains benzophenone). **Generic name:** zinc oxide; **trade name:** ROC factor 10 A+B Total Sunblock (also contains cinnamate).

SKIN CHECK
Examine your skin ALL OVER once a month, checking for patches, and considering these seven points: **1** Was it there last month? **2** Does it itch? **3** Is its size increasing? **4** Has it changed colour, or become variable in colour? **5** Is the border irregular in shape? **6** Is there spontaneous bleeding or ulceration? **7** Has it become nodular, or does it extend into the underlying skin? If you answer yes to one or more of these, see your doctor.

Limitation of, and protection from, sun exposure and other risk factors are especially important for those who burn easily. Use a high protection factor sunscreen.

Caution: some sun screens can cause staining of clothes, occasional allergic reactions or even photosensitivity reactions. Those with oil of bergamot (which contains 5-methoxypsoralen) have been implicated in causing skin cancer, but this is not proved.

WHAT IS SKIN CANCER?

– A malignant growth on or in the skin; some can spread to and damage other sites. There are many different types, which vary considerably in local aggression and ability to spread.

The commonest cancer is the **basal cell carcinoma,** alternatively known as a **rodent ulcer.** It varies in appearance, but is frequently a pearly-margined nodule, which may or may not be ulcerated and form a deep scab. The overlying skin often carries an increased number of small, superficial blood vessels. These nodules normally grow slowly and commonly occur on sun-exposed sites, particularly the head and neck, but can appear anywhere. Basal cell carcinomas are locally destructive and will slowly enlarge, but do not normally spread elsewhere.

Squamous cell carcinoma is the next commonest. It usually presents as an unexplained ulcer or nodule on the skin. It occurs frequently on sun-exposed sites, and has the potential to spread. These tumours are uncommon, but there is real risk in neglecting them.

Malignant melanoma is one of the most aggressive skin malignancies and, because of its ability to spread rapidly, always requires urgent treatment. These are usually, but not always, dark brown or black in colour, and can occur at any site, but again sun-exposed areas are the commonest. They occasionally develop in pre-existing moles. Some families seem more prone than others to problems with moles, and should therefore be especially vigilant. See SELF-HELP.

Growths on the skin which have the potential, given time, to turn into skin cancers, are known as **pre-malignant skin conditions.** The commonest is the **solar keratosis,** which occurs in middle age. It usually manifests itself as a rough, darkened, scaly area of skin in a sun-exposed area, frequently the head and neck, or backs of the hands. Each patch of keratosis is small, less than about $\frac{1}{2}$ in (1 cm) in diameter, and there are often several of them. The risk of one of these lesions developing into skin cancer is about one in a hundred per year. They sometimes spontaneously resolve, but can be treated as a preventive measure. If the lesion becomes thickened, it is presumed to have become malignant and needs treatment.

A similar condition, **Bowen's disease,** usually occurs as a red-brown or orange scaly patch, which varies in size and frequently occurs on sun-exposed sites.

With early diagnosis, most skin cancers are

treatable. However, recent studies show that deaths from skin cancer are increasing, possibly because of the numbers of people vacationing in the sun.

CAUSES The main factor is cumulative exposure to sunlight; while there is evidence that short intensive exposures can be harmful, it is the total exposure over the years that matters. In general, the fairer the skin, the greater the risk. Other factors are X-ray therapy, radiation exposure, ingestion of arsenic-containing tonics and certain types of immune suppressing drugs. Light-skinned people are especially at risk – a factor sometimes called the Celtic skin syndrome outside US.

QUESTIONS TO ASK THE DOCTOR

- Is my skin problem benign or malignant?
- What are the risks of it spreading?
- Is my skin cancer curable?
- What is the treatment?

TREATMENT

Basal and squamous cell carcinomas are, for preference, removed surgically; X-ray therapy is an alternative under certain circumstances. Occasionally other methods such as cryotherapy or lasers are used. Cryotherapy uses a freezing spray, usually liquid nitrogen. Malignant melanomas are always removed surgically as a matter of urgency. Solar keratoses are removed surgically, either by excision or by curretage – scraping off. Cryotherapy is an alternative, as is application of **5-fluorouracil cream** which destroys abnormal cells. Bowen's disease is treated in the same way as solar keratoses, but surgical removal may be preferred.

OVER-THE-COUNTER TREATMENTS

Sun screens have their role in limiting sun exposure, especially for those with fair skins. *See* **sunburn,** *page 278.* It is especially important to protect children.

SIDE EFFECTS

Some sun screens can cause staining of clothes, occasional allergic reactions or even photosensitivity reactions. Those with oil of bergamot (which contains 5-methoxypsoralen) have been implicated in causing skin cancer, but this is not proved.

SELF-HELP

Prevention is of course the key: follow the routine suggested in the opposite margin.

PATIENTS' EXPERIENCE

"I lived in a sunny climate until I was 20 years old. Like my father, I have a fair skin. When he was in his forties, he noticed a small black mark on his back, but did nothing about it, as it didn't cause any trouble. Several years later it enlarged to form a nodule, which bled and seemed to leak a black colour into the surrounding skin. The doctors diagnosed a malignant melanoma and quickly arranged its removal, but it was too late: it had already spread to other parts of the body; Dad died a few months later. My mother, now in her fifties, has had several skin cancers develop on her face. Her doctor said that these were rodent ulcers and arranged for them to be removed. She hasn't had any more trouble, but the doctor keeps a check on her and freezes the occasional rough patch of skin on her face or the backs of her hands. Three years ago, I noticed a small dark brown mole appear on my leg. I was suspicious because I hadn't noticed it before and it seemed to be getting bigger. My doctor sent me to a dermatologist who thought it was a melanoma and arranged for it to be removed. Fortunately, it was still very thin, and I've been assured that there is every chance I won't have further trouble with it. The dermatologist told me that as a family we were prone to skin cancer because of our fair skin and degree of sun exposure abroad. Now in sunny weather, I wear a broad-rimmed hat and cool loose clothing that covers most of my body including arms and legs. On the exposed areas, I apply a factor 15 sun screen. Although I try not to be too neurotic about the sun, I avoid being out at midday and I no longer sunbathe. My dermatologist says this helps prevent further skin cancers, and also sun-induced aging of the skin: reasonable advice for anyone."

INDEX

Main references are in bold type.

B

C

D

E

F

G

CONTRIBUTORS

Dr. D.N. Bateman, Consultant Physician, The Wolfson Unit, Newcastle upon Tyne (Parkinsonism); Dr. N.D.S. Bax, Consultant Honorary Physician, Royal Hallamshire Hospital, Sheffield (Migraine); Dr. P. Belchetz, Consultant Physician Endocrinologist, The General Infirmary at Leeds (disorders of the pituitary gland); Dr. Mary Belshaw, Liverpool (period problems, hay fever); Dr. M.J. Brodie, Consultant Physician and Clinical Pharmacologist, Gardiner Institute, Western Infirmary, Glasgow (epilepsy); Dr. M. Burke, Consultant Obstetrician and Gynaecologist, North Tyneside General Hospital (infertility); Dr. P. Campion, Senior Lecturer, Department of General Practice, University of Liverpool (indigestion, diarrhoea, constipation, haemorroids, obesity, middle and external ear infections, sinusitis); Dr. P. Carey, Consultant in Genito-Urinary Medicines, Royal Liverpool Hospital (sexually transmitted diseases, AIDS); Dr. I.S. Casson, Senior Registrar, General Medicine, Royal Liverpool Hospital (diabetes); Dr. Clare Connolly, general practitioner, Bradford (fungal infections, skin parasites); Dr. Jean Coope, General Practitioner, Bollingham, Cheshire (problems of menopause); Dr. Regina Curley, Senior Registrar in Dermatology, St. George's Hospital, Tooting (eczema); Dr. T.K. Daneshmend, Lecturer in Therapeutics, The University of Nottingham (jaundice, cirrhosis); Dr. J.M. Davies, Consultant Haematologist, Royal Liverpool Hospital (adult and childhood leukaemias, anaemia); Dr. Margaret Dodson, Consultant Anaesthetist, Royal Liverpool Hoaspital (anaesthetics); Dr. H. Elliot, Senior Lecturer in Clinical Pharmachology, Stobhill General Hospital, Glasgow (disorders of heart rhythm); Dr. Peter Elliot, General Practitioner, Denbigh (hyperthyroidism, hypothyroidism, strains and sprains, back pain); Dr. Christine Evans, Consultant Urologist, Royal Liverpool Hospital (impotence); Dr. Ronald Finn, Consultant Physician, Royal Liverpool Hospital (food intolerance); Dr. Katy Gardiner, General Practitioner, Liverpool (irritable bowel); Dr. Ian Gilmore, Consultant Gastroenterologist, Royal Liverpool Hospital (malabsorbtion, ulcerative colitis); Dr. R.M. Graham, Senior Registrar, Department of Dermatology, Royal Liverpool Hospital (viral warts, skin cancers, psoriasis); Dr. Susanna Graham-Jones, Lecturer, Department of General Practice, The University of Liverpool (stress, fatigue, dizziness, headache); Dr. John Green, Senior Lecturer in Medical Oncology, Clatterbridge Hospital, Wirral (lung cancer); Dr. G. Grennan, Hope Hospital, Salford (osteoarthritis); Dr. M. Grimmer, Senior Registrar, University of Liverpool (angina, heart failure); Dr. J. Guillebaud and Dr. Gillian Robinson, The Margaret Pyke Centre, Soho Square, London (contracepion); Mr. S. Harding, Senior Registrar in Ophthalmology, St. Paul's Eye Hospital, Liverpool (chronic glaucoma, red eye/dry eye); Dr. P. Humphrey, Consultant Urologist, Walton Hospital, Liverpool (multiple sclerosis); Dr. D.H. Jones, Consultant Dermatologist, Raigmore Hospital, Inverness (acne); Dr. Denise Kitchener, family doctor, Liverpool (nausea and vomiting, pneumonia and pleurisy, cough, senile dementia, common cold, influenza, shingles, meningitis, drugs in pregnancy, urinary incontinence, drugs in children, disorders of eating, vitamin deficiencies, rheumatoid arthritis, ankylosing spondylitis, deafness, laryngitis, bites and stings); Mr. S. Leinster, Consultant Surgeon, Royal Liverpool Hospital (breast cancer); Dr. J.L. Maddocks, Reader in Clinical Pharmacology and Consultant Physician, Royal Hallamshire Hospital, Sheffield (lymphomas); Dr. J. Martin, Consultant Paediatrician, Alder Hey Children's Hospital, Liverpool (childhood leukaemias); Dr. J.P. Miller, Consultant Gastroenterologist, University Hospital of South Manchester (lipid disorders); Dr. M.E. Molyneux, Liverpool School of Tropical Medicine (malaria); Dr. A.I. Morris, Consultant Physician, Royal Liverpool Hospital (alcoholism); Professor Michael Orme, Reader in Pharmacology, University of Liverpool (introduction, myocardial infarction); Dr. Julia Parker, Senior Registrar in Psychiatry, Bristol and Western Health District (drug misuse, shizophrenia); Dr. David Roberts, Senior Registrar, University of Liverpool (hypertension); Dr. A. Scott, Senior Lecturer in Chemical Pharmacology, The University of Liverpool (problems of the circulation, blood clots); Mr. R. Sells, Consultant, Renal transplants, Royal Liverpool Hospital (organ transplants); Dr. M. Serlin, Consultant Physician, Southport General Infirmary (bronchitis and emphysema); Dr. E. Szabadi, Reader in Psychiatry, University of Manchester, and Honorary Consultant Psychiatrist, Withington Hospital (depression); Mr W.R. Tyldesley, Director of Dental Education, University of Liverpool (conditions of the mouth); Dr. C. Wells, Consultant in pain relief, Walton Hospital, Liverpool (pain); Dr. P. Winstanley, Senior Registrar, University of Liverpool (peptic ulcer, asthma); Dr. A.A.A. Zurek (cramp).

Acknowledgements

Editorial

Editorial Director	Andrew Duncan
Editorial assistance	Rosemary Dawe, Fiona Hardwick, Laura Harper
Index	Judy Batchelor

Susan Golombok's help in formulating the concept is acknowledged with thanks.

Design

Art director	Mel Petersen
Designer	Lyn Hector
Design assistants	Chris Foley, Gene Cornelius, Alastair Pether
Illustrations	Sandra Pond, Wil Giles, Andrew Popkiewicz, Paul Saunders, Tony Graham